Fertility and Infertility in Veterinary Practice

Edited by

J. A. LAING PhD, BSc, MRCVS
Emeritus Professor of Animal Husbandry,
University of London, London, UK

W. J. BRINLEY MORGAN DSc, PhD, BVSc, DipBact, MRCVS
Formerly Deputy Director, Ministry of Agriculture, Fisheries and Food,
The Central Veterinary Laboratory, Weybridge, Surrey, UK

W. C. WAGNER DVM, PhD, Diplomate, American College of Theriogenologists
Professor and Head, Department of Veterinary Biosciences,
College of Veterinary Medicine, University of Illinois,
Urbana, Illinois, USA

Fourth Edition

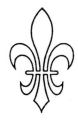

Baillière Tindall
London   Philadelphia   Toronto   Sydney   Tokyo

Baillière Tindall   24–28 Oval Road
W. B. Saunders   London NW1 7DX, England

West Washington Square
Philadelphia, PA 19105, USA

1 Goldthorne Avenue
Toronto, Ontario M8Z 5T9, Canada

Harcourt Brace Jovanovich Group (Australia) Pty Ltd
Post Office Box 300,
North Ryde, NSW 2113, Australia

Harcourt Brace Jovanovich Japan Inc.
Ichibancho Central Building, 22–1 Ichibancho
Chiyoda-ku, Tokyo 102, Japan

© 1988 Baillière Tindall

First published 1955
Second edition 1970
Third edition 1979
Fourth edition 1988

Filmset by Eta Services (Typesetters) Ltd, Beccles, Suffolk
Printed and bound in Great Britain at the University Press, Oxford

British Library Cataloguing in Publication Data
Fertility and infertility in veterinary
   practice.—4th ed.
   1. Livestock. Fertility
   I. Laing, J. A.   II. Brinley Morgan, W. J.
   III. Wagner, W. C.   IV. Fertility and infertility in veterinary
   practice
   636.089′26
ISBN 0-7020-1264-5

Preface

This book is intended primarily for veterinarians in general practice and senior veterinary students. It is based on the third edition of *Fertility and Infertility in Domestic Animals*, but has been completely rewritten to meet the needs of current veterinary practice and much American experience incorporated. The sections dealing with embryo transplantation and artificial insemination have been brought up to date and new chapters written on the breeding of dogs and cats.

Where possible, each species has been dealt with separately. In the case of infectious disease this cannot be done without undue repetition. But the accounts of non-specific infection of the uterus in cattle and horses, and also that of contagious equine metritis, have been combined with the general chapters on infertility in these animals. The index allows ready cross-reference to other types of infectious disease.

Our best thanks are due to those who have given us permission to reproduce illustrations, to the very large number of veterinarians in general practice who have provided the investigational material on which much of the information in this book is based, to the publishers for their care and expertise in its production, to Mrs M. J. Lees for her expert assistance in its initial planning and to Dr P. J. Goddard for advice on the use of ultrasonic techniques for diagnosis.

J.A.L.
W.B.M.
W.C.W.

Contributors

G. W. BeVier DVM, MS
Assistant Professor, Department of Veterinary Biosciences, College of Veterinary Medicine, University of Illinois, Urbana, Illinois, USA

M. J. Corbel BSc, PhD, DScMed, MRCPath, CBiol, FIBiol
Formerly Senior Research Officer, Ministry of Agriculture, Fisheries and Food, Central Veterinary Laboratory, Weybridge, Surrey, UK

M. Dawson BVetMed, MSc, MRCVS
Senior Research Officer, Ministry of Agriculture, Fisheries and Food, Central Veterinary Laboratory, Weybridge, Surrey, UK

G. D. Dial DVM, PhD
Assistant Professor, Department of Food, Animal and Equine Medicine, School of Veterinary Medicine, North Carolina State University, Raleigh, North Carolina, USA

S. Edwards MA, VetMBMSc, MRCVS
Senior Research Officer, Ministry of Agriculture, Fisheries and Food, Weybridge, Surrey, UK

Ronnie G. Elmore DVM, MS, Diplomate, American College of Theriogenologists
Head, Section of Theriogenology, Department of Large Animal Medicine and Surgery, College of Veterinary Medicine, Texas A & M University, College Station, Texas, USA

D. B. Galloway BVSc, MVSc, PhD
Senior Lecturer and Head, Animal Reproduction Unit, Department of Veterinary Clinical Sciences, School of Veterinary Science, University of Melbourne, Princes Highway, Werribee, Victoria, Australia

C. J. Gaskell BVSc, PhD, DVR, MRCVS
Small Animal Hospital, Department of Veterinary Clinical Science, University of Liverpool, Crown Street, Liverpool, UK

R. M. Gaskell BVSc, PhD, MRCVS
Department of Veterinary Pathology, University of Liverpool, Veterinary Field Station, Neston, Wirral, UK

B. K. Gustafsson DVM, PhD
Chairman and Professor, Department of Veterinary Clinical Medicine and Surgery, College of Veterinary Medicine, Washington State University, Pullman, Washington, USA

J. W. Harkness MSc, BVM&S, MRCVS
Senior Research Officer, Ministry of Agriculture, Fisheries and Food, Central Veterinary Laboratory, Weybridge, Surrey, UK

T. H. Howard DVM, PhD
Director of Veterinary Services, American Breeders Service, DeForest, Wisconsin, USA

Shirley D. Johnston DVM, PhD, Diplomate, American College of Theriogenology
Associate Professor, Department of Small Animal Clinical Science, College of Veterinary Medicine, University of Minnesota, St Paul, Minnesota, USA

J. A. Laing PhD, BSc, MRCVS
Emeritus Professor of Animal Husbandry, University of London, London, UK

K. P. Lander PhD, BVM&S, DipBact, MRCVS
Department of Veterinary Services, Veterinary Research Laboratory, PO Box 8101, Causeway, Harare, Zimbabwe

T. W. A. Little PhD, BVM&S, DipBact, MRCVS, FIBiol
Deputy Director, Ministry of Agriculture, Fisheries and Food, Central Veterinary Laboratory, Weybridge, Surrey, UK

R. M. Lofstedt DVM, MS
Associate Professor, Section of Theriogenology, Department of Health Management, Atlantic Veterinary College, University of Prince Edward Island, Charlottetown, Prince Edward Island, Canada

M. Lucas BVSc, DipBact
Senior Research Officer, Ministry of Agriculture, Fisheries and Food, Central Veterinary Laboratory, Weybridge, Surrey, UK

W. J. Brinley Morgan DSc, PhD, BVSc, DipBact, MRCVS
Formerly Deputy Director, Ministry of Agriculture, Fisheries and Food, Central Veterinary Laboratory, Weybridge, Surrey, UK

D. E. Noakes PhD, BVetMed, MRCVS
Professor of Obstetrics and Diseases of Reproduction, Royal Veterinary College, Hawkshead House, North Mymms, Hatfield, Hertfordshire, UK

Randall S. Ott DVM, MS, Diplomate, American College of Theriogenologists
Professor of Theriogenology, Chief, Field Service and Theriogenology Section, Department of Veterinary Clinical Medicine, College of Veterinary Medicine, University of Illinois, Urbana, Illinois, USA

M. M. Pace PhD
American Breeders Service, DeForest, Wisconsin, USA

W. C. Wagner DVM, PhD, Diplomate, American College of Theriogenologists
Professor and Head, Department of Veterinary Biosciences, College of Veterinary Medicine, University of Illinois, Urbana, Illinois, USA

A. E. Wrathall PhD, BVM&S, MSc, MRCVS
Head, Diseases of Breeding Department, Ministry of Agriculture, Fisheries and Food, Central Veterinary Laboratory, Weybridge, Surrey, UK

Raymond W. Wright Jr BS, MA, PhD
Professor of Animal Sciences, College of Agriculture, Washington State University, Pullman, Washington, USA

R. S. Youngquist DVM, Diplomate, American College of Theriogenologists
Professor and Chief, Section of Theriogenology, College of Veterinary Medicine, University of Missouri, Columbia, Missouri, USA

Contents

1

The Normal Genital Organs

D. E. NOAKES

In order to diagnose abnormalities of the genital organs with accuracy, it is important to have a good understanding and appreciation of their normal structure and function.

Many comprehensive textbooks describe in detail the normal anatomy and physiology of the reproductive system of domestic animals. It is not the purpose of this chapter to copy these but to consider the normal genital system from the point of view of its clinical examination. Assessment of the functional status of the reproductive system has also been enhanced by the ability to measure various reproductive hormones in blood, serum, plasma or milk. These are routinely measured in laboratories and relatively simple 'on-farm' test kits have been developed recently. It is important to stress that, because many hormones are released in a pulsatile fashion, the assay of single isolated samples in the circulation can be of limited value and the significance of the result needs careful interpretation.

THE MALE ANIMAL

The male reproductive system comprises three components:

1. The primary sex organs or gonads: the testes.
2. The accessory sex organs: the epididymides, ductus deferens, vesicular glands, prostate gland and bulbourethral glands.
3. The copulatory organ: the penis.

The presence of certain of the accessory sex organs varies among species.

Puberty

Puberty occurs when the male is capable of producing spermatozoa. Prepubertal animals will frequently show evidence of mounting behavior and penile erection. The time of onset of puberty is primarily dependent upon the individual reaching a weight threshold, which varies both among species and within species, but is between about one-third and two-thirds of mature body weight. Other factors, such as age, genotype, climate, season of year, and social factors, such as isolation from other males and females, play an important role in timing. Full sexual maturity, as measured by maximum fertility, occurs sometime after the time of puberty.

Endocrine Changes

The main male gonadal steroid, testosterone, is produced by the interstitial or Leydig cells of the testis. Production of this hormone is primarily under the direct influence of luteinizing hormone (LH), which itself is released from the anterior pituitary gland as a result of gonadotropin releasing hormone (GnRH) secreted by the hypothalamus.

Testosterone concentrations in the peripheral circulation of the juvenile are relatively low; as the young male progresses towards puberty testosterone concentrations gradually rise as the frequency and amplitude of LH pulse release increases. Once puberty occurs testosterone concentrations in the peripheral circulation remain elevated, although it must be stressed that, because of its pulsatile release, there are considerable fluctuations in absolute concentrations which can be seen if frequent blood samples are taken. Even after puberty there is evidence of seasonal variations, especially in seasonal breeder species such as the sheep and goat, declining when the females of the species are acyclic and resulting in decreased sperm production and testis weight. Even in species such as cattle, where there is no very obvious seasonality of reproduction, there are several reports of seasonal variations in plasma LH and testosterone.

Spermatogenesis and its Control

Spermatozoa are produced by the germinal epithelium of the seminiferous tubules from before the onset of puberty. Daily sperm production in mature males per gram of testicular tissue ranges from as low as 13×10 in some bulls and up to 31×10 in some boars; other domestic species are intermediate.

The seminiferous tubules are composed of a basement membrane and germ cells that give rise to spermatozoa. Sertoli cells provide both a supportive role for the germ cells and an endocrine function. Waves of sperm production occur along the length of the seminiferous tubules (spermatogenesis) as a result of division of the germ cells, progressing from spermatogonia through primary and secondary spermatocytes to spermatids and finally, spermatozoa (Fig. 1.1). During spermatogenesis the number of chromosomes is reduced from the diploid number to half this, the haploid number. The time taken for spermatogenesis varies between species, but is about 60 days in the bull and slightly shorter in the boar.

Spermatogenesis is induced and controlled directly by follicle stimulating hormone (FSH) and indirectly by LH, the latter acting via testosterone produced by the Leydig cells. The seminiferous tubules are exposed to higher concentrations of testosterone than other peripheral tissues, in part because of the transfer of steroid from vein to artery in the pampiniform plexus in the spermatic cord. The germ cells do not have receptors for testosterone, but the Sertoli cells which do may have a role in mediating its effect upon spermatogenesis. There is also evidence that the Sertoli cells produce a nonsteroidal hormone, inhibin, which exerts a negative feedback upon FSH production. The Leydig cells may also respond to prolactin stimulation (see Fig. 1.1).

While seminal characteristics, including sperm production, can vary widely in seasonal breeders such as the ram, goat and stallion, there are also fluctuations in the bull, cat and dog. In the latter species it may be in response to high ambient temperatures which cannot be compensated for sufficiently by scrotal relaxation, thus resulting in some inhibition of spermatogenesis.

Clinical Examination

Clinical examination of the male reproductive system should be performed in three stages. First, libido should be assessed and normal copulatory behavior and erection of the penis should be observed. Second, the external genital organs including the penis, prepuce, scrotum, testes and epididymides should be examined visually and by palpation. Finally, where possible, rectal palpation of the internal genital organs should be performed. In a fractious or difficult animal it may be necessary to use a tranquilizer drug or general anesthesia to facilitate a thorough and detailed examination. Where necessary a semen sample may be collected and evaluated (see Chapter 2).

Stallion

Development of the Male Reproductive Tract and Puberty

Testicular descent occurs in the colt foal towards the end of fetal life, although complete entry into the scrotum may not occur until just after birth. Puberty occurs at about 12–18 months of age although it is very much dependent upon the breed of horse and the growth rate. Full sexual maturity is not usually attained until 2–3 years of age.

Clinical Examination

Unlike the bull, it has been less customary to examine stallions to evaluate potential reproductive capacity. There has been a tendency to exclude any reference to fertility when selecting sires, and only attributes such as conformation or racing performance have been considered. There has also been a tendency for horse breeders to fail to recognize that a stallion might be responsible for poor fertility in a stud, particularly if he mounts mares and copulates vigorously. It is certainly advisable to subject stallions to a critical appraisal of reproductive function at the beginning of the breeding season.

It is important to observe normal copulatory behavior in a familiar environment, using the usual methods of restraint and control. It is also necessary to provide a mare of suitable size which is in estrus and adequately restrained to prevent injury to the stallion.

Precopulatory behavior is more prolonged than

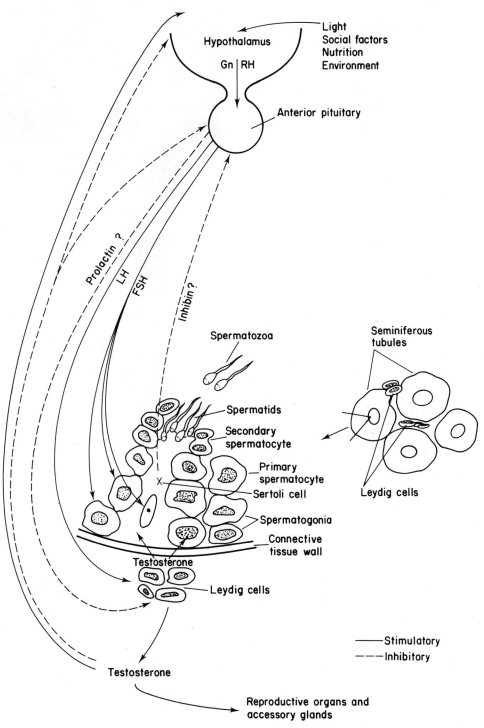

Fig. 1.1 Spermatogenesis and its hormonal control.

in the bull, the time interval between the first introduction of the stallion to the mare and subsequent mounting, the reaction time, varying among individuals and with the season of the year. Times as short as 1 min in May and June have been reported as compared with 10–15 min during November to February.

When ejaculation occurs, the contractions of the pelvic urethra cause the characteristic 'flagging' of the tail. The contractions can also be palpated if the base of the penis is held soon after intromission. Ejaculation normally occurs within 2–3 min, the duration of coitus being 3–5 min. When the stallion dismounts, although erection is reduced, the corona glandis is still enlarged.

If a semen sample is required it can be obtained before intromission by means of an artificial vagina or condom (see Chapter 2).

External Genitalia

Scrotum and Testes   The scrotum of the stallion is less pendulous than the bull's and is best palpated from the side. Critical visual inspection is often difficult and it may be preferable to do so under general anesthesia. The skin of the scrotum should be soft and thin; the testes when fully descended lie with their longitudinal axes almost horizontal, but when they are retracted towards the external inguinal ring the longitudinal axes become almost vertical. The testes vary in size depending upon the type of horse, measuring an average 10 × 5 × 5 cm and weighing 200 g. There is frequently some disparity in size, particularly in some pony breeds.

The epididymis is closely attached to the dorsal border of the testis, hence palpation is difficult. When the testis is fully descended and the cremaster muscle relaxed, palpation of the spermatic cord is possible although identification of the ductus deferens is difficult.

Penis   Many stallions, because of their familiarity with the procedure of washing the penis and prepuce during grooming, will readily accept manual extraction of the penis. This is performed by introducing the hand into the prepuce, grasping the penis and applying constant but gentle traction. In many cases it is easier to tease the stallion and visually inspect the erect penis. This can also be tried when bacteriological swabs need to be taken from the urethral fossa for the identification of venereal pathogens. If this is not possible the penis can be examined, to the level of the preputial reflection, following relaxation obtained with the administration of a tranquilizer drug such as acetyl

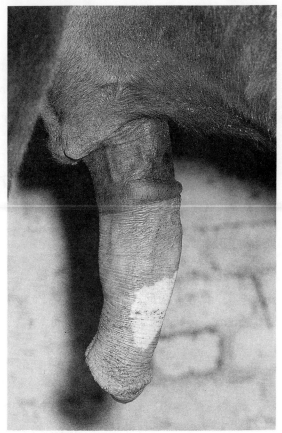

Fig. 1.2   Flaccid penis of a pony stallion.

promazine (Fig. 1.2), although the owner should be warned of the slight risk of permanent paralysis.

The surface of the penis is frequently covered by a grayish-brown caseous or creamy material known as smegma; in some animals it dries forming flakes. The integument is soft, slightly wrinkled and usually pigmented. The distal end of the penis is enlarged to form the glans penis which has a convex surface, the ventral part of the glans having a distinct depression or fossa from which the urethral process protrudes for about 2–3 cm. Running along the ventral surface of the penis is the retractor penis muscle which can be palpated as a thin band of tissue.

Erection of the penis occurs due to engorgement of the erectile tissue (corpus cavernosum penis). As a result of normal erection the penis increases in length by about 50%.

The nonerect, free portion of the penis is about 20–30 cm in length, so that the fully erect penis of the stallion often protrudes 45 cm from the prepuce. The corona glandis becomes swollen and the end of the glans enlarged (Fig. 1.3).

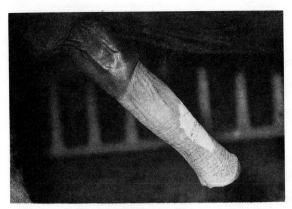

Fig. 1.3 Erect penis of a pony stallion.

Internal Genitalia

These are shown in Fig. 1.4. Rectal palpation of the internal genital organs is not often performed and adequate restraint is necessary. The pelvic urethra can be readily identified running cranially along the midline of the pelvic floor as a muscular cylinder 4–6 cm in diameter. The prostate gland can be palpated at the cranial end of the urethra surrounding the neck of the bladder. It is possible to identify the two lateral lobes and the isthmus, which connects them, running across the width of the urethra.

The vesicular glands can be identified with difficulty as paired flask-shaped structures extending cranially and laterally from the base of the urethra. They are smooth and not lobulated as in the bull. The ampullae of the ductus deferens can be palpated as two pencil-sized tubular structures, 1–2 cm in diameter passing upwards and backwards between the vesicular glands and over the neck of the bladder.

Bull

Development of the Male Reproductive Tract and Puberty

Testicular descent occurs in the bull calf midway through fetal life. However, the age at which the young bull reaches puberty is dependent upon the breed, previous growth rate and the present body condition. The normal age of puberty is 9–10 months, and in some cases mounting efforts occur before spermatozoa are present in the ejaculate. Before puberty the mucosal surface of the penis is partially adherent to the penile part of the prepuce. These gradually separate so that by about 32 weeks of age it is complete and the penis can be extruded normally.

Although young bulls may be fertile at this age full sexual maturity is not reached until 2–3 years of age. It is therefore important to use the immature bull less intensively during the first 1–2 years.

Clinical Examination

In order to study normal copulatory behavior it is necessary to provide a cow or a heifer which is in estrus and, where possible, to allow the normal mating routine to be followed in a familiar environment with nonslippery floor surfaces.

Precopulatory activity is normally brief. However, interest in the cow and the reaction time before mounting will provide a good measure of libido. Frequently, before mounting, small quantities of a clear, watery fluid will escape from the preputial orifice. This secretion is produced by the bulbo-urethral glands and it is believed to irrigate the urethra before the passage of the sperm-rich fraction of the ejaculate. Movement of the penis within the prepuce usually can be observed before the bull mounts and is indicative of penis erection; in the bull this is mainly due to the pumping of blood by the ischiocavernosus muscle from the cavernous spaces of the crura into the rest of the corpus cavernosum penis, from which there is no venous drainage distally. This results in an increased pressure causing obliteration of the sigmoid flexure with erection and protrusion of the penis; there is little enlargement of the penis (Fig. 1.5).

As the bull mounts and the penis is protruded, it can be examined visually. After intromission, ejaculation occurs almost immediately, and is associated with a vigorous thrusting movement of the pelvis. Pain or discomfort associated with injuries or lesions to the hind limbs, feet or lumbosacral region may prevent the bull from thrusting, resulting in failure of ejaculation. The bull soon dismounts and the penis is quickly retracted into the sheath. If the bull is allowed to remain with the cow he will normally attempt copulation several times in quick succession.

At this stage the collection of a complete ejaculate can be attempted using an artificial vagina (see Chapter 2); if this is performed then the semen sample should be evaluated before proceeding with the next stage of the examination.

External Genitalia   The degree of resentment to palpation varies between individual bulls. Palpation of the scrotum and testes is best performed in a warm environment so that the scrotum is well relaxed and the testes fully descended. A bimanual approach from behind is preferable (Fig. 1.6) so that the two testes can be compared for size and consistency. The

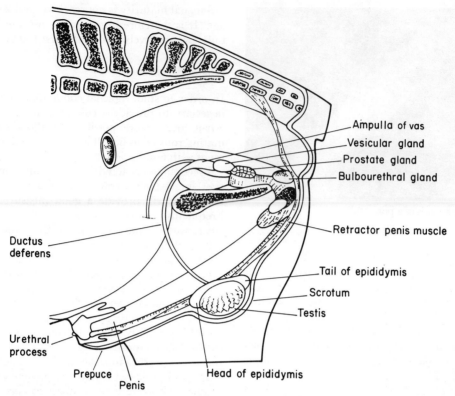

Fig. 1.4 Stallion's genitalia (after Ashdown, R. R. and Hancock, J. L. in Hafez, *Reproduction in Farm Animals*).

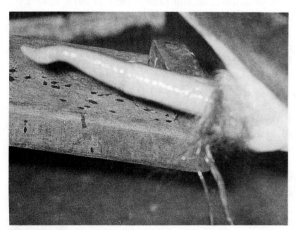

Fig. 1.5 Erect penis of the bull.

scrotum is covered with a soft, almost hairless integument and the testes should be freely mobile within the scrotum so that it is possible to push them well up towards the external inguinal ring (Fig. 1.7). The bull should not show signs of pain or discomfort.

The testes should be of similar size, normally 13 × 7 × 7 cm and approximately 350 g in weight, and the longitudinal axis is vertical when they are fully descended. They should feel tense on palpation but capable of slight compression; too hard or flaccid are signs of abnormality. Progressive changes which result in an increase or decrease in size are best determined by measuring the maximum scrotal circumference, usually 35–42 cm in an adult bull depending upon breed (see Chapter 5).

The epididymis is closely attached to the surface of the testis. The tail of the epididymis can usually be palpated as a soft swelling at the most dependent part of the scrotum.

The spermatic cord can easily be identified as a thick band of tissue present in the neck of the scrotum and containing the spermatic vessels, cremaster muscles, vaginal tunics and the ductus deferens. The latter structure can frequently be palpated as a hard, cordlike structure.

The tip of the nonerect penis is usually palpated within the prepuce 10–15 cm cranial to the scrotum and should be freely mobile within the sheath. It is possible to palpate the penis caudally to the base of the scrotum; the diameter of the penis, apart from the tapered tip, is the same along its entire length. Any increase in size, swelling or discomfort, especially related to the point of insertion of the retractor penis muscle, should be considered signi-

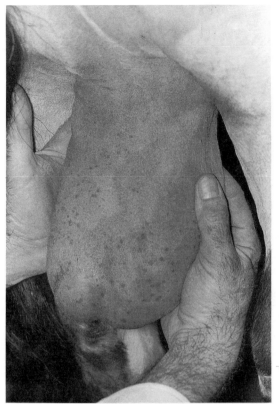

Fig. 1.6 Bimanual palpation of the scrotum and testes of the bull.

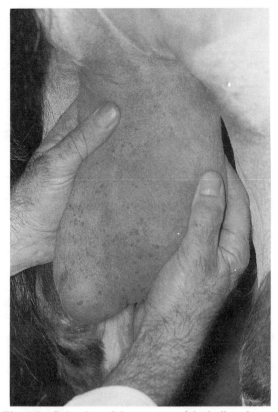

Fig. 1.7 Palpation of the scrotum of the bull to demonstrate mobility of the right testis.

ficant and indicative of injury. It is possible to exteriorize the penis for detailed examination by a number of techniques. A regional block of both pudendal nerves is a very useful procedure since the penis, as well as becoming relaxed, is also desensitized. General anesthesia, anterior epidural anesthesia or deep sedation can also be used. The penis should normally protrude 25–45 cm in the mature bull; its mucosal surface is normally pink in color and smooth.

The preputial orifice is situated 5–10 cm caudal to the umbilicus. The size of the opening varies in different breeds and individuals; in most dairy breeds it is possible to insert three fingers of one hand.

Internal Accessory Genitalia   These are shown in Fig. 1.8. Rectal palpation of the accessory organs is not a difficult procedure although insertion of the hand into the rectum can present problems because of the tight anal sphincter and surrounding retractor penis muscle.

The pelvic urethra is identified as a hard tubular structure 3–4 cm in diameter extending cranially along the pelvic floor for a distance of 10–15 cm.

The urethra suddenly terminates and at this point is surrounded by a hard collar of tissue, the body of the prostate gland. Laterally and cranially to the prostate gland it is possible to palpate paired soft, spongy, saccular structures, the vesicular glands. The ampullae of the ductus deferentes can be readily identified as two parallel tubular structures, 1–1.5 cm in diameter, which enter the pelvic urethra cranial to the prostate gland. The bulbourethral glands cannot be palpated per rectum because they are covered by muscles at the base of the penis.

Ram

Development of the Male Reproductive Tract and Puberty

Testicular descent occurs in the fetal lamb midway through fetal life, and puberty occurs at 6–8 months of age. Full sexual maturity does not occur in rams until about 2 years of age and they should be used sparingly during the first breeding season, when they are frequently only 9–10 months of age.

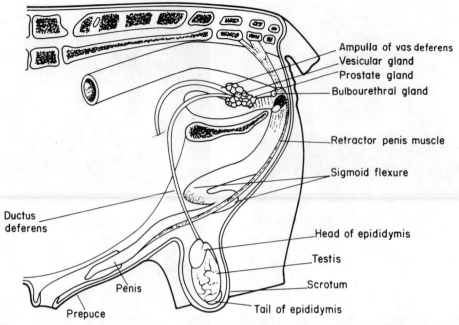

Ampulla of vas deferens
Vesicular gland
Prostate gland
Bulbourethral gland
Retractor penis muscle
Sigmoid flexure
Ductus deferens
Head of epididymis
Testis
Scrotum
Penis
Tail of epididymis
Prepuce

Fig. 1.8　Bull's genitalia (after Ashdown, R. R. and Hancock, J. L. in Hafez, *Reproduction in Farm Animals*).

Clinical Examination

Precopulatory behavior in the ram is short, copulation and ejaculation being completed within a few seconds. The ram will frequently mate a ewe repeatedly in quick succession. When the penis is erect, the urethral process (Fig. 1.9) becomes engorged and ejaculation occurs as a spray on to the external os uteri. The mechanism of erection is similar to that of the bull (see page 5).

External Genitalia　The scrotum is well-developed and pendulous and is covered with wool. Normal fully developed testes have their long axes vertical in the scrotum, weigh about 275 g each and measure $10 \times 6 \times 6$ cm. They are normally of similar size and freely mobile in the scrotum. Palpation of the epididymis is similar to that described for the bull.

The penis can be palpated as a freely mobile structure within the prepuce and the glans penis can be examined by protruding the penis from the sheath. As in the bull, the surface of the penis and the penile part of the prepuce are fused at birth, complete separation occurring from about 10 weeks of age. The mucosa of the penis is pink, moist and smooth, with a free portion of about 4 cm. A characteristic feature is the presence of the well-developed urethral process (see Fig. 1.9) which is normally 4 cm in length.

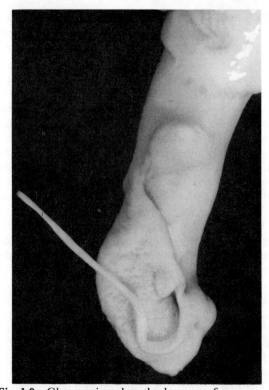

Fig. 1.9　Glans penis and urethral process of ram.

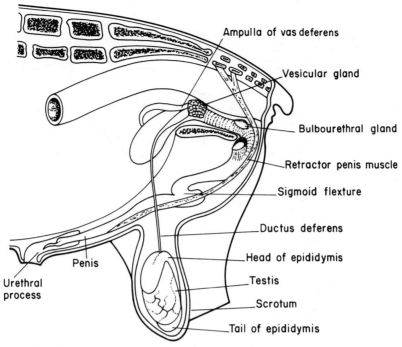

Ampulla of vas deferens

Vesicular gland

Bulbourethral gland

Retractor penis muscle

Sigmoid flexure

Ductus deferens

Head of epididymis

Testis

Scrotum

Tail of epididymis

Penis

Urethral process

Fig. 1.10　Ram's genitalia (after Ashdown, R. R. and Hancock, J. L. in Hafez, *Reproduction in Farm Animals*).

Internal Genitalia　These are shown in Fig. 1.10. The internal reproductive organs are very similar to those of the bull. It is not possible to palpate them per rectum. Semen can be collected by electro-ejaculation or with an artificial vagina.

Male Goat

The anatomy and method of clinical examination of the male goat are very similar to that of the ram. Puberty occurs from about 5 months of age but is influenced by body weight, breed and time of year. Semen is best collected in an artificial vagina, although if this fails electroejaculation can be used (see Chapter 2). Seasonal variations in libido and sperm production closely parallel the breeding season of the female goat (see page 29).

Boar

Development of the Male Reproductive Tract and Puberty

Testicular descent occurs during the last quarter of fetal life; puberty occurs at 5–8 months with full sexual maturity attained by the young boar at 9–10 months. The epithelium of the penis and the penile part of the prepuce separate completely at about 20 weeks of age.

Clinical Examination

The penis becomes erect, similarly to that described for the bull, protrudes from the prepuce before intromission and shows characteristic spiraling movements as it seeks out the vulva. Following intromission the ejaculation of the first semen fraction is associated with vigorous thrusting movements, the second fraction is discharged without obvious external signs, while the thrusting movements are repeated as the third fraction is ejaculated. The act of coitus lasts about 6–7 min. It is likely that the spiraled, erect penis engages the cervical canal and becomes 'locked' into the folds.

External Genitalia　The preputial orifice is small, will accept one to two fingers in the adult boar, and is surrounded by long stiff hairs. A spherical diverticulum leads from the dorsal wall of the prepuce and frequently becomes distended with urine, cell debris and secretions. The size of the cavity varies among individuals.

The penis is spiraled and has no glans, the mucosa is smooth, pale pink in color and moist. Examination of the penis is difficult except at coitus or under general anesthesia. Normally it is freely mobile within the sheath and the sigmoid flexure is situated cranial to the scrotum.

The scrotum is not as pendulous as in other do-

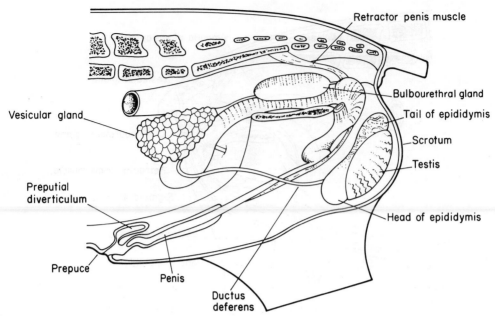

Fig. 1.11   Boar's genitalia (after Ashdown, R. R. and Hancock, J. L. in Hafez, *Reproduction in Farm Animals*).

mestic species and is situated subanally. The testes are positioned with their longitudinal axis directed dorsad and caudad so that the tail of the epididymis is uppermost. They are soft, freely mobile within the scrotum, with dimensions of 13 × 7 × 7 cm and weighing approximately 360 g. The tail of the epididymis can be palpated as a blunt, conical projection at the posterior pole of the testis.

Internal Genitalia   These are shown in Fig. 1.11. In larger boars it is possible to examine the internal genital organs by rectal palpation. There is a very obvious difference in size of the organs compared with the castrate. The paired bulbourethral glands are large, cylindrical structures which lie partially over the pelvic urethra, and are approximately 12 cm long and 3 cm wide in the mature animal.

The vesicular glands are large, lobulated pyramidal structures, 15 cm in length and 5 cm in width extending cranially over the pelvic brim into the abdominal cavity. The prostate gland has a large body 2.5 cm in diameter which covers the junction of the neck of the bladder and urethra; the disseminate part surrounds the pelvic urethra and is largely covered by urethral muscle.

Male Dog

Development of the Reproductive Tract and Puberty

The testes of the dog normally descend into the scro-

tum just before or just after birth. The time of onset of puberty varies from breed to breed with the smaller breeds being more precocious and ranging from 5 to 12 months of age.

Clinical Examination

Copulation in the dog is prolonged, frequently lasting 20–30 min. The behavior of the dog is peculiar amongst domestic species in that after the initial mounting and intromission the male steps over its penis and turns so that the dog and bitch assume a copulatory tie while facing in opposite directions.

Erection primarily involves elongation of the glans penis, the bulbus glandis remains anchored rigidly to the os penis and the pars longa glandis rides forward over the os. During the copulatory tie the penis becomes flexed through 180° at the level of the scrotum and proximal to the os penis (Fig. 1.12). It has been suggested that the turning causes occlusion of the emissary vein of the glans, preventing detumescence thus assisting in the transfer of semen into the uterus and preventing its escape and leakage.

External Genitalia   The soft and thin walled scrotum of the dog lies just ventral to the ischial arch. The testes are oval in shape and usually similar in size. There is much disparity between large and small breeds with an average measurement of 3 × 2 × 1.5 cm and an average weight of 11 g. The longitud-

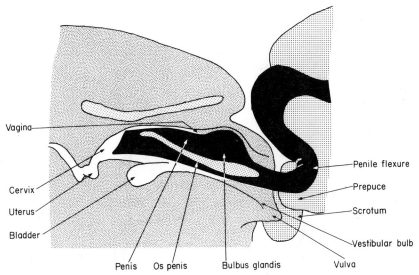

Vagina

Cervix

Uterus

Bladder

Penis   Os penis   Bulbus glandis

Penile flexure

Prepuce

Scrotum

Vestibular bulb

Vulva

Fig. 1.12   The penis of the dog during the copulatory tie (after Grandage, 1972).

inal axis of the descended testis is almost horizontal, the epididymis is closely opposed to the dorsolateral surface and the physical position of the testes often appears to be almost tandem. Occasionally one or both testes descend from the inguinal canal but subsequently occupy an ectopic site in the inguinal region on the medial aspect of the thigh or close to the prepuce.

The penis can be readily examined by manual protrusion from the prepuce and the surface is smooth, pink and moist. The preputial orifice should be large enough to admit the nonerect penis readily. The glans penis consists of two parts: the distal pars longa glandis 5–6 cm in length, and the thicker proximal bulbus glandis. The latter structure becomes considerably enlarged during erection which can be readily induced by applying digital pressure to the penis just proximal to the bulbus glandis.

In young dogs a creamy yellow preputial discharge is often apparent and can be regarded as normal unless it becomes excessive in volume and is associated with discomfort.

Internal Genitalia   These are shown in Fig. 1.13. The dog has no vesicular or bulbourethral glands. However, the prostate gland is relatively large and well-developed and can be palpated per rectum using the gloved middle finger. It is present at the junction of the neck of the bladder and urethra as a bilobed structure. Enlargement of this organ is common; this renders it easier to identify if slightly enlarged although it can drop over the brim of the pelvis, and hence out of reach, when it is grossly enlarged.

Male Cat

Development of the Reproductive Tract and Puberty

The testes are normally descended at birth although in some kittens they may not be evident in the scrotum until 4–12 weeks of age. Spermatozoa are usually present in the seminiferous tubules by 6–7 months although puberty does not occur until 9–12 months; the pure breeds are less precocious.

Clinical Examination

Male cats are capable of copulation and are fertile throughout the year. Observation of normal copulatory behavior is difficult because mating occurs most frequently at night. The act of coitus is short, lasting about 10 s and is often repeated at intervals of 5–15 min.

External Genitalia   These are shown in Fig. 1.14. The scrotum, not a very prominent structure, is a few centimeters below the anus; the skin is completely covered with hair. The testes have average measurements of 1.6 × 1.1 × 1.10 cm; the longitudinal axis is positioned obliquely, similarly to that described for the boar (page 10).

The penis is short and is directed both caudally and ventrally. In some cases an os penis is present but it is only 3–4 mm in length and is mainly rudimentary. There is no glans penis or bulbus glandis but a terminal cap approximately 1 cm in length which contains numerous papillae or spines directed towards the base of the organ.

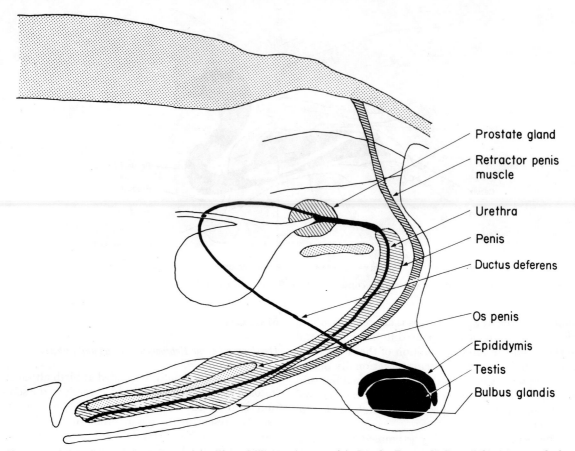

Fig. 1.13   Male dog's genitalia (reproduced from Miller's, *Anatomy of the Dog*, by Evans, H. E. and Christensen, G. C.).

Internal Genitalia   These are shown in Fig. 1.14. Examination by digital rectal palpation is not possible. The cat has a prostate gland at the junction of the bladder and urethra, and bulbourethral glands. There are no vesicular glands.

THE FEMALE ANIMAL

The female reproductive system consists of two main components:

1. The primary sex organs or gonads; the ovaries.
2. The tubular genital tract consisting of vulva, vestibule, vagina, cervix, uterus and uterine tubes.

Puberty

In the female the onset of puberty is shown by a phase of sexual receptivity, known as estrus or heat, which is repeated cyclically in most domestic species. The onset of puberty is largely related to the attainment of a critical body weight, although age,

genotype, climate, social environment and photoperiod are important. In female cattle, beef heifers reach puberty when they are about 50% of mature body weight, dairy heifers at about 35% of mature body weight. In sheep 40–63% body weight is appropriate, depending upon breed.

Before puberty there is follicular growth to a size where the oocyte is surrounded by a layer of thecal cells (Fig. 1.15) followed by atresia, the stimulus being intraovarian. Further development to mature Graafian or antral follicles does not occur until puberty since this is dependent upon the stimulus of both follicle stimulating hormone (FSH) and luteinizing hormone (LH). Secretion of both hormones is minimal, but as puberty approaches there is increased episodic and pulsatile release.

Endocrine Control

FSH and LH are secreted by the anterior pituitary in response to the stimulation of gonadotropin releasing hormone (GnRH), a peptide produced by

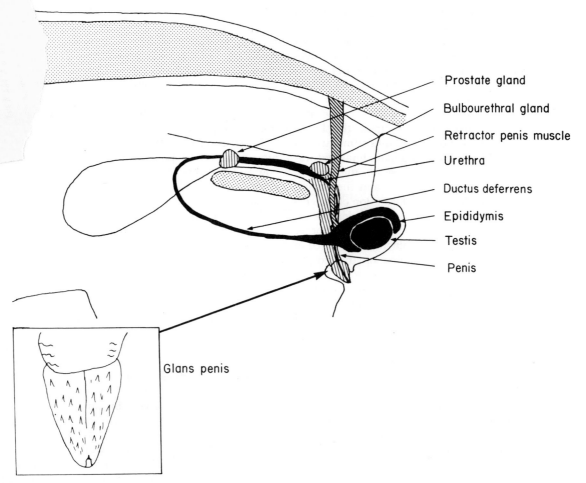

Prostate gland

Bulbourethral gland

Retractor penis muscle

Urethra

Ductus deferrens

Epididymis

Testis

Penis

Glans penis

Fig. 1.14 Male cat's genitalia.

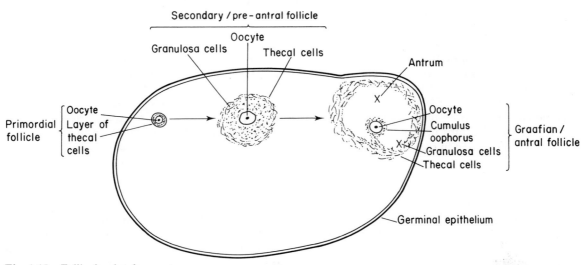

Secondary / pre-antral follicle

Oocyte

Granulosa cells

Thecal cells

Antrum

Primordial follicle

Oocyte
Layer of thecal cells

Oocyte

Cumulus oophorus

Granulosa cells

Thecal cells

Graafian / antral follicle

Germinal epithelium

Fig. 1.15 Follicular development.

the hypothalamus. FSH promotes the growth and differentiation of follicles and stimulates conversion of androgens to estrogens by the granulosa cells. LH increases ovarian blood flow and increases the synthesis of steroids by those cells that have LH receptors, especially theca interna and granulosa cells of the preovulatory follicle. Estradiol levels rise, resulting in the physical and behavioral changes of estrus, and exert a positive feedback upon the hypothalamus and anterior pituitary, thus stimulating a sudden surge of LH, which stimulates final maturation and ovulation with release of the oocyte. Following ovulation the granulosa and thecal cells give rise to luteal cells with the formation of the corpus luteum (CL). This is generally under the influence of LH, although in some species another anterior pituitary hormone, prolactin, is involved in the formation and maintenance of the corpus luteum.

The corpus luteum produces progesterone which exerts a negative feedback upon the anterior pituitary gland suppressing the secretion of FSH and LH. The corpus luteum, by virtue of its progesterone secretion, is largely responsible for controling cyclical activity. In the absence of pregnancy, in all domestic species except the dog, the uterus eventually produces a luteolysin (presumably prostaglandin $F_{2\alpha}$) which causes regression of the corpus luteum. It appears also that the corpus luteum produces oxytocin which is carried to the uterus and stimulates the production of prostaglandin. A decline in progesterone secretion occurs which removes the negative feedback upon the hypothalamus and anterior pituitary. As a consequence GnRH secretion results in the secretion of FSH and LH thus stimulating follicular growth and maturation. There is now evidence that certain endogenous opioid peptides can inhibit the release of GnRH and thus prevent gonadotropin release.

The pineal gland has an important role in controlling the timing of cyclical activity in those species that are seasonal breeders. The pineal is sensitive to the photoperiod and, via the secretion of the indoleamine hormone melatonin, modulates the secretion of the gonadotropic hormones.

The interrelationships between the various hormones are summarized in Fig. 1.16.

Stages of the Estrous Cycle

Traditionally the pattern of cyclical activity is divided into four phases: proestrus, estrus, metestrus and diestrus. Proestrus, a period of follicular growth, occurs before the onset of estrus. Estrus is when the female will accept coitus and is the only truly definable phase of the cycle. Metestrus is when the corpus luteum is developing; and diestrus is when the corpus luteum is present and functional. Apart from estrus, there is no distinct separation of the phases of the cycle and it is generally accepted that it is perhaps best considered from the aspect of hormone dominance—the follicular or estrogen-dominated phase, and the luteal or progesterone-dominated phase.

Anestrus refers to the periods of sexual quiescence after puberty. In polyestrous species, such as the cow and sow, repeated cyclical activity is only interrupted by pregnancy except for pathological reasons.

The puerperium is the period after parturition during which the reproductive system is returning to its normal, nonpregnant state.

Mare

The mare is seasonally polyestrous, the stimulus necessary to initiate cyclical activity being the increase in the length of daylight and, to a lesser extent, the improvement of nutrition and warmth in spring. The breeding season of horses is largely influenced by the rules concerning the registration of thoroughbreds which gives a birthdate of January 1. The natural breeding season will vary depending on the latitude of the region. In the United Kingdom this would be May to October, while in the United States it may begin in March to May depending on location. Fillies reach puberty between 12 and 18 months of age, although in most cases regular cyclical activity does not occur until they are 2 years old. It is possible to advance the seasonal onset of cyclical activity by subjecting mares to additional artificial lighting; if they are housed in lighted conditions during the winter months some will maintain continuous cyclical ovarian activity.

The duration of the estrous cycle, that is, the interval between the start of successive estrous periods, is on average 21 days. However, at the beginning and end of the breeding season the cycle is frequently prolonged and irregular. The duration of estrus is 5–6 days with ovulation occurring about 1–2 days before the end; ovulation does not have a fixed relationship to the onset of heat. Anovulatory heats can occur with the subsequent regression of the follicle. The hormonal changes in the peripheral circulation during the estrous cycle are shown in Fig. 1.17. Unlike other domestic species a single FSH peak is shown towards the end of diestrus. There is controversy about when a second peak associated with the LH peak occurs.

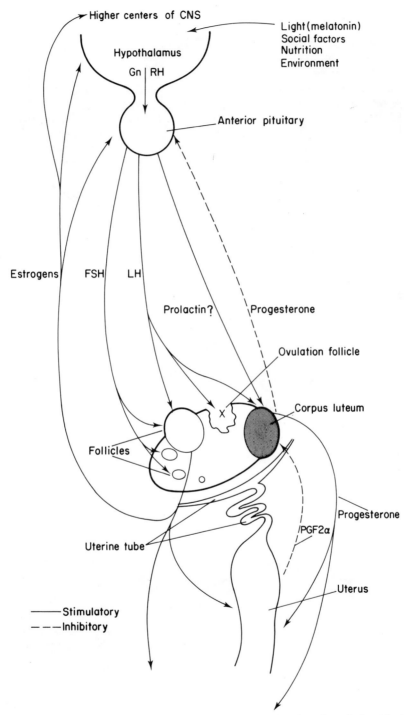

Fig. 1.16 Endocrine control of cyclical reproductive activity in the female—the relationship between the hypothalamus, anterior pituitary and genital system.

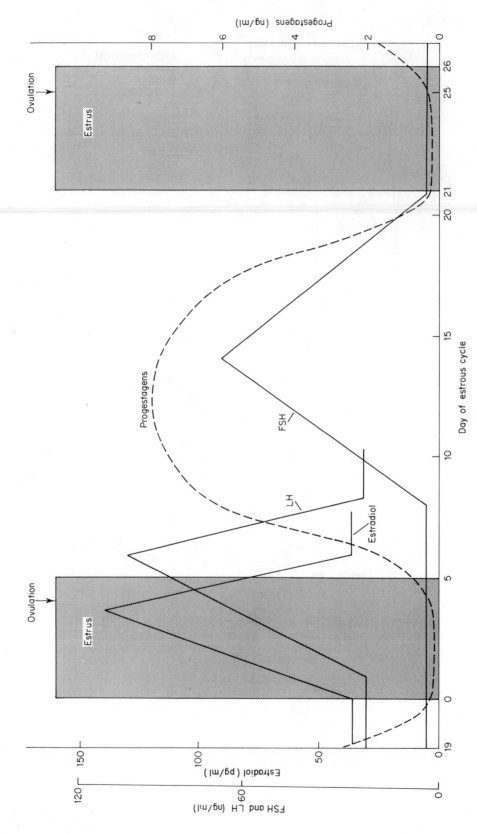

Fig. 1.17   Hormone concentrations in the peripheral blood of the mare during the estrous cycle.

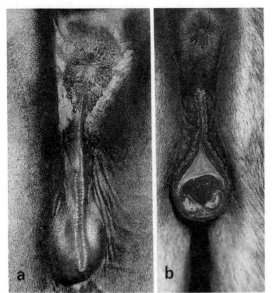

Fig. 1.18 Vulva of mare: (a) showing conformation of the labia; (b) showing eversion of the clitoris at estrus.

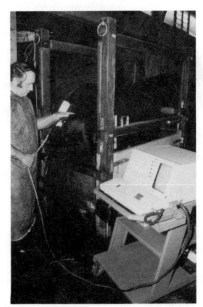

Fig. 1.19 Use of B mode ultrasound in a mare using a transrectal approach.

Signs of Estrus

In the absence of the stallion many mares will not show very obvious signs of estrus, although some will 'show' to other mares and geldings. There may be changes in temperament, crouching, urination, eversion of the vulval labiae and exposure of the clitoris (Fig. 1.18). These signs are more obvious when the mare is 'teased' with a stallion, and for this reason good stud practice requires the regular and routine use of a stallion for this purpose. A mare that is not in estrus will usually kick out and squeal when approached by the stallion; and some mares, when accompanied by their foal, will not show a positive response even though they are in estrus.

Clinical Examination

Careful examination of the genital organs of the mare can provide information about its reproductive status. In all cases it is necessary to ensure that the mare is adequately restrained to prevent injury to the clinician before a rectal or vaginal examination is made. This is best afforded with the mare in stocks but since in most cases these will be unavailable, examination around a wall, door or partition is possible; with a very fractious mare the use of tranquilizer drugs should be considered.

External Genitalia　The vulva of the mare should be symmetrical, positioned almost vertically in the perineal region with both labia closely opposed (see Fig. 1.18). No obvious changes can be detected at estrus although eversion of the clitoris or 'showing' is a characteristic behavioral sign of sexual receptiveness (see Fig. 1.18).

Internal Genitalia　These can be examined either visually, with the aid of a vaginal speculum, by palpation per rectum or per vaginum or the comparatively recent development of brightness mode (B mode) direct imaging using a rectal transducer probe (Fig. 1.19).

Vaginal Examination

The appearance of the vaginal mucous membrane and the cervix can provide information about the reproductive status of the mare. Adequate cleansing of the perineum and vulva is necessary and a clean hand with a bland lubricant or sterile speculum should be used. The urethra opens ventrally at the vestibular/vaginal junction and can be identified by the presence of soft folds 10–15 cm cranial to the vulva. It readily dilates in mares and will accept the insertion of one to two fingers.

Several types of vagina specula are available; those illustrated in Fig. 1.20 are particularly useful. Type (a) has the advantage of having a soft, interchangeable outer tube which can be replaced after the examination of each mare, and its own light source. Type (b) is a simple device, self-retaining when opened and which, with the aid of a torch or

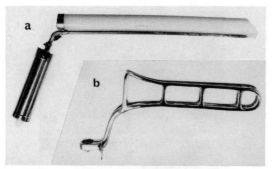

Fig. 1.20 Two types of vaginal specula which can be used in the mare and cow.

light source, enables good visual examination of the cervix and vagina.

Cyclical Changes During estrus the vaginal mucosa is moist, hyperemic and glistens when illuminated. The cervix is edematous with the external os partially dilated so that it will readily admit the insertion of two or three fingers. In diestrus, when the genital tract is under the dominance of progesterone, the mucosa is pale and dry; the cervix loses the edema associated with estrus, and the external os becomes closed so that it will admit the insertion of one finger. The vagina is covered with sticky mucus becoming progressively thicker as pregnancy advances and filling the cervix which is thus closed. During anestrus, when the mare ceases to have cyclical ovarian activity, the vaginal mucosa is very pale and dry, the cervix is nonedematous, can appear opened or closed, and will readily admit the introduction of two or three fingers.

Rectal Palpation

Practical Procedure The mare tends to resent rectal examination more than the cow. It is necessary to insert carefully a well-lubricated hand through the anus and into the rectum and then to remove feces carefully. Rectal examination of a mare before she is presented for mating can occasionally be hazardous since the relaxed anal sphincter can result in the stallion performing intromission into the rectum which may cause rupture of the rectum.

In performing the procedure it is necessary to follow a definite examination routine. Identification of the vagina is difficult since it is a thin-walled structure with only a potential cavity; but creating a pneumovagina by inserting the hand into the vagina facilitates its identification. The cervix can be identified as a distinct but soft tubular structure,

3–4 cm wide and 5–7 cm in length lying caudal to the brim of the pelvis (Fig. 1.21).

The body of the uterus, 15–20 cm in length, is a well-defined structure which extends cranially and ventrally. The uterine horns join the uterine body at almost a right angle (see Fig. 1.22) and extend cranially, dorsally and laterally (see Fig. 1.21). The point of separation of the two horns can be identified as an obvious cleft or depression. The uterine horns end somewhat blindly since the uterine tube opens into the extremity of the uterine horn through a distinct papilla.

The uterus can be palpated by grasping each horn between thumb and fingers and following it along its length, compressing it against the shafts of the ileum or gently palpating the cranial border with a partially cupped hand.

The ovary is attached to the distal pole of each horn by a tough, fibrous band, the utero-ovarian ligament (Fig. 1.22). The ovaries are characteristically lima or broad bean-shaped with a distinct depression, the ovulation fossa. The size varies considerably depending upon the reproductive status and breed of the individual. In general, during cyclical activity the ovaries are larger, especially when mature follicles are present, than during sexual quiescence or anestrus.

Identification of the ovaries by rectal palpation is not difficult. They are suspended from the sublumbar region by the mesovarium (the anterior part of the broad ligament) which can be identified due to its close proximity to the shaft of the ilium and tuber coxae (see Fig. 1.21). Critical examination of the ovaries may require the use of both hands, especially in large mares since palpation of the left ovary is much easier with the right hand, and of the right ovary with the left hand. By fixing the ovary between the thumb and fourth finger it is possible to palpate the ovarian structures with the index and middle fingers, at the same time estimating their dimensions.

Cyclical Changes of Ovaries The follicle is a fluid-filled structure which, when of sufficient size and position, can be identified on palpation as a smooth, rounded structure projecting from the surface of the ovary (Figs 1.23 and 1.24); it yields slightly when digital pressure is applied. Follicles can usually be palpated when they are 1 cm or more in size. They rarely ovulate when less than 3 cm in diameter and can grow to 7 cm in diameter when fully ripe in large breeds of horses. Just before ovulation the follicle usually becomes softer and less tense, which is a good indication that ovulation will occur within 24 h. In most cases only one follicle reaches maturity

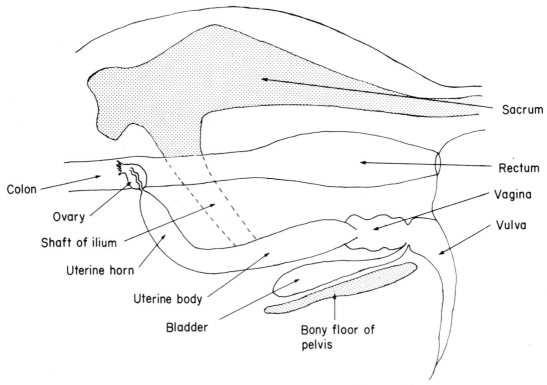

Fig. 1.21 The position of the genital organs within the pelvic cavity and abdomen of the mare.

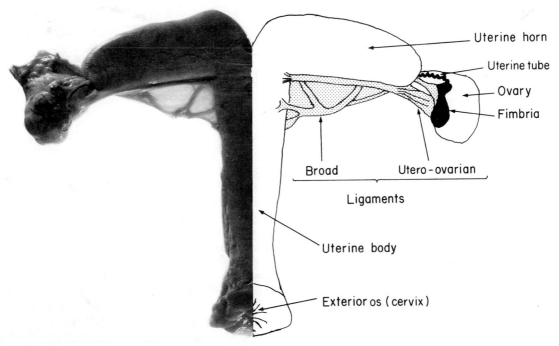

Fig. 1.22 Genital organs of the mare.

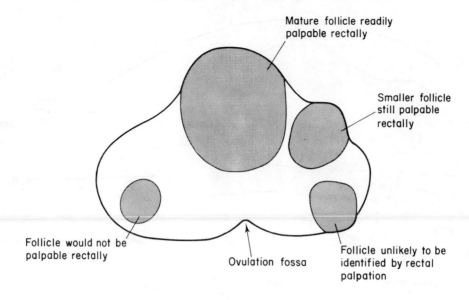

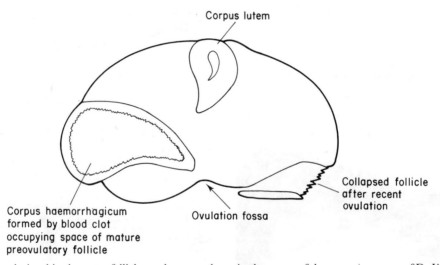

Fig. 1.23   The relationships between follicles and corpora lutea in the ovary of the mare (courtesy of Dr W. E. Allen).

and ovulates. However, twin ovulations do occur, particularly in thoroughbreds. An annual incidence of 15–25% has been recorded. In pony mares it is less common. Twin pregnancies rarely go to term because of fetal death and abortion. While it is possible to diagnose twin conceptuses very early in pregnancy using B mode direct imaging (see Chapter 4, p. 68) and destroying one conceptus or terminating the pregnancy, it is preferable to prevent twins being conceived. This can be done using B mode ultrasound and a rectal transducer probe to monitor follicular growth and ovulation (see Figs

1.19 and 1.24). In some mares ovulations occur on the same day (synchronous), where there would be a greater chance of twin conceptions compared with ovulations on different days (asynchronous), or during diestrus.

Just after ovulation it is possible to palpate the depression which was previously occupied by the mature follicle. However, it is quickly filled with a blood clot which is ultimately replaced by luteal cells to form the corpus luteum (see Figs 1.23 and 1.24). It is often possible to confuse a softened follicle just before ovulation with the blood-filled follicular

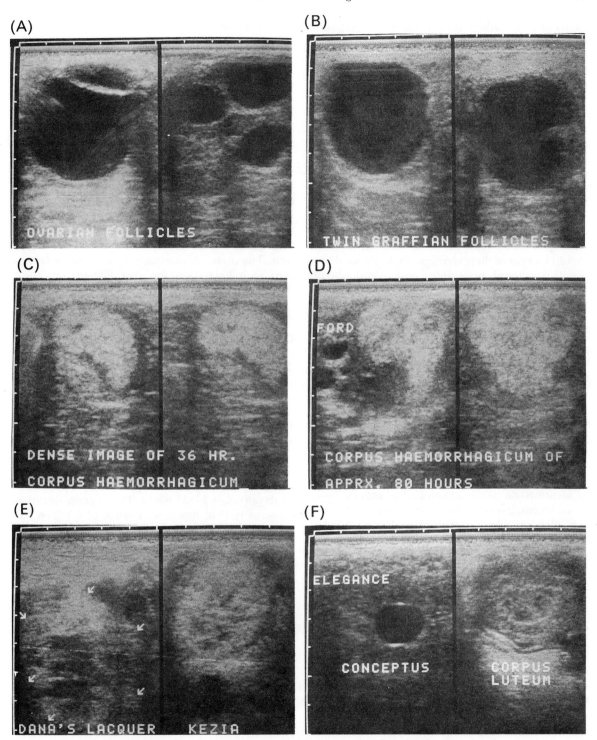

Fig. 1.24 Transrectal ultrasound scan of the mare's ovaries at various stages of the estrous cycle. (A) Ovaries at estrus, left ovary with 5 cm follicle, right ovary with three 2–2.5 cm follicles. (B) Ovaries at estrus each with a mature 4 cm follicle. (C) Two photographs of the same ovary containing a Corpus Hemorrhagicum 36 h after ovulation. (D) Two photographs of the same ovary containing a Corpus Hemorrhagicum 80 h after ovulation. (E) Ovary with a 3 day corpus luteum (Dana's Lacquer) and an ovary with a 7 day corpus luteum (Kezia). (F) Ovary of pragnant mare with 13 day corpus luteum. (Courtesy of Mr J. R. Newcombe.)

cavity after ovulation. Many mares resent palpation of the ovary immediately after ovulation.

It is usually possible to identify the developing corpus luteum for 2–3 days after ovulation but in most cases, unlike the cow, it is difficult after this time (see Figs 1.23 and 1.24). It has been described as palpable in Welsh mountain ponies for an average of 8.5 days after ovulation in nonpregnant mares. The corpus luteum does not protrude from the surface and tends to feel similar to the rest of the ovarian stroma. Although part of the mature follicle develops superficially, ovulation always occurs at the ovulation fossa (see Fig. 1.23).

Sequential examinations are valuable in assessing changes in reproductive function. It is important when performing such examinations that a record should be kept of these changes. To facilitate this, a simple, shortened, preferably personal code should be devised. For example, by reference to the length and breadth of thumb and fingers the dimensions of the ovaries should be measured and recorded. The presence of follicles and their consistency, for example, tense or soft, should be noted and their diameters estimated. Recording the position of the follicles can be done by labeling the poles of the left ovary A and B and the right ovary C and D: so a follicle of 3 cm in diameter which is at the lateral pole of the left ovary can be labelled 3A, one placed in the middle of the ovary A3B, and one at the medial pole of the ovary 3B.

During anestrus the ovaries are small, hard and frequently do not contain any structures which can be identified on rectal palpation. Towards the onset of the breeding season the ovaries become softer and it is often possible to identify several small follicles. These may grow to 3–4 cm in diameter but do not ovulate and eventually regress and become atretic. Once ovulation has occurred most mares assume a fairly regular cyclical pattern.

Cyclical Changes of the Uterus and Cervix During estrus the uterus is flaccid with little tone and feels 'thin-walled'; during diestrus there is some increase in tone and the uterine horns feel more tubular although not as marked as during early pregnancy (see Chapter 4). In anestrus the uterus feels very flaccid.

The cervical changes which can be identified by means of a vaginal speculum (see above) can also be detected on rectal palpation. During diestrus, pregnancy and pseudopregnancy the cervix is readily identified as a narrow firm tubular structure but at estrus it is soft and broad; the creation of a temporary pneumovagina assists in this examination (see page 18).

The Puerperium

Return to cyclical ovarian activity is rapid after foaling, with most mares returning to estrus 5–9 days postpartum—the 'foal heat'. It may be anovulatory, or not associated with estrous behavior. However, many mares conceive when covered at this time. Sometimes the foal heat is followed by a period of anestrus.

The physical shrinkage or involution of the uterus is rapid. In pony mares it is usually possible to palpate the whole of the uterus per rectum within 12 h of foaling although it may be slightly longer in thoroughbreds. There is some disorganization of the endometrium, particularly of its subepithelial layers, but it does not necessarily prevent conception. The uterus of most mares becomes contaminated with bacteria at or after foaling, but these usually disappear after the foal heat (see Chapter 9).

Cow

The cow is normally polyestrous with recurrent and regular cyclical activity throughout the year. However, the periodicity can be suppressed as a result of poor nutrition and perhaps by high milk yields. Heifers normally reach puberty at 6–10 months of age and, apart from pregnancy or functional abnormalities, have continuous regular estrous cycles. The average length of the estrous cycle or the interval between the start of successive estrous periods, is 21 days (range 17–25 days). The average duration of estrus is 15 h; however, a range of 0.5–25 h has been recorded, and 20% of the cows found to be in estrus for less than 6 h. Cows are atypical amongst domestic species in that ovulation occurs on average 12 h after the end of estrus. Because of its relatively short duration, estrus detection can be a problem. In many cases it is doubtful if detection is better than 60%. It can be significantly improved if the frequency and duration of observations is increased. Various methods to assist estrus detection, especially in heifers, have been tried, such as teaser bulls with marking devices, heat mount detectors or tail paint. The most reliable single sign of estrus in the cow is standing to be mounted by other cows; however, a few pregnant cows will also show this behavior. Other signs are:

1. Mounting of other cows.
2. The presence of roughening or abrasions on the rump.
3. The grouping of sexually active cows, particularly at night, in fields or yards.

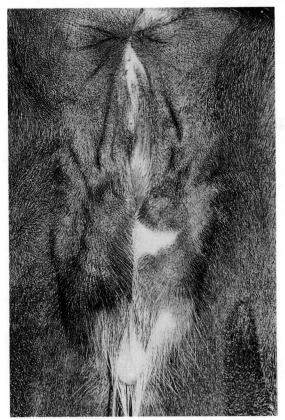

Fig. 1.25 Vulva of cow.

4. Reduced food intake.
5. Reduced milk yield and bellowing if isolated.

The significance of vulval and vaginal mucus is described below.

Clinical Examination

Detailed clinical examination of the reproductive system is possible in most cows and provides valuable information about the reproductive status of the individual animal. With greater emphasis on ensuring optimum reproductive efficiency, especially in dairy herds, routine examinations of cows are frequently performed and an appreciation of the normal genital organs is important.

External Genitalia The vulval labia are covered with soft, thin skin and they are symmetrical and closely opposed to ensure closure of the vestibule and vagina (Fig. 1.25). The vulva shows no obvious cyclical changes apart from the presence of the characteristic clear, elastic mucus which hangs from the ventral commissure at estrus. In a number of cows and heifers some bloodstained mucus is apparent

during the first few days after the end of estrus and is referred to as metestrual bleeding. In many cases the mucus becomes adherent to the tail or hindquarters.

Vaginal Examination of Internal Genitalia It is possible to inspect the vagina and cervix with the aid of a speculum, although the procedure is not routinely used in the cow. The types of specula previously described for the mare (page 18) can be used; the vulva should be thoroughly cleansed and a sterile instrument used. The speculum is inserted initially upwards at an angle of approximately 30° before passing over the ischial arch when it is directed forwards in a horizontal plane.

Cyclical Changes Visual inspection of the mucosa during the luteal phase of the cycle reveals a pale pink mucous membrane, dry apart from small amounts of sticky, tenacious mucus; the cervix is tightly closed. Towards the end of the luteal phase the mucous membrane becomes a light pink color with an increase in the amount of mucus. At estrus the mucosa is bright pink in color and moist, the external os uteri is dilated and pools of clear, elastic mucus accumulate in the floor of the anterior vagina. The mucus is frequently discharged from the vagina and hangs as a distinct strand from the ventral commissure to form the 'bulling string', which is a reliable sign of estrus. During anestrus the vaginal mucous membrane appears pale and dry.

Since the degree of mucus secretion and the appearance of the vaginal mucosa are obviously under the cyclical influence of ovarian hormones, attempts have been made to measure the changes as an aid to estrus detection. The appearance of arborization or fernleaf patterns in smears of unstained, dried cervical and vaginal mucus has been used to detect estrus. Similarly the elasticity of cervical mucus and changes in electrical conductivity and potential have been determined. It is of no practical assistance. Changes in the hormone concentrations during the estrous cycle are summarized in Fig. 1.26.

Rectal Palpation

Palpation of the reproductive organs of the cow per rectum is used to assess the reproductive status of the animal and to determine the presence of any abnormalities. In most cases it is a relatively simple and safe procedure both for the animal and operator, although it is necessary to have adequate restraint. A gloved, lubricated hand is gently inserted into the rectum, feces are best evacuated by gentle stimula-

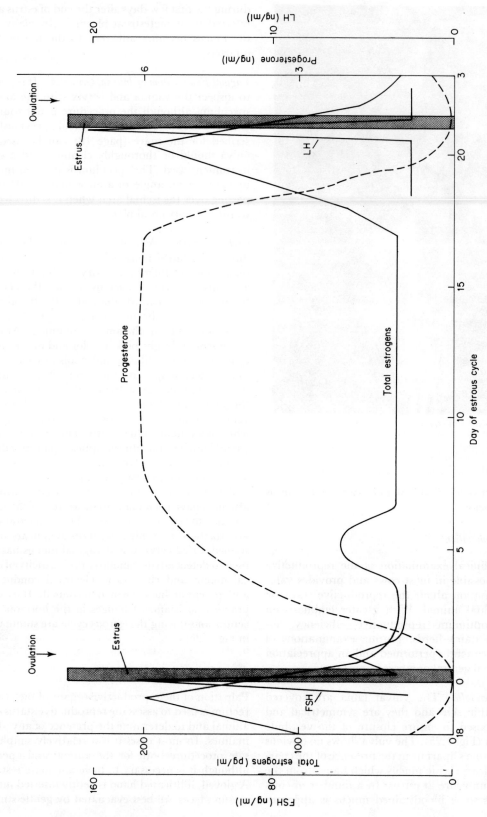

Fig. 1.26 Hormone concentrations in the peripheral blood of the cow during the estrous cycle.

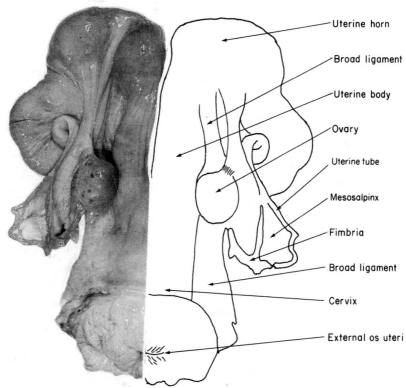

Uterine horn

Broad ligament

Uterine body

Ovary

Uterine tube

Mesosalpinx

Fimbria

Broad ligament

Cervix

External os uteri

Fig. 1.27   Genital organs of the cow.

tion of a normal defecation reflex rather than vigorous actions which tend to stimulate peristalsis and increase rectal tone. The ease of palpation varies between breeds and individuals. It is easier in dairy breeds, especially the Jersey than in the beef breeds such as the Hereford and Charolais, particularly if they are fat. It is also easier when the cows are fed on dry preserved feed during the winter rather than fresh spring grass because of increased peristalsis and rectal tone. It is possible to palpate all the reproductive organs of the heifer since they are within the pelvic cavity. However, in the large multiparous cow it is often difficult because the uterine horns and ovaries are within the abdominal cavity and hence out of reach. In these animals it is necessary to retract the uterus into the pelvis to facilitate complete examination.

A strict, systematic routine must be followed and the findings recorded.

Vagina and Cervix   Identification of the normal vagina is difficult as it is soft and thin-walled. Careful palpation along the floor of the bony pelvis in the midline should reveal the cervix as a hard, slightly irregular, tubular structure. In heifers it is 2–3 cm in diameter and 5–6 cm in length resting on the pelvic floor. In multiparous, nonpregnant cows it is slightly larger and may well rest upon or over the pelvic brim. In the nonpregnant or early pregnant animal it is mobile and can be grasped through the rectal wall and moved from side to side within the pelvic cavity. The cervix increases in size as a result of pregnancy. It is also possible to identify the annular folds which are present in the mucosa, and which frequently cause partial obstruction to the insertion of an intrauterine catheter.

Uterus   Since the uterine body is so short in the cow (4–5 cm in length) the bifurcation of the two horns can be identified as a slit-like depression just cranial to the cervix. The uterine horns curve initially downwards and forwards; then, after forming the greater curvature, they pass backwards and upwards with the tip of the horn 5–6 cm from the cervix (Fig. 1.27). The sizes of the uterine horns and body vary and are dependent upon the parity of the animal and whether it is gravid, nongravid or puerperal. In the nongravid cow they are 35–40 cm in length and 4–5 cm in diameter. On palpation it is usually possible to identify the base and curvature of the horns, but not so readily the extremities.

The uterine horns gradually merge into the uter-

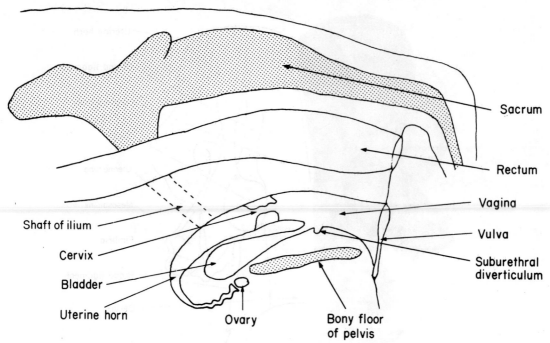

Sacrum

Rectum

Vagina

Vulva

Suburethral
diverticulum

Shaft of ilium

Cervix

Bladder

Uterine horn

Ovary

Bony floor
of pelvis

Fig. 1.28   The position of the genital organs within the pelvic cavity of the cow.

ine tubes (see Fig. 1.27), convoluted structures 20–25 cm in length opening into the abdominal cavity at the ostium. The normal uterine tube is rarely possible to identify on rectal palpation, although if thickened and indurated it can be recognized.

The ovarian bursa, a pocket formed between the mesovarium and utero-ovarian ligament, can be palpated per rectum with difficulty and is normally free from the surface of the ovary.

Uterine Cyclical Changes   The uterus undergoes distinct changes associated with the estrous cycle. A few days before the onset of estrus it is possible to identify an increase in uterine tone which becomes more pronounced at estrus. At this time the uterus becomes turgid, erect and coiled, particularly in response to palpation. The tone diminishes after estrus but persists for about 2 days. During this phase of the estrous cycle identification of the entire length of the horns becomes much easier. In the luteal phase the uterine horns return to their soft, flaccid state which renders palpation more difficult.

Ovaries—Location and Palpation   Location and identification of the ovaries of the cow requires repeated practice. They are probably most readily located by following the uterine horns from their bases to just beyond their curvatures, and then gently sweeping backwards with the fingers towards the cervix.

Another method of locating them is to palpate the cervix and bifurcation and then to sweep downwards on either side with the fingers since the ovaries are positioned within a few centimeters of the cervix (see Figs 1.27 and 1.28). In pluripara it is often necessary to palpate beyond and below the pelvic brim.

The ovaries vary in size and shape depending upon the stage of the estrous cycle, usually being 2–4 cm in length by 2–3 cm in width and 2–3 cm thick. Identifying structures on the ovary requires the ability to 'pick up' the ovary through the rectal wall with thumb and fingers, using one or more free fingers to palpate the surface of the ovary. Occasionally this can be difficult if the ovary is situated behind the broad ligament, in which case it is necessary to manipulate the ovary so that it is no longer enclosed by the structure.

Ovaries—Cyclical Changes   The ovaries of the prepubertal heifer are small, smooth and inactive but with the onset of puberty they show distinct cyclical changes. Most observers report that the right ovary is more active than the left.

Throughout the estrous cycle there are continuous phases of follicular growth and regression. Around the start of estrus several follicles will continue to grow and one, or occasionally two, will reach a diameter of 2–2.5 cm, and be capable of subsequent ovulation. Thus at most stages of the estrous

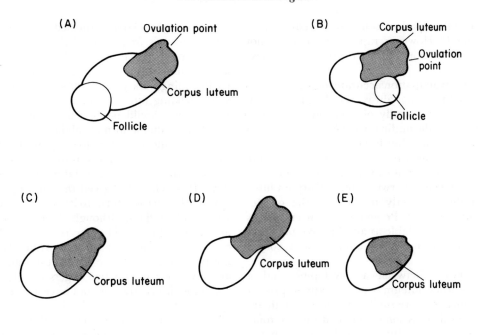

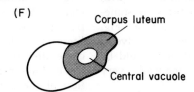

Fig. 1.29 The relationships between follicles, corpora lutea and the ovary of the cow. A, Follicle on opposite pole to corpus luteum thus readily identifiable on rectal palpation. B, Follicle adjacent to corpus luteum thus not readily identifiable on rectal palpation. C, D, Corpus luteum has a distinct protuberance thus readily identifiable on rectal palpation. E, Corpus luteum encompassed more within ovarian stroma and thus difficult to identify on rectal palpation. F, Corpus luteum with central fluid-filled vacuole incorrectly referred to as a 'cystic' corpus luteum.

cycle follicles up to about 1.2 cm in diameter are present in the ovaries; it is this follicular growth and regression that is responsible for some of the variations in ovarian size during the cycle. The ability to palpate accurately and identify follicles usually depends upon their physical relationship to the corpus luteum of diestrus (Fig. 1.29). When follicles are present they can be identified as tense, smooth structures protruding from the surface of the ovary which yield slightly when compressed (see Fig. 1.29). Towards the time of ovulation, which occurs about 12 h after the end of estrus, the follicle becomes softer and less turgid.

The corpus luteum of the cow is readily identifiable, and changes in corpus luteum size are largely responsible for the major changes in ovarian size throughout the estrous cycle. Immediately after ovulation the ovary feels flattened, soft and yielding and sometimes it is possible to palpate a small depression at the site of ovulation. During the next 3–4 days the corpus luteum develops at the site of ovulation from the granulosa and theca interna cells. This results in the ovary becoming larger and it is often possible to palpate the corpus luteum as a firm, slightly yielding structure. By 7–8 days the corpus luteum is fully formed measuring 2–2.5 cm in diameter. Frequently the corpus luteum produces a distinct protuberance from the surface of the ovary (see Fig. 1.29) which makes identification of the structure much easier. However, it may be encompassed within the stroma of the ovary and be more difficult to identify (see Fig. 1.29).

The corpus luteum becomes slightly harder and firmer with age and it is possible to determine, by sequential rectal palpation, some slight reduction in size after day 17. However, rapid regression does not occur until 24–48 hours before the onset of the next estrus.

At a single examination accurate identification of ovarian structures is not always possible. It has been recorded that, in a study of 180 cows examined before slaughter, the findings were correct in 83% of the ovaries examined but in only 67% of the cows. Nearly half of the incorrect interpretations were due to the failure to determine the presence of follicles in ovaries which were otherwise empty. Corpora lutea were identified correctly in 89% of the ovaries which contained them. Progesterone concentrations of milk are now available as an objective measurement of the presence and function of a corpus luteum.

Differentiation between a developing and a regressing corpus luteum can sometimes present problems since they are similar in size and both are present when there is some increased uterine tone. The developing corpus luteum yields slightly on palpation while the regressing corpus luteum is harder.

Postmortem examination of ovaries reveals a number of corpora lutea which contain a central fluid-filled cavity. While these structures are sometimes referred to as 'cystic' corpora lutea (see Fig. 1.29), they are normal and usually have no adverse effect on function. It is doubtful if they could be identified on rectal palpation unless the wall is very thin and the vacuole large.

The normal ovaries of older pluriparous cows are larger than those of nulliparous or primiparous heifers. Frequently small nodular structures can be identified in old cows due to the remnants of the many regressed corpora lutea and especially the remnants of the corpora lutea of pregnancy which are prominent, white in color due to the presence of connective tissue, and called corpora albicantes. The incidence of twinning varies between breeds and within breeds; the average number of twins born is between 1 and 3%. However, the incidence of double ovulations is higher and probably reflects a high rate of early embryonic death associated with this occurrence.

The Puerperium

Ovarian activity is usually in abeyance for 1–2 weeks after parturition. However, in some cows follicular development occurs with subsequent regression. In a few cases maturation and ovulation can occur as early as 10 days postpartum although in most of these there are no signs of behavioral estrus. In dairy cows the first ovulation after calving is at 3–4 weeks, slightly later in suckled beef cows; the first luteal phase is frequently slightly shorter with an interestrous interval of 15 or 16 days. A number of factors influence the return to cyclical ovarian activity including milk yield, bodily condition, season of year, suckling intensity, nutrient intake and genotype. Cows should not normally be served before 45–50 days after a normal calving.

The uterine size decreases rapidly following the expulsion of the calf, and it is usually possible to define the whole uterus on rectal palpation after 7–10 days. It is generally agreed that in a normal puerperium the uterus returns to its normal nonpregnant size by 42–46 days, although changes after 25 days are imperceptible. The cervix is fully dilated to enable expulsion of the calf, but within 24–36 h it is not possible to introduce a hand through the cervix and it will accept only two fingers after 4 days.

Although the cow does not have a true deciduous placenta, there is considerable loss of maternal tissue after parturition. The upper two-thirds of the uterine caruncles become necrotic and are completely sloughed by about the 12th day postpartum. The sloughing and liquefaction of the maternal tissue is largely responsible for the persistent lochial discharge which is seen as a normal feature in the postpartum cow. In some pluriparous animals up to 2 liters of discharge can be voided but this should cease after 10–12 days. Eventually the integrity of the endometrium is reestablished by epithelialization of the denuded caruncles, usually by 25–30 days in normal cows. Mucopurulent exudate on the endometrial surface can delay this regrowth of the epithelial layer.

In most cows the uterus becomes contaminated with bacteria from the environment during or after a normal calving. The flora is mixed and fluctuates, but is generally readily eliminated around the time of the first postpartum ovulation when estrogen concentrations are high (see Fig. 1.26). The uterus subsequently becomes sterile (see Chapter 6).

Ewe

The ewe is typically seasonally polyestrous. In most breeds the onset of cyclical activity is dependent upon the decline in day length. Puberty is usually reached at 8–9 months of age although genotype, growth rate and social factors exert a major influence. Many ewe lambs will conceive in the autumn of the same year in which they are born. A minimum body weight as a percentage of mature body weight is necessary for the attainment of puberty, and this must be reached during the first

Table 1.1 Adult ewe body weights

Breed or cross	kg
Lowland ewes	
Masham	70
Grey face	69
Mule	72
Welsh halfbred	58
Scotch halfbred	76
Romney halfbred	75
Clun × Welsh	62
Clun × Suffolk	74
Upland ewes	
Grey face	68
Scotch blackface	52
Swaledale	50
Welsh Mountain	38
Clun	61

breeding season (Table 1.1). If not, then the first estrus will be delayed until the next breeding season.

The interestrous interval is 16–17 days and estrus normally lasts 24–36 h with ovulation occurring towards the end of this period. At the beginning of the breeding season both silent and anovulatory estrus can occur. Hormonal changes in the peripheral circulation are summarized in Fig. 1.30.

Signs of Estrus

The ewe does not normally show overt signs of estrus in the absence of the ram. Where possible she will seek out the ram and will permit him to mount and serve.

Clinical Examination

Vaginal examination is readily performed with the aid of a speculum and is a useful technique. However, digital exploration and palpation of the vagina and rectum are of little value.

Genitalia

The vulva is 2–3 cm in length, the labia are thick and frequently pigmented, the ventral commissure is characteristically pointed and projects downwards. The vagina is approximately 8 cm in length. The cervix is 3–4 cm in length, and the cervical canal is closed by the presence of interdigitating projections and crypts which make it virtually impossible to introduce a catheter. The uterus is similar in appearance to that of the cow; the uterine body is short and the two cornua, 10–12 cm in length, are coiled and taper to join the uterine tube. The caruncles are smaller than those of the cow and have a concave surface.

The ovaries of the ewe are oval in shape, their size depending upon the reproductive status of the individual.

Cyclical Changes

During the periods of the year when the ewe is not pregnant and anestrous there is some follicular growth followed by atresia; ovulation rarely occurs.

In the breeding season the ovaries show obvious cyclical changes. Follicular growth and atresia occurs throughout the luteal phase of the estrous cycle with follicles not usually exceeding 0.5 cm in diameter. At the commencement of estrus there is rapid growth so that just before ovulation one or more follicles have grown to be about 1 cm in diameter. The follicular fluid gives a characteristic purple coloration to the ripe follicle. The corpora lutea reach a maximum mean size of 0.9 cm at 6–7 days after ovulation, remaining for about 13 days after the previous estrus before starting to regress. The mature corpus luteum is salmon pink in color.

Apart from slight edema of the vulva, and slight hyperemia in nonpigmented breeds there are few external changes associated with estrus. The cervical mucus and vaginal epithelium undergo cyclical changes. Cervical mucus increases in amount just before and during estrus. When samples collected with the aid of a glass rod or pipette are placed on a slide and allowed to dry in air they show the typical fern pattern. Interpretation of the cellular changes in vaginal smears is more difficult, the most typical change being the appearance of a large percentage of acidophilic cells 3 days after the onset of estrus.

The Puerperium

The changes are similar to those previously described in the cow. Degenerative changes occur in the uterine caruncles just before parturition and become more extensive afterwards with the necrosis of the upper position of the caruncle by the 7th day postpartum. There is liquifaction and sloughing of the tissue followed by regeneration of the epithelium by 30 days. Involution of the uterus to its nonpregnant state is complete by about 35 days.

Female Goat

The goat is seasonally polyestrous, the stimulus for the onset of cyclical activity being declining day length. The breeding season in the northern hemi-

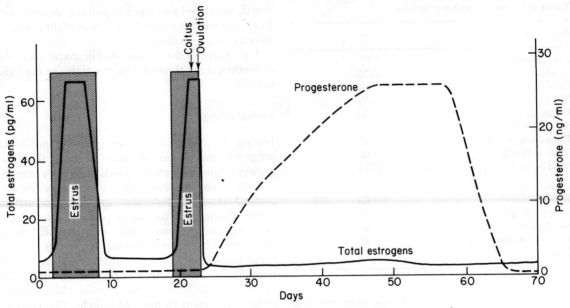

Fig. 1.30 Hormone concentrations in the peripheral blood of the ewe during the estrous cycle.

sphere is from September to February although genotype and social factors exert an influence on the timing.

Puberty occurs as early as 5 months. The inter-estrous interval ranges from 19 to 21 days with estrus lasting about 36h although wide variations are reported. Ovulation probably occurs towards the end of estrus although there are reports of it occurring afterwards.

The detection of estrus in the absence of the male is difficult. There can be some edema and hyper-emia of the vulva and frequently rapid tailwagging.

Sow

The sow is truly polyestrous and puberty is attained at 6–8 months of age with most gilts giving birth to their first litter at about 12 months of age. The average duration of the estrous cycle is 21 days, estrus lasts 2–3 days, usually being shorter in gilts than sows. Ovulation occurs over several hours with the release of 20 or more ova, beginning 38–42 h after the start of estrus. Hormonal changes during the estrous cycle are summarized in Fig. 1.31.

Signs of Estrus

The vulva becomes swollen, edematous and hyper-emic a few days before the sow will accept the boar, and this will quite often pass its peak at the time of acceptance. A clear, watery mucus may be dis-charged. The sow will respond to the haunch or back pressure test.

Clinical Examination

Vaginal examination with the aid of a speculum can be performed although the information that is obtained is of minimal value. Palpation of the internal genitalia is possible per rectum and, although not frequently performed, can provide valuable information on the reproductive status of the sow, particularly changes involving the cervix and ovaries.

Genitalia

These are shown in Fig. 1.32. The vulva labia are thick and are covered with a wrinkled integument, the dorsal commissure is rounded, the ventral commissure forms a long pointed projection. The vagina extends forwards and horizontally for a distance of 10–12 cm before merging imperceptibly with the cervix. There is no distinct os uteri in the pig. The cervix, 10–20 cm in length, is poorly defined and is characterized by a thickened wall and numerous transverse folds. During estrus, edema of the wall reduces the lumen of the cervical canal and facilitates the 'locking' of the spiraled boar's penis during coitus.

The uterine body is short but the uterine horns are long and convoluted measuring up to 1.5 m in length in a large multiparous sow.

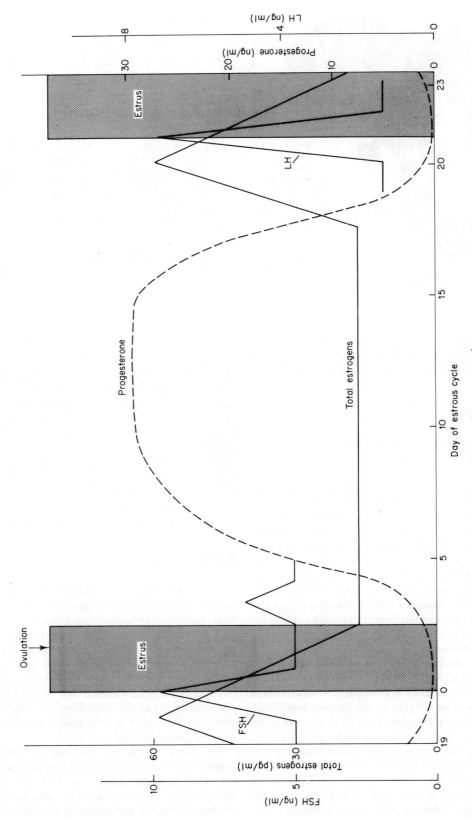

Fig. 1.31 Hormone concentrations in the peripheral blood of the sow during the estrous cycle.

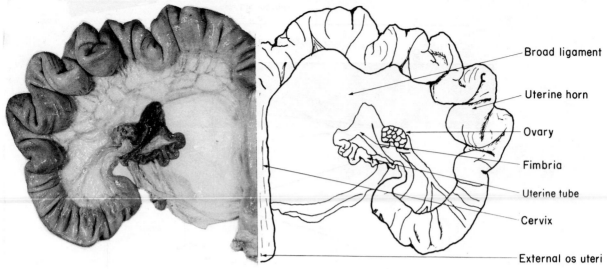

Fig. 1.32 Genital organs of the sow.

Cyclical Changes

A watery vulval discharge is characteristic of sows a few days before the onset of estrus. Smears of this secretion show arborization due to crystal formation and have been used to determine the stage of the estrous cycle. The vaginal epithelium is also sensitive to the influence of ovarian steroid hormones. During the follicular phase of the cycle up to 20 cell layers are present. However, during the luteal phase the number of layers is reduced to three or four. Vaginal pH determinations have also been made to assess the optimum time for artificial insemination with a decrease from pH 7.2 to 6.3 during estrus; the lowest figure is recorded during the height of acceptance. The hormonal changes during the estrous cycle are summarized in Fig. 1.31.

There is continuous development and subsequent atresia of follicles so a pool of proliferating follicles 2–6 mm in diameter is maintained. At about days 14–16 of the estrous cycle, as the corpora lutea start to regress, there is recruitment of 20 or more of these follicles which grow and mature under gonadotropin stimulation. The fully mature follicle attains a size of 7–8 mm in diameter just before ovulation. The corpora lutea reach a maximum size of 0.8–1.1 cm in diameter after 7–8 days and undergo fairly rapid regression 16–17 days after the previous estrus.

The Puerperium

The uterine horns return to normal nonpregnant size by 21–28 days after farrowing. There is some lochial discharge for about a week after parturition but there is no degeneration and sloughing of endometrial tissue. The epithelium is reduced in size and leukocyte infiltration of the subepithelial layers is a feature. At about 21 days the epithelium lining the endometrium has returned to a normal columnar type and the leukocytic infiltration has subsided. A few sows have an anovulatory estrus a few days after farrowing, but in most animals cyclical ovarian activity is suppressed until 5–10 days after weaning.

Bitch

The reproductive pattern of the bitch differs from that of the larger domestic species in that successive heat periods are interspersed with a prolonged period of sexual quiescence—anestrus. On average the interestrous interval is 7 months so that bitches come into heat approximately twice per year. Some bitches are more frequent, but some come into estrus only every 12 months. The effect of prolonged domestication has eliminated any seasonal influence although there is an appearance of greatest activity in early spring and autumn.

The bitch has a very definite proestrus which heralds the onset of reproductive activity, and a very prolonged luteal phase traditionally described as metestrus. The term diestrus, usually applied to the luteal phase, is not normally used in this species.

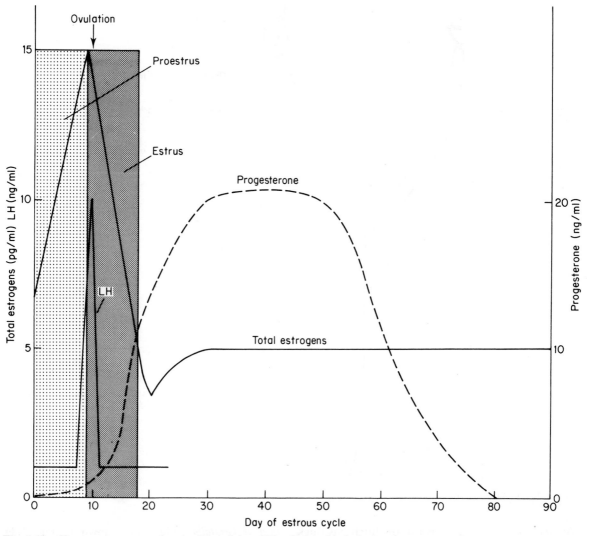

Fig. 1.33 Hormone concentrations in the peripheral blood of the bitch during the estrous cycle.

During metestrus many bitches show overt signs of pseudopregnancy with mammary development, increased body weight and behavioral changes. Most bitches show some signs although their intensity is very variable; it should not be considered abnormal.

The age at which bitches have their first estrus depends to some extent upon the breed, the smaller breeds tending to be more precocious and able to reach puberty at 6 months of age.

The duration of the various stages of the estrous cycle is variable. Traditionally proestrus is considered to last 9 days and estrus 9 days. However, the transition between the two stages is gradual with the total length of the two usually amounting to 18–19 days. Metestrus lasts 8–12 weeks which, in the absence of overt signs of pseudopregnancy, passes imperceptibly into anestrus. The hormonal changes are summarized in Fig. 1.33.

Clinical Examination

The uterus can be examined by abdominal palpation, radiography or B mode direct imaging, although it is not usually necessary other than for pregnancy diagnosis (see Chapter 4) or where pathological conditions such as pyometra are suspected (see Chapter 17). Examination of the vagina by speculum is of very limited value. Visual inspection of the vulva and any discharges that may be present are very helpful in assessing the reproductive status of the bitch.

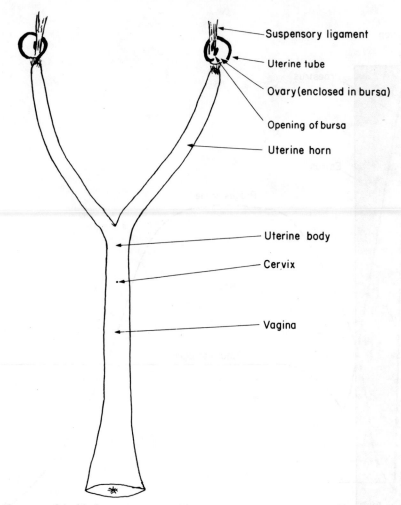

Fig. 1.34   Genital organs of the bitch.

External Genitalia   The vulva of the bitch has thick labia which form a distinctly pointed ventral commissure; the skin is smooth and sometimes pigmented.

The vulva undergoes fairly obvious and distinct changes during the estrous cycle. Frequently, a few days before the onset of the bloodstained discharge of proestrus, there is some enlargement of the labia and perilabial tissue. At proestrus the labia become turgid and edematous. At the start of estrus, the period of acceptance, the vulval swelling starts to diminish and the tissues become less turgid. The vulval discharge changes in appearance becoming paler than at proestrus. During metestrus there is a further decline in labial swelling and the discharge becomes thicker, brown and less obvious before eventually disappearing completely. However, some bitches have a persistent, clear metestral discharge; whether this is normal or not is questionable.

Internal Genitalia   These are shown in Fig. 1.34. Vaginal examination by means of a speculum or digital exploration is tolerated, although in a fractious animal, particularly if there is some degree of vulval hypoplasia, sedation or general anesthesia may be required. The vestibule is directed forwards and upwards before continuing as the vagina, which passes over the pelvic brim and then runs cranially and horizontally. Palpation of the cervix is difficult except in small breeds because of the length of the vagina which ranges from 8 to 14 cm. The cervix cannot be inspected visually with the aid of a conventional speculum because the direction of the longitudinal axis of the vestibule and posterior vagina enables only the dorsal wall of the vagina to be examined. This is possible using a fiber optic endoscope.

The uterine body is short (2–3 cm in length) and the two horns diverge and pass cranially and dor-

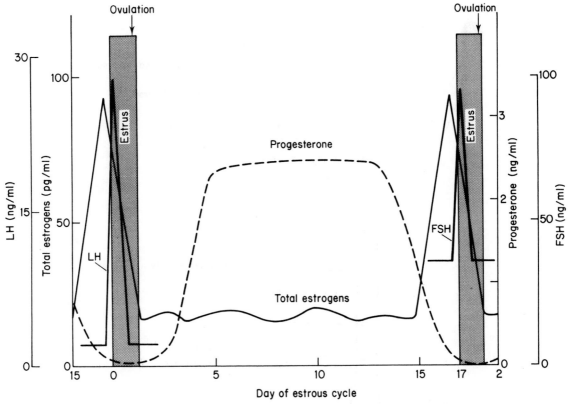

Fig. 1.35 Hormone concentrations in the peripheral blood of the cat during the estrous cycle.

sally towards each kidney. It is possible to palpate the bifurcation per rectum in small breeds.

The ovaries of the bitch are almost completely enclosed within the ovarian bursa which opens ventrally through a small slit-like orifice. Visual examination of the ovaries by laparotomy requires the surgical opening of the bursa. The ovaries are roughly oval in shape and 1–2 cm in length, the size being dependent upon the reproductive status of the animal; each ovary lies just posterior to each corresponding kidney.

Cyclical Changes

During proestrus follicular growth occurs which causes enlargement and irregularity of the ovaries. The number of follicles which reach maturity varies with the age and breed of the bitch; the larger breeds and more mature individuals produce more, the average number being four and five on each ovary. At the onset of true estrus the largest follicles measure 3–5 mm in diameter, normally containing a single oocyte. When fully mature, follicles are 0.6–1.0 cm in diameter; preovulatory luteinization is a feature resulting in an increase in progesterone (see Fig. 1.33). Ovulation occurs 1–2 days after the onset of estrus, the oocyte having to complete meiosis with extrusion of both polar bodies within the uterine tubes. The rupture site of the follicle appears as a small red pinpoint on the surface of the ovary.

The corpora lutea reach a diameter of 0.6–1.0 cm in diameter when fully formed and have a characteristic pink coloration. Histological evidence of regression can be seen as early as 42 days after mating, however, macroscopic evidence is apparent from about 56 days. Complete regression is a slow process and sizable remnants of the corpora lutea can be seen 6 months later.

The vaginal epithelium undergoes distinct cellular changes in relation to the estrous cycle; smears of these together with other cellular components from the uterus and cervix can be used to identify the stage of the reproductive cycle. The method that is most frequently used involves the introduction of small amounts of physiological saline into the vagina and its immediate aspiration. A glass rod and syringe are convenient to use. A smear is made from the fluid, fixed immediately with an ethanol/ether mixture and stained with a trichrome stain, such as Shorr's; alternatively a conventional blood

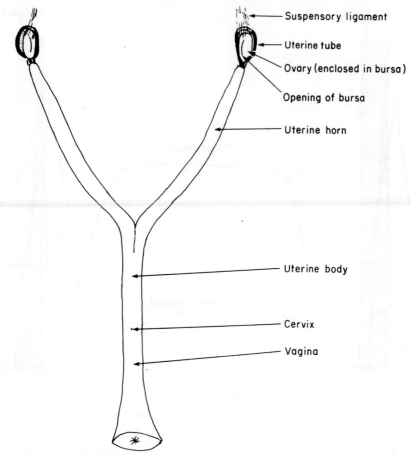

Suspensory ligament

Uterine tube

Ovary (enclosed in bursa)

Opening of bursa

Uterine horn

Uterine body

Cervix

Vagina

Fig. 1.36 Genital organs of the female cat.

smear stain can be used. The interpretation of cell types requires practice. During proestrus the dominant cell type will be the erythrocyte, together with basal cell types of the stratified squamous epithelium. Towards the end of proestrus and early estrus the number of erythrocytes will decrease and superficial squamous epithelial cells will become the dominant cell type. These will become abundant during estrus. Towards the end of estrus and the start of metestrus large numbers of neutrophils appear together with cells from the deeper layers of the epithelium. However, it must be stressed that the transition from one stage to another is a gradual one.

The Puerperium

The uterine horns return to the nonpregnant dimensions after 4–5 weeks. Slightly pigmented cylindrical zones can be identified up to 3 months postpartum which indicate the sites of previous pla-

cental attachment. Desquamation of endometrial tissue and regeneration is complete by about 12 weeks postpartum.

Female Cat

The queen cat is seasonally polyestrous, with a period of anestrus in the autumn and winter, and is obviously influenced by the photoperiod since it is possible to shorten the length of anestrus by increasing the artificial daylight regimen. There are suggestions that cats also have another period of anestrus in early summer but this may well be an artifact associated with pregnancy and lactational anestrus.

Puberty is usually reached at 5–9 months of age. The cat is an induced ovulator usually requiring coitus or other form of cervical stimulation; as a result the duration of estrus and the interestrous interval is greatly influenced by this function. If ovulation occurs, estrus lasts about 4 days with maximum receptivity on day 3; if ovulation does not

Table 1.2 Reproductive data for domestic animals*

	Cattle	Horses	Pigs	Sheep	Goats	Dogs	Cats
Male							
Age at puberty (months)	9–10	12–18	5–8	6–8	5–7	5–12	9–12
Usual age at first service (months)	12	18–24	12	9–12	9–12	12	12
Female							
Age at puberty (months)	6–10	12–18	6–8	4–15	4–15	6–9	5–9
Usual age at first service (months)	14–22	24–38	8–10	9–18	12–18	12–18	12–18
Breeding season	Year-round	Most, spring to autumn; some year-round	Year-round	Breed variation from autumn–winter to year-round	Autumn–winter	Twice yearly	Spring, summer, early autumn
Estrous cycle							
Type	Polyestrous	Polyestrous	Polyestrous	Polyestrous	Polyestrous	Monestrous	Polyestrous
Length (days)	21	21	21	16.5	20	—	14–21
Duration of estrus	15 h	5–6 days	40–60 h	24–36 h	1–2 days	9 days	10 days if unmated
Time of ovulation	12 h a.e. e	24–48 h b.e. e	38–42 h a.b. e	18–40 h a.b. e	24–48 h a.b. e	24–72 h a.b. e	27 h postcoitum
Gestation length (days)	280	336	114	147	151	63	63
First postpartum ovulation	10–20 days (80% silent) 28–36 days (55%) silent	7–9 days	3–7 days after weaning (estrus 2–3 days post-partum usually anovulatory)	Next breeding season or after weaning	Next breeding season	Next breeding season	Next breeding season
First postpartum estrus used for breeding	1st after 42 days	1st or 2nd	1st after weaning	Varies with breed and methods of husbandry	1st	1st	1st

*Working averages or ranges are given. Due allowance must be made for breed and individual variations.
Abbreviations: a.b. e = after beginning of estrus; a.e. e = after end of estrus; b.e. e = before end of estrus.

occur, then estrus lasts up to 10 days and is associated with atresia of the anovulatory follicles. The unmated (usually anovulatory) cat will return to estrus every 2–3 weeks, the nonpregnant cat that has ovulated (pseudopregnant) will return to estrus in 7–8 weeks. There is evidence that ovulation can occur following stimulation of sensory receptors in the skin as might occur when the cat is stroked. The endocrine changes in the peripheral circulation are summarized in Fig. 1.35.

The signs of estrus are confined almost completely to changes in behavior. The queen emits a characteristic 'call', she will rub around her owner's legs, roll over on her back and become more affectionate. She will frequently assume a squatting position with hindlimbs abducted, or maintain the hindlimbs extended and elevated while lying partially on her sternum. The latter position is often accompanied by treading movements of the hindlimbs and rapid tail movements.

Clinical Examination

Apart from abdominal palpation to diagnose pregnancy, examination of the genital system (Fig. 1.36) is not performed.

The vulval labia are small and less obvious than in the bitch; digital exploration of the vestibule and vagina is difficult except in the parturient animal. The tubular genital tract is similar to that described for the dog, with a relatively long vagina, short uterine body and long narrow uterine horns running cranially and laterally towards each kidney.

The ovaries of the cat are suspended by the suspensory ligament beneath the 4th lumbar vertebra. They are partially enclosed within the ovarian bursa. The size of the ovaries varies with the stage of the estrous cycle.

Cyclical Changes

At the beginning of estrus the follicles, of which there are usually three or four on each ovary, are 1–2 mm in diameter and reach a maximum size of 3–4 mm 24 h after coitus. Ovulation occurs 24–54 h after coitus, the corpora lutea which are formed reaching a maximum size of 3 mm after 17 days. In the pseudopregnant cat some evidence of regression is evident from about 24 days after ovulation. It continues gradually and is complete by 37 days.

The vaginal epithelium undergoes cyclical changes which are related to the estrous cycle. However, they are rather more subtle than those of the bitch. Material can be obtained in a similar way to that described for the bitch. The main changes are:

1. Proestrus: mainly noncornified and a few cornified epithelial cells, few leukocytes and red blood cells.
2. Estrus: the dominant cell type is a cornified epithelial cell.
3. Metestrus: a few cornified cells with ragged edges but also leukocytes, bacteria and nucleated epithelial cells.
4. Anestrus: mainly dark staining, nucleated epithelial cells with smooth, oval borders.

Complementary References

Allen, W. E. (1974) The palpability of the corpus luteum in Welsh pony mares. *Equine vet. J.*, **6**, 25.

Allen, W. E. & Newcombe, J. R. (1977) Anoestrous conditions in the mare, their diagnosis and treatment. *Vet. Rec.*, **100**, 338.

Dawson, F. L. M. (1975) Accuracy of rectal palpation in the diagnosis of ovarian function in the cow. *Vet. Rec.*, **96**, 218.

Esselmont, R. J. (1973) *Economic and husbandry aspects of the manifestation and detection of oestrus in cows in large herds.* PhD thesis, University of Reading.

Getly, R. (ed.) (1975) *Sisson and Grossman's, The Anatomy of the Domestic Animals*, 5th edn. Philadelphia: W. B. Saunders.

Grandage, J. (1972) The erect dog penis: a paradox of flexible rigidity. *Vet. Rec.*, **91**, 141.

Meredith, M. J. (1977) Clinical examination of the ovaries and cervix of the sow. *Vet. Rec.*, **101**, 70.

Popesko, P. (1968) *Atlas der Topographischen Anatomie der Haustiere*, Vol. 3. Jena: Fischer.

Prickett, B. W. & Voss, J. L. (1973) Reproductive management of the stallion. *Proc. 18th Ann. Conv. Am. Equine Practrs.*, 501.

Rossdale, P. D. & Ricketts, S. W. (1974) *The Practice of Equine Stud Medicine*, p. 36. London: Baillière Tindall.

Roszel, J. F. (1975) Genital cytology of the bitch. *Vet. Scope*, **19**, 3.

Williamson, N. B., Morris, R. S., Blood, D. S. & Cannon, C. M. (1972) A study of oestrus behaviour and oestrus detection methods in a large commercial dairy herd. *Vet. Rec.*, **91**, 50.

2

Seminal Evaluation and Artificial Insemination

T. H. HOWARD and M. M. PACE

Complete evaluation of the seminal donor for purposes of artificial insemination (AI) should include an estimate of the fertilizing capacity of his spermatozoa and determination that his semen is free from specific semen-transmissible pathogens (SPF status). The only true measure of fertilizing capacity is to inseminate sufficient females to obtain a reliable estimate. The large error component in the binomial analysis of variance necessitates the number of females that must be exposed to the semen be very large. Analysis of 300 inseminations will provide preliminary information about the fertilizing capacity of bovine semen, while 500–1000 inseminations are needed to detect small differences among bulls or seminal treatments. Because of the costs involved in gathering this information, several characteristics of spermatozoa have been used by clinicians to estimate fertility. Elaboration on the techniques described in this chapter can be found in the complementary references.

Use of the appropriate techniques for storage, thawing and insemination of frozen–thawed semen is second in importance only to detection of estrus for the successful employment of artificial insemination. Reproductive health management of herds that are artificially inseminated must include attention to the field storage of frozen semen as well as use of correct methods of thawing of semen, hygienic insemination, and correct placement in the female.

Fertility may also be impaired by semen-borne

infectious disease, and the techniques of AI with frozen semen eliminate the constraints of time and distance on transmission of etiologic agents of disease as well as spermatozoa. Such agents may be introduced by infected semen into previously uninfected livestock populations, there to resume a more typical epidemiologic pattern.

COLLECTION OF SPERMATOZOA

The characteristics and fertility of spermatozoa can be affected by the collection techniques employed. Depending upon the species being collected, one of three basic techniques is used to obtain spermatozoa: use of an artificial vagina; digital manipulation or pressure on the glans penis by a gloved hand; and electroejaculation.

Several variables may affect spermatozoal quality: the age of the donor; the frequency of prior ejaculations; and environmental stresses such as the prevailing ambient temperature, concurrent disease, and the presence of foreign material in the semen.

Species which are spontaneous ejaculators (bull, ram, male goat) must be sexually stimulated by active restraint and mounting without collection, called false mounting, in order to obtain a high quality, concentrated ejaculate. Species such as the horse, pig, and dog that do not ejaculate until after an extended period of intromission tend to produce inferior quality ejaculates if subjected to such sexual stimulation.

Artificial Vagina

The artificial vagina is constructed to mimic the vagina of the female: most designs include a firm outer case and inner latex liner. Ejaculation is the result of nervous stimulation of the glans penis that elicits reflexive muscular contractions of the reproductive tract. To produce the proper nervous stimulation the artificial vagina must be at or above body temperature and some pressure must be exerted on the penis. The liner of the artificial vagina must be of intrinsically low friction or be lubricated with a substance that is not toxic for spermatozoa. Otherwise, there will be damage to the glans penis when it enters the artificial vagina.

The temperature of the collection tube on the liner must be maintained close to that of the body. Elevated temperatures cause rapid deterioration of spermatozoal quality, while temperatures much below body temperature may cause cold shock to the spermatozoa. Cold shock is an irreversible physiologic condition of spermatozoa that have been subjected to rapid cooling, resulting in the bending of the flagellum, loss of intracellular components, and diminished fertilizing capacity.

Gloved Hand

Special care must be taken when using the gloved hand collection technique never to employ spermicidal chemicals for sterilization or lubrication of the glove. Surgical gloves are often found to be unsuitable for this use because of the presence of such contaminants. Particular attention should be paid to the temperature of the receptacle and to environmental microbial contamination of the semen.

Electroejaculation

Seminal collection by electroejaculation is often employed in clinical settings for purposes of breeding soundness evaluations. The utility of this method for purposes of AI is limited by a number of factors, usually including a diminished harvest of spermatozoa and less consistent seminal characteristics. Ejaculates obtained by electroejaculation are typically more dilute because of the increased volume of fluid from the accessory glands, and spermatozoal motility is frequently lower, particularly if epididymal reserves of spermatozoa are poorly depleted or there is contamination by urine.

To avoid misleading evaluation of the animal's breeding potential, emphasis is usually placed on seminal characteristics that are least affected by the collection method or that can be most objectively measured. For example, the Society for Theriogenology scoring system for breeding soundness evaluation of bulls assigns only 20% of the score to spermatozoal motility, while 40% results from the spermatozoal morphology count and another 40% from a scrotal circumference measurement.

While sedation or anesthesia is necessary for successful and humane electroejaculation of the boar, collection of the bull, ram and male goat can be accomplished without undesirable side-effects by an experienced operator utilizing the equipment now available. Ventrally oriented rectal electrodes and a low amperage ejaculator eliminate most of the side-effects that were associated with more primitive equipment. However, inexperienced operators should never be entrusted with seminal collection by this method. Use of finger electrodes is particularly helpful for collection of nervous or incapacitated large animals.

Use of electroejaculation to compensate for failure of young males to demonstrate normal libido is contraindicated. The genetic implications of such impotence are disquieting, and it can be predicted with assurance that such animals will be less productive of semen and should be replaced.

INITIAL EVALUATION OF THE EJACULATE

Gross Assessment

After collection there should be a visual evaluation to verify that the ejaculate is of the appropriate volume and color for the species being collected, and that it is free of foreign material such as blood or pus. The semen of the boar and stallion contains a gel that should be separated by fractionation or filtration. During this and all subsequent components of the evaluation procedure, the semen and all items that contact it should be maintained at 37 °C.

Concentration of Spermatozoa

The number of spermatozoa in the ejaculate is dependent on such factors as age, the size of testes, sexual preparation, and method of collection. Table 2.1 shows the species variation in spermatozoal concentrations. The number of spermatozoa in the ejaculate can be obtained by use of a hemocytometer, measurement of the optical density of the semen, or use of an electronic particle counter.

Table 2.1 Ranges of normal values for volume and spermatozoal concentrations of whole ejaculates produced by several species

	Volume (ml)	Concentration (spermatozoa × 10⁶ per ml)
Cattle	3–15	500–2500
Goat	0.3–2	2000–4000
Sheep	0.3–2	2000–4000
Horse	25–200	100–800
Pig	100–400	50–300
Dog	3–25	100–500
Turkey	0.2–1	3000–8000

Techniques used to measure spermatozoal concentration should be very precise, since small errors translate into large differences when dilution factors are considered. The diluent of the seminal aliquot used for this measurement should stop movement and prevent clumping of the cells. A high osmotic pressure solution such as 4% sodium chloride (NaCl) works well for this purpose. Appropriate dilution ratios for hemocytometry are 1:20 for stallion, boar, and dog semen; 1:200 for bull semen; and 1:400 for ram and male goat semen. The hemocytometer is used in laboratories where only a small number of samples are being evaluated. The variation of this method is higher than that of optical density or electrical counting. Therefore, repeated hemocytometer counts should be incorporated if high accuracy is required, such as that necessary for calculation of a standard curve for spectrophotometric analysis of spermatozoal concentration.

Motility

Initial motility estimates are made by microscopy of either undiluted or diluted semen. Motility estimates of neat semen attempt to grade the vigor of the swirls and wave formation. Many isotonic diluents have been used to assess the individual movement of spermatozoa: 2.9% sodium citrate solution is often employed. Motility evaluations should be performed at 37 °C on a microscope equipped with a temperature-controlled stage. Spermatozoal movement is slowed at temperatures below 37 °C, while these cells are rapidly destroyed at higher temperatures. If motility estimates cannot be made immediately after dilution, the dilution medium should contain macromolecules such as the yolk lipoproteins used in seminal extenders: prewarmed yolk-buffer solutions or scalded skim milk are suitable if a phase contrast microscope is avail-

able for the evaluation. In AI laboratories the extender used to preserve the spermatozoa is used as the diluent for motility estimation. Visual estimation of spermatozoal motility is very subjective: differences of 20% between experienced estimators are not rare. Some of this variation is reduced if uniform preparations are employed. Two 15 µl drops of extended or diluted semen should be prepared on a warm slide, coverslipped, and independently evaluated at 100–300 × magnification by two observers, each of whom views five or six fields under each coverslip.

Morphology

Some spermatozoa in every ejaculate are morphologically abnormal. Morphological evaluation attempts to determine whether the sample is outside the normal range for the species, and whether the physiological function of the testes and epididymides is changing. The structure of spermatozoa can be evaluated with one of several staining methods, examination of fresh mounts of immobilized spermatozoa under a phase contrast or differential interference contrast microscope, or by electron microscopy. The fixed smears commonly utilize such stains as eosin-nigrosin and basic fuchsin, although their resolution is inferior to that of unstained wet mounts of seminal specimens fixed in 0.2% glutaraldehyde. If acrosomal integrity is to be evaluated, either glutaraldehyde-fixed or freshly collected specimens are essential.

Care must be taken with all methods that artifacts are not produced and that sufficient cells are observed to make an accurate assessment. At least 100 cells per smear should be counted; if greater precision is desired, a second preparation should be made. The practice of differential counting of living and dead cells after use of a vital stain such as eosin is of very limited usefulness since the distribution of living and dead cells in seminal smears has been shown to be nonrandom, producing differing ratios from one end of the smear to the other.

Since there are some abnormal spermatozoa in every ejaculate, the relationship between seminal morphology and fertility is complex. High frequencies of abnormal spermatozoa or the presence of a single specific abnormality have been shown to reduce fertility. Researchers have classified spermatozoa in several ways. Some classifications divide the abnormalities according to the region of the cell where they occur, such as head, midpiece, and tail. Others simply divide them into major and minor defects. When using either procedure it is important to be consistent since some cells will exhibit more than one defect.

Morphological evaluations also identify cells in the ejaculate other than spermatozoa. Such cells can give indications of infection, damage to the testes, or testicular degeneration. Interpretation of spermatozoal morphology is always retrospective, since the process of spermatogenesis and maturation requires several weeks and transit through the epididymides another 1–2 weeks. Therefore, the cause of a clinical abnormality may have occurred days or weeks earlier. Repeated collections are helpful for accurate interpretation of the significance of morphological abnormalities, particularly if the epididymal reserves of spermatozoa are replete as the consequence of infrequent ejaculation.

PROCESSING OF SEMEN FOR ARTIFICIAL INSEMINATION

The suitability of a male as a donor for semen preservation is different from his fitness to initiate pregnancy under natural conditions. Since some spermatozoa are damaged or destroyed by the preservation method, selection of donors is necessary to maintain high fertility. The capability to survive cryopreservation is an exquisitely sensitive measure of reproductive fitness, since the spermatozoa of some donors do not survive cryopreservation even though all their functional and morphological attributes are apparently normal.

After collection, semen for cryopreservation is placed into an extender solution. There are many extenders, but all have two basic functions: maintenance of fertility during cryopreservation, and extension of the ejaculate to achieve the appropriate number of spermatozoa in each insemination unit. The basic components of extenders are: a buffer solution that can maintain the necessary osmotic pressure and pH; macromolecules such as lecithin, proteins, lipoproteins or their complexes to prevent cold shock and stablize membranes during freezing; a cryoprotective agent; and antibiotics.

The extender best suited for a species or AI laboratory is dependent upon several factors, and the choice may be dictated by the availability of a reliable source of components. Some combinations of extender components reduce fertilizing capacity. Cryoprotective agents are implicated in reducing the fertility of the semen of some species. Glycerol appears to have no effect on the fertility of bovine spermatozoa but depresses fertility of the ram, boar, stallion, and turkey. Consequently, the extender chosen must be carefully analyzed for its intended use.

After the ejaculate has been mixed with the extender, the extender interacts with the spermatozoa to enable them to survive cooling. This interaction is called equilibration. During the initial cooling to 5 °C the spermatozoa are very sensitive to cold shock. Therefore, the rate of cooling during equilibration is only 0.1–0.5 °C/min. A volume of the extender containing the final portion of cryoprotectant is usually added after the seminal temperature reaches 5 °C. The commonly employed cryoprotectant additives are glycerol, dimethylsulfoxide, and disaccharides.

Further equilibration is needed after the spermatozoa reach 5 °C before the freezing process begins. After equilibration semen is packaged into individual doses; the most frequently used method for many species is the plastic straw. In some instances the glass ampule or pellet are used. There are advantages for each system, and the choice will depend on a number of considerations. The plastic straw, which has a large ratio of surface area to volume of extender, yields a uniform and rapid transfer of heat during freezing and thawing. This attribute is a disadvantage when semen is handled and transferred because of the risk of overexposure to ambient temperature (Fig. 2.1). The glass ampule has the best seal, eliminating contact of liquid nitrogen (LN_2) with semen, but is more difficult to freeze properly. The pellet method of freezing employs small depressions in dry ice or plastic plates as a low cost method of freezing, but identification of semen is difficult and it can become contaminated with microbes or other spermatozoa in the liquid nitrogen.

Extended semen is not always frozen. Very successful AI programs utilizing extenders that preserve spermatozoa at temperatures between 5 °C and ambient are employed in parts of the world where distances and breeding seasons are short. Because losses due to freezing are eliminated, more spermatozoa are available for insemination, enabling very efficient use of a few donor sires and intense genetic selection. However, such semen can only be used for a few days because of the progressive loss of fertility after collection.

When semen is frozen, the rate of freezing is dependent upon several variables, including species, extender, level of cryoprotectant, and the packaging system. The most critical portion of the freezing curve is between the heat of fusion and −40 °C. Freezing rates are usually between 1 and 10°/min.

A number of assays of spermatozoal quality have been developed to predict the fertility of semen that

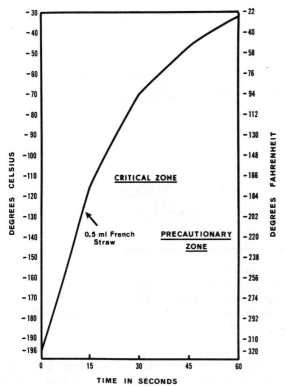

Fig. 2.1 Warming of an individual 0.5 ml straw will reach −120 °C within 15 s after exposure to ambient temperature, initiating irreversible damage to the spermatozoa.

has been frozen and thawed. Some of these assays require elaborate equipment. The reliability of the prediction will depend upon the accuracy and precision of the assay. There is often some art or technique associated with development of a repeatable procedure, which accounts for the lack of complete agreement among laboratories.

Spermatozoal quality assays have been based on the use of physiological characteristics that evaluate the motor mechanism, metabolism, and cell membrane integrity. The spermatozoal quality assays that are used include various methods of measuring motility, membrane integrity, metabolic activity, release of intracellular substance, and penetration of cervical mucus or ova. These assays have also been conducted after spermatozoa have been subjected to the stress of incubation at 37 °C, altered osmotic pressure or pH, cold shock and freezing without cryoprotective agents.

Some investigators believe that the fertilizing capacity of an ejaculate can best be estimated by analysis of the percentage of spermatozoa with a particular characteristic, such as progressive motil-

ity. However, when bovine ejaculates varying in their percentages of progressively motile spermatozoa are extended and frozen such that each insemination dose contains the same number of motile cells, the motility percentage has no correlation with fertility. Any perceived relationship between fertility and the percentage of motile spermatozoa is in fact a relationship between fertility and the total number of motile spermatozoa inseminated.

In order to establish the minimum number of spermatozoa with a characteristic that is necessary to obtain optimum fertility, breeding trials must be conducted that utilize differing numbers of cells. Such trials conducted at our laboratory have found the relationship between fertility and the number of motile spermatozoa inseminated is not linear, but instead is an exponential regression (Fig. 2.2). When plotted, this relationship becomes asymptotic—that is, no further increases in fertility result from insemination of additional motile spermatozoa. The shape of this nonlinear regression line is the same for individual bulls and different thawing methods. However, the asymptotes are different for each line, reflecting the differing fertility of each bull and the capability of each thawing method to preserve that fertility.

Most assays have a positive relationship with fertility, but the characteristics measured are independent of one another. In our hands, no assay has given a more accurate estimation of fertility than the number of progressively motile spermatozoa in a sample immediately after thawing. Use of a time-exposure photographic technique with dark-field microscopy has proven to be a precise and repeatable method of assay. In the choice of a viability assay, consideration should be given to the accuracy and precision of the procedure as well as its adaptability to the laboratory. Caution must be exercised when evaluating a single characteristic of spermatozoa from a species where fertilizing capacity is unknown. For example, the mere addition of stallion spermatozoa to a hydrogen ion extender, or the addition of glycerol to boar spermatozoa, depresses fertility in both species without adversely affecting motility. There is no doubt that fertility can be impaired without affecting some of the viability characteristics of spermatozoa.

PACKAGING AND STORAGE OF FROZEN SEMEN

A number of methods of packaging of extended semen for storage and distribution have been employed, but the most widely adopted is the

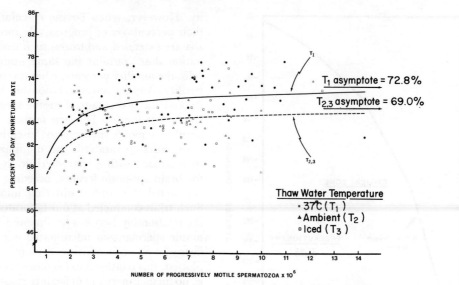

Fig. 2.2 Thawing of bovine spermatozoa in 37 °C water produces consistently higher fertility regardless of the number of spermatozoa inseminated. Once the threshold number of spermatozoa required for optimum fertility is reached, further increases in the number of spermatozoa per insemination do not result in additional improvements in fertility. From Pace *et al.* (1981), with permission of the editors, *Journal of Animal Science.*

paillette or straw. Several sizes and types of straws are in use internationally, but the most widely adopted deliver either 0.25 or 0.5 ml of extended semen, sufficient for one insemination. A single field refrigerator may contain several hundred straws, stored within metal racks or plastic storage goblets. Swine semen is usually frozen in pellets that are stored within small metal or plastic cylinders.

Cryogenic refrigerators are double-walled vacuum-insulated vessels designed to maintain liquid nitrogen-preserved semen successfully for up to 8 months without replenishment (Fig. 2.3). If a vessel's integrity is compromised by neglect or abuse, either a gradual or sudden loss of refrigerant will result. The most vulnerable elements of the refrigerator are the outer shell, which is subject to puncture and corrosion, and the fragile fiberglass necktube suspending the inner reservoir. Refrigerators should be stored upright in a clean, well-ventilated area. A piece of wood or heavy cardboard beneath the vessel will control scratching and corrosion of the outer shell.

Care must be taken to avoid tipping and jarring of the vessel when it is moved, as the inner nitrogen reservoir may swing in a pendulum-like motion that will fracture the necktube. When the reservoir is refilled care must be taken not to dispense into the refrigerator large amounts of warm nitrogen vapor that could damage the semen within. The necktube should remain plugged when the vessel is unused to control both nitrogen loss and entry of environ-

mental contaminants. Liquid nitrogen (LN_2) will preserve any microorganisms or debris that fall into the vessel and also accumulate frozen condensate; periodic emptying and cleansing of the refrigerator will prevent accumulation of such contaminants.

Refrigerant levels should be regularly measured, as failure of most refrigerators is preceded by a period of increased LN_2 consumption. If a refrigerator failure is suspected, the refrigerator should be refilled with LN_2 immediately, or the semen transferred to a reliable refrigerator. The only exception occurs when a thermocouple is immediately available that will permit a measurement of the temperature within the failing vessel. So long as any LN_2 remains in the vessel the fertility of the semen will be preserved, but if the reservoir temperature rises above − 120 °C, irreversible damage to the spermatozoa will result. Temperature-sensitive monitor ampules that indicate whether such warming has occurred should be present in the refrigerator (Fig. 2.4).

If seminal damage is suspected, representative doses of semen should be evaluated by a laboratory competent in evaluation of frozen semen. Such evaluations are best made by the original processor, since seminal evaluation techniques and standards are not uniform among laboratories. Veterinary practitioners should not attempt to evaluate processed, frozen–thawed semen unless it is suspected that the semen has been completely thawed, in which case all spermatozoa will be dead.

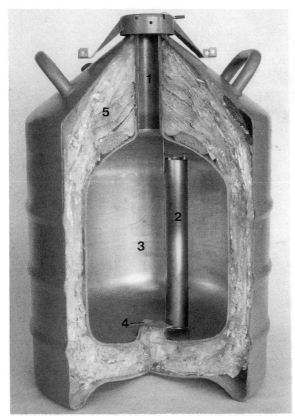

Fig. 2.3 A cutaway view of a cryogenic refrigerator. Access to stored semen is through a fiberglass necktube (1) into which storage canisters (2) are lifted from the LN$_2$ reservoir. (3) Canisters are held in place by an index spider (4). Insulation is provided by a vacuum (5) between the reservoir and outer shell. Perforation of the shell or fracture of the necktube will result in loss of insulation and rapid LN$_2$ depletion.

HANDLING AND THAWING OF FROZEN SEMEN

Great diversity exists in the methods of extension, cooling, glycerolization and freezing of semen. Consequently, recommendations for thawing of semen are equally diverse, since important interactions may exist among these methods and those used to thaw the semen. Further diversity is added by the size and geometry of the seminal packages: those of small volume and large surface area-to-volume ratios (straws or pellets) thaw much more rapidly than larger containers such as glass ampules. Precise instructions for the handling, thawing and insemination methods that are obtained from the processor must be strictly observed.

Damage to frozen spermatozoa during storage in field refrigerators is more often the cumulative result

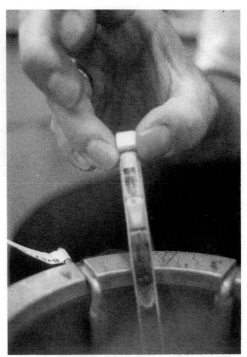

Fig. 2.4 Temperature-sensitive monitor ampules are placed in LN$_2$ refrigerators to identify seminal damage before catastrophic infertility results. If the liquid within the upper inverted ampule melts and refreezes, the semen should be evaluated before use. Melting of the lower inverted ampule indicates a high probability of seminal damage.

of a series of improper manipulations rather than one catastrophic event. When individual doses are removed from field refrigerators care must be taken to avoid repeated warming of other semen that may remain in the refrigerator for months or years before use. If semen is transferred between refrigerators, the danger of overexposure is greatest when individual straws are transferred. Repeated abuse of frozen straws by lifting the necktube for 1 min periods has been shown to induce dangerous warming of straws stored in plastic goblets empty of LN$_2$. Complete metal racks are superior to racks with plastic goblets because the heat gained by exposure in the necktube will be more rapidly transferred away from the frozen units in the all-metal racks. The recommended procedure is to employ forceps to remove straws from the storage goblet, to lift the canister no more than 30 s, to withdraw or transfer doses within 10 s (Fig. 2.5).

Damage to semen packaged in straws when stored in active field refrigerators has been demonstrated. Semen intended for longterm storage should not be stored in such containers. Persistent inatten-

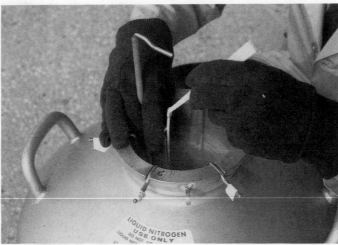

Fig. 2.5 The correct procedure for removal of a single dose of frozen semen from a storage refrigerator. Forceps are used to grasp the straw, and the storage rack is held at the level of the frostline in the refrigerator necktube. Removal of the straw should be accomplished in 10 s or less.

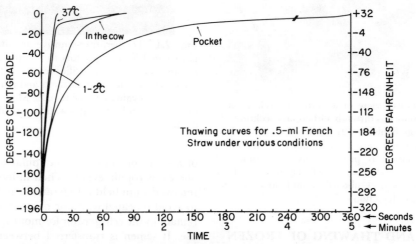

Fig. 2.6 The time required for thawing of spermatozoa packaged in 0.5 ml straws increases dramatically if a thawing bath is not used. The rapid thawing resulting from a water bath thaw is essential for optimum survival of the spermatozoa.

tion to instructions to keep semen packages below the frostline in the refrigerator necktube or failure to lower canisters for sufficient cooling after exposure undoubtedly contribute to such seminal damage. Some of the worst offenses by inseminators include use of the fingers to remove straws, transfer or removal of semen in exposed or windy locations, and the use or transfer of semen from a refrigerator containing only a small amount of liquid nitrogen.

While no universal procedure for the thawing of frozen semen has been adopted, the use of water-bath thawing is strongly preferred over thawing in air because of the rapid thawing rate produced by the water (Fig. 2.6). Laboratory studies indicate that greater survival of spermatozoa is obtained when the water bath temperature is at least 37 °C. If a 37 °C water bath is used, semen packaged in straws should be thawed for at least 30 s. Reliable thawing is assured if the water bath temperature is verified with an accurate thermometer. Pelleted semen is thawed by transferring pellet(s) to a container of buffer or extender or to a teflon-coated metal block.

If a water bath is used to thaw semen, the water

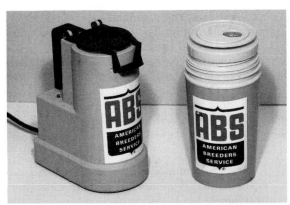

Fig. 2.7 Field thawing of frozen semen at body temperature is facilitated by either a thermostatically controlled electric thawing bath or a simple insulated glass-lined bottle with an added thermometer.

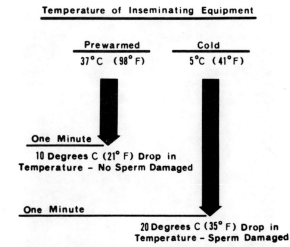

Fig. 2.8 The effect of 5 °C (41 °F) air temperature upon the temperature of semen. The temperature will drop rapidly in an unprotected insemination syringe. All insemination equipment should be prewarmed and protected against exposure. Insemination must be performed as rapidly as possible after the syringe is assembled.

must be replaced at least daily to avoid contamination of the seminal packages (Fig. 2.7). If the 37 °C bath temperature is employed, semen thawed in this manner should be inseminated within 15 min after thawing. The practice of thawing large numbers of straws simultaneously in a small field thawing container will significantly reduce the thawing rate and is likely to result in lowered fertility. Body temperature water thawing of semen can be employed in cold weather without loss of fertility if the thawed semen and prewarmed insemination equipment are protected from exposure during and after assembly by shelter and the use of paper insulating wrap (Fig. 2.8). Consideration must be given to possible inclement weather when insemination facilities are designed.

Semen packages must be thoroughly dried after thawing. Straws are opened by a perpendicular cut below the ultrasonic weld or other seal at the tip after positioning the air space at the end of the straw. The opened straw is then snapped into the disposable insemination sheath and assembled into the insemination syringe. The proper combination of straw, sheath, and syringe is essential to successful insemination. The plastic sheaths are easily warped if left in direct sunlight, closed insemination kits, or vehicles and exposed to temperatures above 50 °C. Sterile, individually wrapped sheaths or pipettes are essential to the highest possible level of hygiene. Lubricants used for insemination must not be spermicidal.

INSEMINATOR PERFORMANCE

Inseminator performance is commonly associated with large variations in the fertility of artificially inseminated herds. Herd health and management programs of such herds should always include regular examinations of inseminator performance, including handling and thawing of semen, hygienic precautions, and placement of dye in extirpated reproductive organs or slaughter-bound females. There is a particularly common tendency for experienced technicians to develop the habit of placing semen too deeply into one bovine uterine horn or the other (Fig. 2.9).

One telltale clue to the development of careless technique by an inseminator is absence of cleanliness and organization of the insemination kit and thawing bath. It is prudent to observe discreetly the steps to insemination whenever such opportunities arise.

Several methods are available to evaluate the anatomical orientation of inseminators, including dye-filled straws, radiography, and an electrical training syringe that sears the extirpated uterus at the site of deposition. Such methods should be employed in retraining at least annually or before seasonal insemination begins. It is quite important to perform such evaluations in a positive educational setting that preserves the morale and self-esteem of the inseminator. Identification of genital tracts by number and use of private scorecards for consultation afterward is an effective approach when evaluation of a group of inseminators is conducted in a public setting.

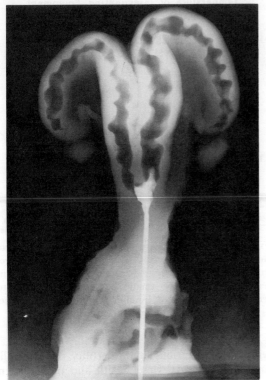

Fig. 2.9   Consistent deposition of semen just anterior to the internal os of the bovine cervix is essential to fertility in artificially inseminated herds. Inseminators should be regularly examined to verify their capability to place semen correctly. Incorrect semen deposition results in reduced fertility and alteration in the distribution of pregnancies between the uterine horns from the usual 60% right/40% left.

SIRE HEALTH AND INTERNATIONAL MOVEMENT OF SEMEN

Methods of infectious disease surveillance and prevention for semen donors have developed concurrently with those of artificial insemination. Disease control programs in AI centers are usually the responsibility of the national veterinary service, and the importance attached to particular diseases often reflects national disease control priorities. Responsible sire health programs must deal both with those infectious agents that are primarily sexually transmissible as well as opportunistically semen-borne infections, transmission of which could be greatly amplified by artificial insemination. Distinction should be made between those methodologies and health certification standards more appropriate to live animal movement and those unique to artificial insemination. Confusion of the two can be very counterproductive: the interval between a particu-

lar diagnostic test and a seminal collection is far less important than the donor or herd being of negative status before and after the collection date.

A very useful classification of the infectious diseases of concern in artificial insemination has been proposed. This organizational framework recognizes freedom from infection, or specific-pathogen-free (SPF) status, based on several criteria, by virtue of:

1. Territorial status.
2. Repetitive immunologic or microbiologic surveillance that demonstrates herd freedom from infection.
3. Hygienic control of environmental contamination.
4. Antibiotic addition to processed semen.

Documentation of the disease-free status of semen donors commonly utilizes each of these levels of SPF certification. Most of the obstacles to movement of semen internationally are found at the levels of national territorial status or herd status, or when national control strategies for important infectious disease are fundamentally different.

SPF STATUS: TERRITORIAL AND HERD CONSIDERATIONS

It is a well-established principle of cryobiology that most, if not all, microorganisms are at least as well-preserved by the cryopreservation process as spermatozoa. Accordingly, the scope of animal contacts of an infected semen donor will be expanded many orders of magnitude over natural mating, can potentially spread over several continents, and will be limited only by the time that the inventory of contaminated frozen semen is kept and used. This risk is balanced by the advantage of the time-stopping effect of the frozen semen process. The capability to hold semen in frozen storage enables precollection and postcollection testing and surveillance of the donor and herdmates for incursion of disease before the semen is released for shipment. This capability does not extend to living animals and is one reason that trade in frozen semen provides an important safeguard against disease transmission in international germ plasm exchange.

The choice of whether or not to adopt immunization as a disease control strategy for seminal donor herds can be a management dilemma. Few currently used vaccines or serodiagnostic tests permit discrimination between immune responses initiated by infection or vaccination, with the result that vaccinated donors find limited acceptance.

However, when a sire population is maintained in an immune status that differs significantly from that of the surrounding national herd, very high disease control security is necessary. International regulatory imperatives have led to the creation of unvaccinated, seronegative semen donor herds among national herds in which widespread use of modified live vaccine or the presence of infection necessitate use of high security housing and complete control of transport, human access, feed and bedding, and precautionary postcollection quarantine of semen. Such viral diseases as classical swine fever, pseudorabies, infectious bovine rhinotracheitis/balanoposthitis, and foot and mouth disease present formidable obstacles to trade because of different national strategies of eradication or vaccination.

Techniques for isolation of infectious agents from semen have been adopted in lieu of or in combination with serological testing when found to be of adequate sensitivity. Seminal virus isolation tests are commonly used to document freedom of semen from bovine herpesvirus-1 (HV1), bovine virus diarrhea virus, bluetongue virus, and foot and mouth disease virus. Seminal specimens have particularly toxic effects on both viruses and cell cultures that may limit the sensitivity of such *in vitro* isolation methods. This limitation may be partially overcome by use of centrifugation or other techniques for reduction of seminal toxicity. Semen is not always the diagnostic specimen of choice even if the agent is potentially semen-borne: concurrently drawn specimens such as blood or esophageal–pharyngeal washings that are of lower toxicity or higher potential virus titer have been used in lieu of semen. One AI center has practiced continuous surveillance for several common pathogenic viruses by inoculating into susceptible test animals pooled aliquots from all ejaculates collected. This method may be more sensitive than *in vitro* techniques and provides surveillance of the entire herd rather than a single donor.

Insect vector-borne viruses have become a unique challenge to traditional regulatory practices and to AI center sire health management on a global scale. Such viruses are seldom more than potential sporadic contaminants of semen during the viremic period of infection. However, the uneven pattern of their international distribution and the seeming unpredictability of epizootics have added a large measure of complexity to germ plasm movement. Notable examples include Akabane virus, bluetongue, ephemeral fever, epizootic hemorrhagic disease, Japanese encephalitis, and vesicular stomatitis viruses. The movement of such agents from enzootic zones in tropical or warmer temperate areas into epizootic or sporadic incidence zones in cooler temperate regions is now believed to be the consequence of movement of infected insects by weather systems, although animal movements can also precipitate epizootics if competent vectors are present.

Identification of those geographic areas at risk because of the presence of transmission-competent native vectors or weather-borne exotic vectors has brought greater understanding of the appropriate regulatory response to such diseases and has reduced some trade barriers. The use of appropriate epidemiologic surveillance techniques is essential to risk assessment. Serologic surveys, establishment of sentinel herds in epizootic zones, and virologic assays of vector pools, combined with seasonal collection of semen, have facilitated movement of some livestock genetics from zones of high prevalence to those of low prevalence or absence. In this context political boundaries are far less important than the suitability of the environment for the insect. Vector-borne infections present the greatest difficulties when tropical or warmer temperate areas incorporate or are adjacent to major livestock breeding populations. Paradoxically, trade in tropically adapted cattle and sheep is attended by the impediment that throughout the world such breeds are native to areas where vector-borne infections of ruminants are enzootic.

SPF STATUS: MANAGEMENT AND TESTING OF DONORS

Reliable control of infectious disease among seminal donors can be achieved only when such animals are subjected to an appropriate period of isolation for testing prior to admittance to a resident donor herd. The disease status and management of each herd of origin should be scrutinized, and each candidate should receive a complete physical and genital evaluation in addition to appropriate tests. In circumstances where the threat of enzootic disease, vaccination practices or seasonal vector transmitted infections are of concern, removal of the sire to the AI center very early in life is often necessary.

Most traditional testing methods for seminal donors have been immunologic. Immunologic tests have the advantage of conveniently amplifying evidence of the presence of agents that may be difficult to isolate. Conventional serologic methods do not, however, discriminate between immunized and convalescent animals or between persistent and nonpersistent infections. Immunologic testing of the entire herd will provide further assurance that the infectious agent of concern was not present during the period of seminal collection. Freedom from infection certified by territorial or herd status is only as meaningful as the commitment to search out, eradicate, and prevent reintroduction of the etiologic agent.

Microbiologic isolation from an appropriate specimen may be employed when serologic response is absent or unreliable, such as in diagnosis of genital trichomoniasis, campylobacteriosis or contagious equine metritis. When such methods are employed, it is imperative to select those of the appropriate sensitivity to detect the minimal infectious dose of the agent of concern. The sensitivity threshold of a single culture of preputial smegma in Clark's transport enrichment medium is reported to be 100 *Campylobacter fetus venerealis* organisms in the inoculum. This sensitivity can be amplified by repeated sampling over a period of up to 6 weeks before permitting newly acquired bulls to enter genital campylobacteriosis-free donor herds.

Resident sires in AI centers should be subjected to repetitive testing with timing and frequency that take into consideration both the sensitivity and specificity of the test methods used as well as the potential rapidity of disease spread if the etiologic agent is introduced. The epidemiologic characteristics of the disease and the high animal density may permit a primary venereal pathogen to spread very rapidly in the environment of an AI center. Accordingly, surveillance for such agents should be performed at least semiannually, while tests for an agent such as *Mycobacterium paratuberculosis* that is unlikely to be transmitted among adult animals, may be done on an annual schedule.

The collection and processing of semen in the environment of a farm or ranch is a high-risk undertaking in the best of circumstances. If such semen is distributed to other properties the practice is indefensible. Very seldom is it possible to ensure the absence of animal and human contacts necessary to control even the sporadic semen-borne diseases, to say nothing of primary sexually transmitted agents. Where this practice is not forbidden it should be strongly discouraged by the attending veterinarian.

The duration of the precollection quarantine applied should be sufficient to permit detection of all infections of concern. In the United States, the admittance isolation of bovine seminal donors entails a minimum of 6 weeks for completion of all required sampling for genital campylobacteriosis and trichomoniasis. Single sampling during isolation is not adequate in most circumstances; for example, the sensitivity of a single caudal fold tuberculin test is reportedly no greater than 80%. Repetition of tests at the appropriate interval will raise this sensitivity to about 96%.

The most sensitive and specific diagnostic methods available should be applied to seminal donors because of the scope of their potential contacts. Conventional diagnostic techniques intended to screen large, unselected populations may not always be appropriate to the high value/high risk setting of an AI center. Complete dependence on serodiagnosis may be misleading, as in the case of failed immune response characterizing persistent bovine virus diarrhea infection. Strategies that combine several testing methods are appropriate if use of any single test has associated sensitivity or specificity limitations.

If donor sires return to breeder herds from the AI center, herd health measures in the center should not be limited to semen-borne infections alone. Nonvenereal infections such as anaplasmosis, babesiosis, or bovine leukosis are easily transmitted within the environment of a donor herd to the detriment of the health of individual sires and any herds to which they may be transferred.

SPF STATUS: SEMINAL MICROFLORA AND ANTIBIOTIC ADDITIVES

Both neat and processed semen may be expected to contain low numbers of vagrant microorganisms originating from the prepuce of the donor. No unequivocal adverse effects of the presence of such organisms on fertility have been demonstrated. However, certain bacteria such as *Corynebacterium pyogenes* in the bull and *Pseudomonas* sp. in the stallion may be associated with opportunistic genital tract infections in the female. Males harboring such bacteria should either be successfully treated or discarded unless effective seminal antibiotic control can be assured.

The presence of a large population of contaminating microbes in processed semen is suggestive of lack of regard for fundamental sanitation during seminal collection and processing. All collection apparatus, glassware and seminal packages should be sterile, and extenders should be prepared and stored under sanitary conditions. Unclean donor housing or laboratories, careless use of electroejaculation as a collection method, processing of semen at ambient temperature, and failure to sterilize seminal packages are all potential sources of seminal contamination.

Antibiotics have been used in bovine seminal extenders for many years, primarily as a control technique for genital campylobacteriosis. However, to be fully effective in this role combinations of bactericidal antibiotics must be added to the semen prior to dilution as well as to the extender. Very significant interactions between some antibiotics and extenders occur that may negate bactericidal or bacteriostatic effects. Antibiotic effectiveness cannot be extrapolated from one extender to another. While campylobacteriosis is now controlled by maintenance of SPF donors, other bacteria such as *Hemophilus* sp., *Mycoplasma* sp., and *Ureaplasma* sp. in the bull and *Pseudomonas* sp. or *Proteus* sp. in the stallion are controlled by antibiotic addition. Antibiotics must be carefully selected for compatibility with spermatozoa. For example, aminoglycoside antibiotics such as streptomycin and gentamycin are far better tolerated by spermatozoa than tetracylines.

INTERNATIONAL SEMEN MOVEMENT IN THE FUTURE

Much international animal trade now emphasizes trade in animals of known genetic merit. Consequently, shipment of frozen semen from progeny-tested males will continue to be the most reliable method to transfer germ plasm internationally.

Some animal health barriers are being overcome by use of new diagnostic technologies: a recent importation into the United States of semen from foot and mouth disease-vaccinated and bluetongue-seropositive donors made use of virologic tests of pharyngeal washings, serologic tests for response to FMD virus core antigen, and bluetongue virus isolation tests. These diagnostic tests replaced serologic methods that are confounded by antibody responses associated with vaccination or nonpersistent infection.

Implementation of better standardized serologic techniques such as enzyme-linked immunoassay as well as use of subunit vaccines that permit later serologic discrimination between vaccinal and convalescent immunity are likely to eliminate some obstacles to trade associated with current serodiagnostic and immunization methods. Successful utilization of such methods will not invalidate the principles of SPF status, but may alter the acceptable certification criteria for some diseases. Well-managed donor herds of known health history that are repeatedly tested and securely housed will continue to provide the greatest disease control security for the international animal breeding community.

Complementary References

American Breeders Service AI Management Manual (1986) American Breeders Service, DeForest, Wisconsin.

Bartlett, D. E., Larson, L. L., Parker, W. G. & Howard, T. H. (1976) Specific-pathogen-free semen: a goal? *Proceedings 6th Tech. Conf. Reprod. Artificial Insemination*, National Association of Animal Breeders, pp. 11–22.

Cole, H. H. & Cupps, P. T. (1969) *Reproduction in Domestic Animals*. New York: Academic Press.

Crowe-Swords, P. & Taylor, J. (1979) *Bovine Semen Collection and Processing Techniques*. Edmonton: Agriculture Alberta.

Hare, W. C. D. (1985) *Diseases Transmissible by Semen and Embryo Transfer Techniques*. Technical series no. 4. Paris: Office International des Epizooties.

Howard, T. H. (1986) CSS sire health: present and future. *Proceedings 11th Tech. Conf. Reprod. Artificial Insemination*, National Association of Animal Breeders, pp. 19–26.

Pace, M. M. (1980) Fundamentals of assay of spermatozoa. *Proceedings 9th Int. Congr. Anim. Reprod. Artificial Insemination*, pp. 133–146.

Pace, M. M., Sullivan, J. J., Elliott, F. I., Graham, E. F. & Coulter, G. H. (1981) Effects of thawing temperature, number of spermatozoa and spermatozoal quality on fertility of bovine spermatozoa packaged in 0.5 ml french straws. *J. Anim. Sci.*, **53**, 693–701.

Salisbury, G. W., Vandemark, N. L. & Lodge, J. R. (1978) *Physiology of Reproduction and Artificial Insemination of Cattle*. San Francisco: W. H. Freeman and Co.

Schultz, R. D., Adams, L. S., Letchworth, G., Sheffy, B. E., Manning, T. & Bean, B. (1982) A method to test large numbers of bovine semen samples for viral contamination and results of a study using this method. *Theriogenology*, **17**(2), 115–123.

Sellers, R. F. (1980) Weather, host and vector–their interplay in the spread of insect-borne virus diseases. *J. Hyg., Cambridge*, **85**, 65–102.

Thacker, B. J., Larsen, R. E., Joo, H. S. & Leman, A. D. (1984) Swine diseases transmissible with artificial insemination. *J. Amer. Vet. Med. Assoc.*, **185**(5), 511–516.

XII Biennial Symposium on Animal Reproduction (1975) eds Zimmerman, D. R. *et al. J. Anim. Sci.*, **47**, suppl. 2.

3

Embryo Collection, Evaluation and Transfer

RAYMOND W. WRIGHT JR

BACKGROUND TO EMBRYO TRANSFER

Walter Heape not only performed the first embryo transfers at the end of the last century but also had a profound influence on other studies of reproduction including uterine environment, sperm–egg interaction, and anatomy of the reproductive tract. Heape's first transfer in 1890 stimulated an interest in embryo transfer both in Europe and the United States.

Gregory Pincus, with his colleague, M. C. Chang, are probably best known for their work in developing the oral contraceptive while at the Worcester Foundation in Shrewsbury, Massachusetts. However, before that time Pincus was a visiting National Research Council Fellow from Harvard University and in 1929 successfully transferred rabbit embryos to recipient does.

Pincus' work stimulated an interest in how this new science might be applied to the genetic improvement of domestic livestock. The Foundation of Applied Research of San Antonio, Texas, founded in 1912 collected over 750 donor cattle over an 8 year period. The results were disappointing, the effort achieving only four pregnancies which all aborted before 8 months. However, much was learned about embryo collection and transfer, superovulation and embryo handling that aided a cooperative effort between the USDA and the

University of Wisconsin in 1951 to achieve the first live birth in cattle from embryo transfer.

Although synchronization and superovulation were relatively routine procedures in the 1950s, embryo transfer success rates remained low in domestic animals. Much interest was centered around the embryo collection and transfer procedures which were patterned after earlier work in laboratory animals. Superior results were being reported in the 1960s using surgical methods in sheep, goats and cattle with the exploitation of this technology into the commercial embryo transfer marketplace. The complications of adhesions, surgical trauma and cost of the procedure limited the application of embryo transfer only to donors of superior genetic or monetary value. In the 1970s laboratories in the United States and Europe developed the nonsurgical embryo collection techniques for cattle still used today. This technological advance allowed the collection and transfer of embryos outside the surgical arena, and a new 'on-the-farm' embryo transfer industry evolved (Fig. 3.1).

The embryo transfer industry is now fully established in over 14 countries with an estimated 13 000 cattle embryos transferred in the United States and over 4000 in Canada in 1979. Although the collection and transfer of embryos is now routine, the related technologies of embryo preservation and micromanipulation for the production of identical

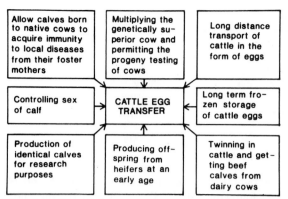

Fig. 3.1 Potential uses and application of embryo transfer in cattle.

Table 3.1   First records of successful embryo transfers

Date	Species	Date	Species
1891	Rabbit	1968	Ferret
1933	Rat	1974	Horse
1934	Sheep	1976	Baboon
1942	Goat*	1978	Man†
1949	Mouse	1978	Cat
1949	Cow**	1979	Dog
1951	Goat	1981	Gaur††
1951	Cow††	1984	Marmoset
1951	Pig	1984	Zebra††
1964	Cow (cervical)	1984	Przewalskis horse††

*Reinsertion.
**Aborted.
†*In vitro* fertilization and reinsertion.
††Interspecies recipient.

twins, and determination of sex and control of genetic makeup of the embryo will result in a reduction of cost and wider application of embryo transfer technology.

The main objective of performing embryo transfer in swine is not the production of genetically superior offspring, but rather the prevention and control of disease. It is known that 43% of commercial embryo transfers were performed to establish new herds from herds with pseudorabies; 26% to make additions to specific-pathogen-free herds; 23% to obtain boars for closed commercial herds; and only 7% for obtaining offspring from genetically superior donors.

TECHNOLOGY OF EMBRYO TRANSFER

Donor and Recipient Selection

There is a multitude of reasons why an animal is selected to be an embryo transfer donor. In cattle, the decision may be based on economics rather than true genetic superiority. The following selection criteria will insure genetic superiority as well as a good probability of producing embryos of high quality.

1. When possible a donor should be selected with a previous record of success in embryo transfer; recent information suggests that certainly in sheep, and perhaps cattle, successful superovulation is related to the total number of oocytes in the ovary before treatment; the number of oocytes present in the ovary is correlated with the breed.
2. Donors should be between the ages of 1 and 4 years in sheep and 3 and 10 years in cattle.
3. Donors should be tested to be free of genetic disease and conformational abnormalities.
4. Donors should exhibit regular estrous cycles and have had at least two regular cycles following a seasonal or lactational anestrous cycle.
5. Selection should include animals with superior production traits of economic importance and above-average production of offspring from previous matings of the same dam and sire.
6. Donors should be tested to ensure absence of disease particularly critical to meet health requirements for the export of embryos.
7. Previous sound reproductive performance including no more than two inseminations per conception or, in cattle, three calves born within 2 calendar years.
8. Donors should be included in a routine herd health program including genetic consultation and production performance of offspring; practitioners should educate clients as to expectations for success and the difficulty of obtaining offspring from problem donors.

Recipient management is an area critical to the success of an embryo transfer program but is commonly overlooked. Generally, recipients should be selected and culled under the same criteria as in superior commercial or purebred cattle operations. Purchase of recipients from the sale barn or recipients open due to infertility or animals previously treated with growth stimulants should be avoided at all costs. New recipients should be calfhood vaccinated and be tested to be free of tuberculosis and brucellosis prior to herd introduction. Upon arrival, recipients should be isolated and retested for tuberculosis and brucellosis, treated for internal and ecto-

Table 3.2 Prostaglandin and prostaglandin analogs

Agent	Trade name	Manufacturer	Dose*
Dinoprost	Lutalyse	Upjohn	25 mg
Cloprostenol†	Estrumate	ICI Pharma	500 μg
Alfaprostol†	Alfave	Hoffman-LaRoche	5.0 mg
Fenprostalene†	Bovilene	Syntex	1.0 mg

*Manufacturers' recommended dose.
†Analog.

parasites, given preventive virus and leptospirosis vaccinations, and identified with both metal and plastic ear-tag identification systems. Recipients can be grazed on pasture but should receive an average of 9 kg of a high-energy grain ration daily while lactating. Recipients in a growing phase of nutrition and with a dystocia-free history can be used as early as 60–90 days after calving.

Recipients which are too thin or too fat will yield poor success rates and should be excluded from an embryo transfer program. Cows, when well managed, can be as equally good recipients as heifers due to a lower occurrence of perinatal mortality and an equivalent conception rate.

Estrus Synchronization—Cattle

A high degree of estrus synchronization between donor and recipient is essential for high conception rates. (An ideal recipient is an animal that exhibited estrus the same day or not more than 1 day before the donor.) An equally important factor for high conception rates is embryo quality. An embryo that is of high quality can adjust to a greater degree of asynchrony compared with an embryo of poor quality.

Prostaglandin $F_{2\alpha}$ ($PGF_{2\alpha}$) or its analogs are the most common luteolytic agents used to synchronize estrus in cattle (Table 3.2). While there are differences in the structure and biological activities of the prostaglandin products, there is no evidence to suggest superiority of a particular product.

Estrus is expected to occur approximately 48 h following luteolytic dose of $PGF_{2\alpha}$. Ideally, recipients should be in estrus 12–18 h before or on the same day as the donor. Poor pregnancy rates may result from recipients which exhibited estrus 60 h or longer after $PGF_{2\alpha}$ injection.

Superovulation—Cattle

Donor cows will respond more predictably when the

superovulatory hormone is given between 8 and 14 days following estrus. Two drugs, pregnant mare serum gonadotropin (PMSG) and follicle stimulating hormone (FSH) are most commonly used to induce superovulation. However, FSH has been shown to increase ovulation rate, embryos recovered and embryos of superior quality compared with PMSG, which may be used for a donor suspected to be refractory to FSH because of repeated stimulation or on other problem donors.

FSH is generally administered twice daily (i.m.) although several studies have shown no decrease in response with once a day injections. Certain donors may require the addition of luteinizing hormone (LH) to FSH at a 1 : 5 ratio; however, it is not added routinely as most commercial preparations of FSH contain some LH. Several superovulation treatment schedules are shown in Table 3.3. Schedule A is used for a donor that does not respond well to FSH treatment. Schedule B is most often used for superovulation of heifers or donors not previously superovulated where the possibility of hyperstimulation exists. Donors previously stimulated with FSH, obese or older cows may respond better with treatment C.

Practitioners should recognize that superovulation is a highly variable event and always be aware of the potential for hyperstimulation (Fig. 3.2). Strict attention to detail is necessary for a successful embryo transfer program including: donor and recipient selections; health and nutrition; timing of injection; and estrus detection with good communication among all individuals involved.

Breeding—Cattle

Little variation in conception rates is observed among fresh semen, natural breeding or artificial insemination when timed correctly with ovulation. Donors may ovulate over 24 h with the interval from estrus to the first ovulation remaining unchanged. Therefore, multiple breedings at 12 h intervals are generally used (see Table 3.3) with some breeders using 2 units of frozen semen at each breeding.

Table 3.3 Superovulation treatment schedules for cattle

Day*	Time	Treatment A	Treatment B	Treatment C
10	a.m.	2500–5000 i.u. PMSG	5 mg FSH	5 mg FSH
	p.m.		5 mg FSH	5 mg FSH
11	a.m.		4 mg FSH	5 mg FSH
	p.m.	Recipients PGF$_{2\alpha}$	4 mg FSH†	5 mg FSH†
12	a.m.	Donors PGF$_{2\alpha}$	3 mg FSH††	5 mg FSH††
	p.m.		3 mg FSH	5 mg FSH
13	a.m.		2 mg FSH	5 mg FSH
	p.m.		2 mg FSH	5 mg FSH
14	a.m.			
	p.m.	Breed	Breed	Breed
15	a.m.	Breed	Breed	Breed
	p.m.	Breed	Breed	Breed

*Day 0 onset of estrus.
†Recipient PGF$_{2\alpha}$.
††Donor PGF$_{2\alpha}$.

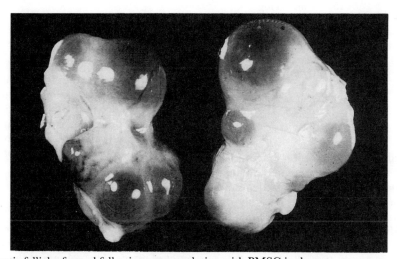

Fig. 3.2 Large cystic follicles formed following superovulation with PMSG in sheep.

Semen should be routinely examined before insemination and particular care given to cleanliness and good insemination techniques. Bull fertility has been shown to be highly correlated with the number of fertilized embryos recovered and may affect the viability of embryos transferred.

Synchronization—Sheep and Goats

Recipients can be synchronized with PGF$_{2\alpha}$, progesterone or intravaginal progestins (Table 3.4.). PGF$_{2\alpha}$ given during the luteal phase of the cycle will show estrus in 1–3 days. A double injection of PGF$_{2\alpha}$ given 8–10 days apart in sheep and 12–14 days apart in goats is useful when the time from last estrus is unknown. Progestin pessaries can be used for estrus synchronization in cycling recipients or for the induction of estrus in anestrous animals (see Table 3.4). PMSG (350–500 i.u.) or 1000 units of LH (i.v.) at the time of pessary removal can be used to aid ovulation for animals treated during anestrus.

Superovulation—Sheep and Goats

Poor ovulation rate and increased number of unovulated follicles associated with the use of PMSG in sheep and goats has made FSH the drug of choice. FSH treatment is initiated 2–3 days before PGF$_{2\alpha}$ injection, or 1–2 days before pessary removal (Table 3.5). Teaser males are useful in the detection of estrus at 12 h intervals starting 12 h after PGF$_{2\alpha}$ injection or pessary removal.

Table 3.4　Synchronization treatment in sheep and goats

Agent	Dose	Comments
Progesterone	10–15 mg i.m.	Duration: 12–14 days (sheep) 14–18 days (goat)
Progestin (Cronolone)	30–45 mg (pessary)	Duration: 12–14 days (sheep) 14–18 days (goat)
PGF$_{2\alpha}$	8–15 mg i.m.	Luteal phase of cycle
Cloprostenol	150–250 g i.m.	Luteal phase of cycle

Table 3.5　Superovulation schedule

	Sheep			Goats	
Day	Time	Treatment	Day	Time	Treatment
10	a.m.	5 mg	14	a.m.	5 mg
	p.m.	5 mg		p.m.	5 mg
11	a.m.	4 mg	15	a.m.	4 mg
	p.m.	4 mg		p.m.	4 mg
12	a.m.	3 mg + PGF$_{2\alpha}$	16	a.m.	3 mg
	p.m.	3 mg		p.m.	3 mg
13	a.m.	2 mg*	17	a.m.	2 mg + PGF$_{2\alpha}$
	p.m.	2 mg		p.m.	2 mg
			18	a.m.	2 mg*
				p.m.	2 mg

*Pessary removal.

Pessary removal or PGF$_{2\alpha}$ injection for recipients should occur 24 h ahead of superovulated donors to ensure estrus synchronization. Like cattle, super-ovulation response in sheep and goats is highly variable due to age and nutritional status of the donor and time of breeding season. Breeds of high fecundity (Finnish Landrace) generally respond better than breeds of low fecundity (Suffolk).

Breeding—Sheep and Goats

Superovulated ewes consistently show a lower fertilization rate compared to female goats, possibly as a result of poor sperm transport through the cervix, endogenous progesterone or residual effect of the progestin pessary. Ewes and goats should be inseminated or hand-mated at 12 h intervals until the cessation of estrus. Fertilization rates are generally higher with natural mating compared to artificial insemination for both goats and ewes.

Estrus Synchronization—Swine

Synchronization can be achieved by weaning a group of sows with estrus occurring in 4–10 days. A high proportion of sows will be in estrus in 4–5 days

when 500–800 i.u. of PMSG are given at the time of weaning. An alternative method is to breed sows and abort them between 16 and 45 days of pregnancy with two injections of PGF$_{2\alpha}$ 12 h apart. A tighter synchrony can be achieved with an injection of 500–800 i.u. of PMSG at the time of the second PGF$_{2\alpha}$ injection.

Superovulation—Swine

Sows can be superovulated with a single injection of 1200–1500 i.u. of PMSG at weaning or at the first PGF$_{2\alpha}$ injection during 16–45 days of pregnancy. The superovulation response ranges from 0 to 45 ovulations and is quite variable among individual females and breeds. If embryos are collected from sows on more than two consecutive estrous cycles, the time of estrus usually is not controlled and superovulation is not used.

Breeding—Swine

Optimum conception is achieved with natural mating or artificial insemination every 12 h from the onset of estrus. The volume of the dose for artificial insemination should be approximately 75 ml and contain at least 5 billion live spermatozoa.

EMBRYO COLLECTION AND TRANSFER

Before 1975 most embryo collections were performed by surgical methods. Nonsurgical approaches are now commonly used for embryo collections in cattle and the horse. Surgical procedures are still being used in the other farm species, primarily due to the difficulty of passing a catheter through the cervix. Nonsurgical techniques avoid the potential damage of the reproductive tract by adhesions, are repeatable, do not require elaborate facilities and can be applied when the embryos have reached the uterus and in animals where the cervix can be penetrated with a catheter.

Cattle

One to eight-cell embryos (1–5 days following estrus) can be collected by flushing media either from the fimbria toward the uterus or from the uterotubal junction toward the fimbria following the insertion of a glass or teflon cannula into the infundibulum. This surgical approach has limited commercial application as it requires general anesthesia and surgical invasion of the abdominal cavity.

Embryos are routinely collected by nonsurgical methods 6–8 days after the onset of estrus. Prior to day 5, the embryos may be in the oviduct and after day 8 may be hatched (escaped from the zona pellucida), difficult to visualize and fragile.

The donor is placed in a restraining chute and the rectum cleared of feces. The front end of the donor should be elevated a minimum of 35 cm to create a positive pressure in the abdomen. The perineal region and vulvar lips are thoroughly washed with water, particular attention being paid to removing all soap from the region. The tail is tied out of the way and an epidural anesthetic is administered. The operator must consciously avoid introducing air into the rectum, a problem frequently encountered in older dairy cows. The ovaries can be palpated to approximate the number of corpora lutea and large unovulated follicles.

Two types of catheters are commonly used for nonsurgical collection in cattle. The Foley catheter is inexpensive, readily available and can be reused following gas sterilization (ethylene oxide). The length of the Foley catheter may be limiting in collecting large dairy cows and the rubber is very flexible which can cause difficulty in threading the uterus. In addition, a stilette is not provided with this catheter and must be manufactured.

The Rausch catheter is 67 cm long with an 18-gauge outside diameter and is supplied with a stilette with a Luer-Lok fitting. It is somewhat stiffer than the Foley catheter which makes threading the uterus simpler. The length from the catheter tip to the cuff is 5.5 cm, longer than the Foley and has four holes to inject and retrieve fluid. The Rausch catheter is expensive and not generally available from medical supply houses but can be reused following gas sterilization.

Two systems are commonly used for nonsurgical collection in cattle: the continuous flow, closed-circuit system, and the interrupted-syringe method. Practitioners may use a combination of these two systems and both are equally effective when done properly. The closed system offers the advantage of cleanliness, sterility and fluid control but requires

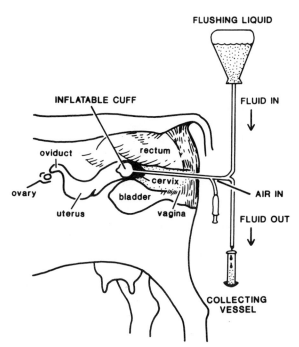

Fig. 3.3 Continuous flow method for the nonsurgical collection of embryos in cattle.

additional tubing and connections. The syringe method is faster and allows embryo searching before the flush is complete (Fig. 3.3).

The sterile catheter with the stilette locked into position is coated with a sterile lubricant, and it is advisable to use a plastic sheath over the catheter to prevent contamination of the uterus. Extreme care should be taken to remove all fecal contamination from the lips of the vulva which are parted wide for catheter insertion. The catheter is passed through the cervix aided by manipulation through the rectal wall and into the right uterine horn while withdrawing the stilette slowly. The catheter is positioned so that the cuff is approximately halfway between the uterine body and the tip of the uterine horn. The cuff is then slowly inflated with saline or air until the cuff completely fills the uterine lumen. Care should be taken to avoid overinflation of the cuff which can result in endometrial damage and loss of flushing medium into the broad ligament. The stilette is removed and a clamp placed on the exteriorized end of the catheter.

A conservative approach to filling the horn with fluid should be used to avoid overdistention and possible rupture of the endometrium. Generally, 25–35 ml of fluid (approximately the size of a 35 day pregnancy) is sufficient to distend the horn and this amount is repeated approximately eight times; 85% of the embryos collected will be found in the first

100–150 ml of fluid. Gentle agitation and lifting of the uterus is performed to ensure that the fluid reaches all areas of the endometrium.

When the collection of the right uterine horn is completed the stilette may be reinserted or the catheter removed completely from the reproductive tract before reinserting the stilette. The latter procedure is advisable for inexperienced practitioners to ensure proper locking of the stilette in the catheter. The flushing procedure is repeated for the left uterine horn.

Following completion of the flush, each uterine horn is infused with 30–50 ml of antibiotic solution using a uterine infusion catheter. $PGF_{2\alpha}$ can be given at this time or within a week of the flush; however, return to estrus can vary from a few days to several weeks.

Most practitioners utilize a flank approach to transfer embryos surgically. The recipient is palpated to determine the side of the corpus luteum which will be the same side as the flank incision. An epidural and local (L-block) anesthesia (Lidocaine) is administered and the surgical site is shaved and cleaned. A 15–20 cm vertical incision is made in the paralumbar fossa, the muscle layers and peritoneum are bluntly dissected. Existence of the corpus luteum is verified and the top of the uterine horn is gently grasped and exteriorized. A small puncture is made into the uterine lumen with the blunt end of a cutting suture needle. The embryo is loaded into a transfer pipette in less than 0.5 ml of fluid which is positioned between two air spaces. The loaded pipette is passed through the puncture into the uterine lumen and the embryo deposited.

Practitioners use a variety of instruments to transfer embryos nonsurgically including telescoping rods, transvaginal surgical techniques and others, but the most commonly used is the Cassou AI gun with a French straw. The recipient is restrained and palpated to determine the presence and location of the corpus luteum. The vulvar area is cleaned and wiped dry with careful attention paid to removal of all fecal contamination. A double sheath is used to reduce contamination from the vagina and the Cassou gun is threaded through the cervix to a position cranial to the external uterine bifurcation. The site of embryo deposition is secondary to an atraumatic placement for good results. The embryo should be deposited with a slow but even pressure from the Cassou gun into the uterine horn ipsilateral to the corpus luteum.

Sheep and Goats

Embryos are collected and transferred surgically in sheep and goats due to the difficulty in passing a catheter into the uterus through the cervix. One to eight-cell embryos can be collected from the oviduct with later stages flushed from the uterus. Surgical collection is performed under general or local anesthesia with the animal lying on its back. A 3–5 cm midline incision is made as near the udder as possible using blunt dissection to reach the peritoneum. The uterus and ovaries are exteriorized onto a sterile field and corpora lutea counted.

The oviduct can be cannulated with a glass or teflon tube (2 mm outside diameter) held in place by plastic clips while a blunt needle is inserted into the uterine lumen a few centimeters from the tip of the horn. The caudal segment is pinched off with thumb and forefinger or intestinal forcep and flushing media gently forced in a retrograde manner through the uterus and oviduct. Caution must be taken to limit the pressure which can rupture the endometrium and force fluid into the broad ligament. The operator must be sure to manipulate the oviduct to remove twists which can occlude fluid flow. This procedure is generally used to collect embryos at the one to eight-cell stage, but has the disadvantage of manipulating the delicate fimbria of the oviduct which often leads to surgical adhesions.

An alternative method which avoids the manipulation of these delicate fimbriae is to place a small pediatric Foley catheter into the uterine lumen at the uterine bifurcation with the cuff gently expanded to secure its position. A blunt needle with syringe is inserted at the top of the uterine horn and fluid forced slowly into the uterus with the operator gently massaging the uterus to insure fluid expansion of the endometrial folds. A simple suture is used to close the site of catheter insertion, and the uterus cleansed with a high molecular weight dextran solution to minimize surgical adhesions. Routine closure of the abdomen is performed and the animal given an antibiotic injection.

Swine

Embryos are collected and transferred surgically in swine. The procedure is performed under general anesthesia; one method is induction with intravenous barbiturate such as thiamylal sodium and maintenance of surgical anesthesia with halothane gas. The midventral area is shaved and washed and a 10 cm incision made. The adjacent ovary, oviduct and 30 cm of uterus is exteriorized on to a sterile field. A small incision is made for cannula insertion in the antimesometrial side of the uterus approximately 20 cm from the uterotubal junction avoiding vascular regions. The cannula, usually made of glass of 12 cm length and 10 mm diameter is inserted a few centimeters into the horn and held in place by a clamp. A blunt needle is inserted into the oviduct and 49–60 ml of fluid is forced through the oviduct, into the uterus and out the cannula. The uterus is gently milked with the thumb and forefinger to remove all the fluid. The cannula is removed and the uterus washed with a dextran solution to minimize surgical adhesions. The abdomen is closed and the entire procedure is repeated for the second uterine horn.

Optimal results are achieved when recipients are in estrus 1 or 2 days after the donor and receive at least twelve good quality embryos. Transfers are performed surgically under general anesthesia using an intravenous barbiturate. A midventral incision is made and the ovaries evaluated for corpora lutea and general condition of the reproductive tract. Embryos can be transferred by depositing the embryos into the lumen of the uterus some 5 cm away from the puncture wound, or by threading a catheter into the oviduct and washing the embryos into the uterus with a minimum amount of fluid. All embryos transferred can be placed in one uterine horn because porcine embryos will become equally distributed in both uterine horns.

EMBRYO EVALUATION

Embryo evaluation is an important determinant of the success of embryo transfer procedures. Gross morphological evaluation of embryos has been shown to be useful in predicting pregnancy rates for groups of embryos, but is of limited value in determining survival on an individual embryo basis. Dye exclusion tests, measures of enzyme activity, glucose uptake and live–dead stains seem to correlate well with morphology and embryo survival following transfer. Several of these methods require complex equipment, a lengthy *in vitro* culture period, or both. Consequently they are of little value for on-the-farm embryo transfer conditions.

Morphological evaluation has been widely used to delineate embryo quality. Several schemes for evaluating embryos have been described and all appear equally reliable when compared with actual pregnancy rates. Parameters commonly used to evaluate embryo quality include shape, color, number and compactness of cells, size of the perivitelline space, number of extruded and degenerated cells, and the number and size of vesicles. Categorization from the most ideal to the poorest embryos varies between operators, some utilizing simple two-way classifications (good and poor)

while others use a more complex system. Systems classifying embryos into good, fair and poor categories appear to be the simplest and most reliable. The most extensively used criterion to evaluate bovine embryos is whether an embryo has attained an expected stage of development based upon day of flush post-estrus. Success appears to be less with embryos retarded 2 days or more when compared to embryos at an expected stage of development. To date, embryo evaluation remains one of the most subjective and qualitative aspects of embryo transfer.

Gross Morphology of Bovine Embryos

Gross morphological characteristics of the bovine embryo have been described by several authors. The overall diameter of the bovine embryo is 150–190 μm including a zona pellucida thickness of approximately 12–15 μm. The overall diameter of the embryo remains virtually unchanged from the one-cell stage until blastocyst expansion. Early cleavage stage embryos are commonly designated by the number of cells present such as one-cell, two-cell, etc., up to the sixteen-cell stage. Estimates only can be made as to the number of cells present for early morulae and beyond. Consequently other morphological criteria must be used. The various developmental stages commonly recovered nonsurgically from superovulated donors are listed and briefly described below:

Morula

Four days of age—this is commonly referred to as a 'ball of cells'. Individual blastomeres are difficult to discern from one another. The cellular mass of the embryo occupies most of the perivitelline space.

Compact Morula

Five days of age—individual blastomeres have coalesced forming a compact mass. The embryo mass occupies 60–70% of the perivitelline space.

Early Blastocyst

Six days of age—the embryo has formed a fluid-filled cavity or blastocele and gives a general appearance of a signet ring. The embryo occupies 70–80% of the perivitelline space. Visual differentiation between trophoblast and the inner cell mass may be possible at this stage of development.

Blastocyst

Seven days of age—there is pronounced differentiation of the outer trophoblast layer and the darker more compact inner cell mass is evident. The blastocele is highly prominent with the embryo occupying most of the perivitelline space.

Expanded Blastocyst

Eight days of age—overall diameter of the embryo dramatically increased (1.2–$1.5 \times$), with a concurrent thinning of the zona pellucida to approximately a third of its original thickness. Embryos recovered at the expanded blastocyst stage frequently appear collapsed, characterized by a complete or partial loss of the blastocele. However, the zona pellucida rarely regains its original thickness.

Hatched Blastocyst

Nine days of age—embryos recovered at this developmental stage can be undergoing the process of hatching or may have completely shed the zona pellucida. Hatched blastocysts may be spherical with a well-defined blastocele or collapsed. Identification of embryos at this stage can be difficult for the inexperienced operator.

Quality of individual embryos can be determined using the following criteria:

1. Excellent: an ideal embryo, spherical, symmetrical with cells of uniform size, color and texture.
2. Good: trivial imperfections such as a few extruded blastomeres, irregular shape, few vesicles.
3. Fair: definite but not severe problems, presence of extruded blastomeres, vesiculation, few degenerated cells.
4. Poor: severe problems, numerous extruded blastomeres, degenerated cells, cells of varying sizes, large numerous vesicles but an embryo mass appearing viable.

Summary

A great deal of variability exists in morphological development and embryo quality within and among donors. Embryo recovery in the superovulated cow commonly results in a range of embryonic cell stages differing in estimated developmental ages of 24–48 hours. Embryo evaluation involves the identification of embryonic cell stage of development and an assessment of quality based on morphological characteristics. Little difference is observed in pregnancy rates between embryos of excellent or good quality. Therefore a system of classifying embryos into good, fair and poor categories appears to be the simplest and as equally reliable as more complex systems. Further assessment of developmental capabilities of poor quality embryos can increase efficiency of embryo transfer. Depending on available facilities, embryos of poor quality can be cultured for 24 h to assess their viability. Postculture embryo evaluation and transfer results in pregnancy rates equal to that of noncultured embryos of similar quality.

Results indicate that recipient–donor estrous cycle asynchrony of 2 days in either direction does not drastically alter pregnancy rates. However, synchronization of embryonic development with recipients may have more stringent requirements. It has been shown that bovine blastocysts can be refrigerated ($4\,^\circ\text{C}$) for up to 2 days without significant losses in viability. This technique can be used to store blastocysts in a dormant state while recipients that exhibit estrus after the donor progress to a more synchronous stage of their cycle.

As evidenced by actual pregnancy rates, microscopic evaluation of embryos, even at high magnifications ($200 \times$), remains a very subjective assessment. Development of a reliable, rapid and practical method of assessing embryo viability would be of great benefit to the embryo transfer industry.

CULTURE MEDIA AND SHORT-TERM STORAGE OF EMBRYOS

Media Components

Culture systems for embryos of major farm species were designed to meet one of two objectives. The first was for longterm culture (days), in which various media, gaseous atmospheres and embryo handling methods could be studied. The second was a short-term culture system (hours), in which embryos could be held for brief periods of time before transfer to recipient females.

Embryos from farm animals have been cultured in a wide variety of defined and undefined media. Defined media, rather than undefined media (in which the composition is unknown and the components can vary considerably), are the media of choice when the objective is to study embryo development. However, when the objective is to provide a system that supports *in vitro* embryo survival, the appropriate medium is the one that is effective.

The ions required for successful embryo development include K^+, Ca^{2+}, Na^+, Mg^{2+}, Cl^-, PO_4^{3-} and HCO_3^-. Optimum levels of these ions in media are similar to serum values except for K^+, which is sometimes found in higher concentration in synthetic oviduct fluid (SOF) and Menezo's medium. The role of individual ions in embryonic development is not well-understood; however, Ca^{2+} is known to be important in membrane stability and permeability and also at the time of morula compaction. It is generally agreed that the role of sodium chloride (NaCl) is primarily for osmotic balance of the medium. The osmolarity of commonly used media is in the range of 250–300 milliosmoles (mOsmol).

It is often difficult, when working under field conditions, to maintain embryos under a controlled gaseous atmosphere. This has led to the use of phosphate-buffered medium, which eliminates the need for CO_2 incubators or alternative gassing systems. This is of some concern because it has been found that mouse embryo development decreased following incubation in phosphate-buffered rather than bicarbonate-buffered medium. Further, it has been established that the mouse embryo utilizes CO_2 as a carbon source during development. However, phosphate-buffered medium is preferred owing to the radical change in pH that can occur with bicarbonate-buffered medium when care is not taken to maintain a 5% CO_2 in air atmosphere.

The most commonly used gas atmosphere for embryo culture is a 5% CO_2 in air. Some investigators have found that reducing the oxygen concentration from 20 to 5% (a total gas phase of 5% CO_2, 5% O_2 and 90% N_2) was beneficial for embryo development. No development occurs in the absence of O_2, and the lower O_2 tensions are probably closer to physiological states. No role of N_2 in this mixture has been found, and it is generally considered to be inert.

The role of the bicarbonate ion in the medium is to control the pH, but it also functions in equilibrium with CO_2 as a carbon source during embryo development. For this reason, longterm storage of embryos in phosphate-buffered medium as compared with bicarbonate-buffered medium is not recommended.

Pyruvate and lactate are preferred energy sources for early preimplantation embryos, while glucose is incorporated into the embryo at all stages of development in much greater amounts than either pyruvate or lactate. There seems to be little benefit in including pyruvate or lactate in media for the culture of embryos of eight cells or greater in development. Glucose should be a component of

phosphate-buffered as well as bicarbonate-buffered medium at a concentration of 0.5–1.0 g/l.

Little benefit is gained by using a concentration of serum greater than 10% in complete culture medium. However, when using a phosphate-buffered medium, serum concentrations of 20% are recommended for holding embryos for several hours. Considerably less serum, from 1 to 10%, can be used for flushing. All serum should be heat-treated (56 °C for 30 min) to remove complement activity and should be sterilized by filtration before being used in any medium. Recent results suggest that both newborn calf and steer serum can be used in place of the more expensive and difficult to obtain fetal calf serum for embryo flushing and transfer. Bovine serum albumin (BSA) can be an effective medium supplement for longterm culture. However, care should be taken to adjust the pH of the medium, particularly when concentrations of BSA are greater than 1%. As a matter of convenience, serum is used more frequently than BSA.

Methods for Short-term Embryo Culture in the Field

Embryos should be stored in the same medium that was used for flushing. It is not desirable to move embryos, for example, from a phosphate-buffered to a bicarbonate-buffered medium because of the possible changes in osmolarity, pH and energy substrates. Precautions should be taken if a bicarbonate-buffered medium is used, to prevent changes in pH due to CO_2 escape into the atmosphere. This can be accomplished by using capped tubes, which have been previously gassed, or by placing embryo vessels in an incubator in which the atmosphere can be controlled. No precautions are necessary with phosphate-buffered medium, and it is recommended that a 20% serum concentration be used if less than this amount was employed for the flush.

Flushing and holding medium should contain antibiotics to prevent bacterial contamination. Also, embryo vessels should be sterilized before use and kept in a dust-free environment. No particular precautions need to be taken to maintain embryos at 37 °C but extremes in temperature should be avoided.

Viability of embryos from all species begins to decline following 12 h of storage in phosphate-buffered medium supplemented with serum. Thus, except for swine embryos which do not survive cold storage, embryos that need to be stored longer than 24 h before transfer should be frozen. If freezing is not possible, embryos from sheep, goats, swine and

Table 3.6   Disease transmission by cattle embryos transferred from diseased donors

Agent	Zona penetration	Results
Foot and mouth virus	Negative	A,B
Brucella abortus	Negative	B
Bovine parvovirus	Not determined	C
Bovine viral diarrhea virus	Only one of many studies showed zona penetration	A,B
Bluetongue virus	Negative	A,B
Bovine leukemia virus	Negative	A,B
Infectious bovine rhinotracheitis (IBR)	Not determined	A,B
Akabane virus	Negative	B
Mycobacterium paratuberculosis	Negative	B

A: recipients/calves seronegative.
B: embryos seronegative.
C: embryos developed normally in culture following exposure to the agent.

cattle should be placed in a bicarbonate-buffered medium with 1 g/l glucose and 10% heat-treated serum or 1.5% w/v BSA and held at 37 °C in a 5% CO_2 in air gaseous atmosphere.

Recent evidence has indicated that cattle embryos will survive for 2–3 days at 4 °C. Basically, embryos in culture medium were placed in a stoppered tube in a water bath in a refrigerator. Survival was very good up to 48 h. This does provide an alternative for transporting embryos or retarding the development of embryos while recipients are allowed to 'catch up'.

Attempts to freeze porcine embryos or even cool them to temperatures below 5 °C have proven unsuccessful. Longterm storage systems for porcine embryos should include a bicarbonate-buffered medium supplemented with glucose and BSA concentration of 1.5% w/v. Porcine embryos should be held at 37 °C in a gaseous atmosphere of 5% CO_2 in air for optimal results.

Shipping unfrozen embryos requires a container that can maintain a temperature of 37 °C for a long period of time. The Trans-Temp Container holds a temperature of 37 °C for 48 h and still offers enough space for an embryo container. In addition, this system is well padded and secure enough for shipment under most conditions. Embryos can be shipped in plastic tubes with tight caps that have been previously gassed with a 5% CO_2 in air mixture. It should be remembered that the gas will leak from the tube and that the atmosphere will not be maintained indefinitely. For this reason, plastic tubes can be placed in a stainless steel anaerobic chamber, which can then be gassed directly with 5% CO_2 in air. Next, the anaerobic chamber is placed in the Trans-Temp Container. This system controls both temperature and gas atmosphere and places the embryos in a secure environment.

Live animals, including their fluids, secretions, excretions and gametes are potential transmitters of disease. This is of great concern when animals, semen (there are 34 pathogens recorded in semen and seventeen have transmitted diseases) and embryos are exported to disease-free regions. Historically, embryos have been accepted for import if the dam and sire of the embryos satisfy the health requirements to enter the country themselves.

For an embryo to transmit an infectious disease to a recipient animal it must have been infected with the disease in utero (environmental infection) or carry the infectious agent on its surface (gametic infection). For an environmental infection to occur the disease organism must penetrate the zona pellucida. Viral infectious agents, because of their small size are of particular concern compared to bacterial, protozoal, chlamydial or rickettsial agents.

Cattle diseases related to embryo infectious agents have received most attention with only little research devoted to other farm species. Table 3.6 shows the results of disease transmission from cattle embryos transferred from infected donors.

As previously noted in this chapter, 93% of commercial swine embryo transfers are performed to control the spread of disease or produce disease-free offspring. Table 3.7 lists the diseases that have been studied.

Contrasted with cattle, several infectious swine agents are known to bind and/or penetrate the zona pellucida. The large number of sperm attached and embedded into the swine zona pellucida and the sperm furrows found may be involved (Fig. 3.4).

Procedures for Disease Control

There would be a tremendous advantage if embryo transfer could be used to move disease-free genetic

Table 3.7 Disease transmission by swine embryos transferred from diseased donors

Agent	Zona penetration	Results
Porcine parvovirus	Binds to zona pellucida	Recipients seropositive
		Embryos positive
Pseudorabies virus	Binds to zona pellucida	Recipients seropositive/seronegative
African swine fever virus	Binds to zona pellucida	Not determined
Swine vesicular disease (SVD) virus	Binds to zona pellucida	Not determined
Foot and mouth disease virus	Binds to zona pellucida	Not determined
Enteroviruses	Binds to zona pellucida	Not determined

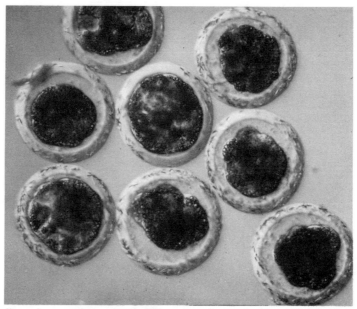

Fig. 3.4 Excellent quality swine morulae and early blastocysts; observe the large number of spermatozoa embedded in the zona pellucida which is characteristic of swine embryos.

material across continents or from diseased parents into disease-free environments.

Extreme care should be taken to use sterile procedures (sterile equipment and solutions) and meticulously clean the perineum and the vulva before collection. All serum used in the flushing medium and semen used for breeding must be tested to be free of mycoplasma and viruses.

Embryos should be washed through ten changes of medium containing antibiotic to reduce the potential of disease transmission from the uterine flushing. It may be possible to dilute out effectively the concentration of the virus some 10-fold if the agent does not bind to the zona pellucida.

Trypsin, pronase and other enzymes and antisera have been used to remove bound infectious agents from the zona pellucida. It is unlikely that these techniques will be approved for the international exchange of embryos. (See page 175.)

Embryos frozen for international shipment offer a greater potential for disease transmission than fresh embryos due to the fracture of the zona pellucida which may occur during freezing. This fracture eliminates the zona pellucida from effectively acting as a barrier to infectious agents entering the embryo. Therefore, extreme care in sterile procedures, health testing of dams and sires before collection and thorough washing of the embryo is imperative for the international exchange of embryos.

Complementary References

Betteridge, K. J. (1977) *Embryo Transfer in Farm Animals.* Canada Department of Agriculture, p. 1079. Monograph no. 16, Ottawa: Agriculture Canada.

Betteridge, K. J. (1981) An historical look at embryo transfer. *J. Reprod. Fertil.*, **62**, 1–13.

Mapletoft, R. J. (1986) Bovine embryo transfer. In *Current*

Therapy In Theriogenology, ed. Morrow, D. A., pp. 54–58. Philadelphia: W. B. Saunders.

Seidel, G. E., Jr & Seidel, S. M. (1981) The embryo transfer industry. In *New Technologies in Animal Breeding*, eds Brackett, B. G., Seidel, G. E. & Seidel, S. M., pp. 41–77. New York: Academic Press.

Singh, E. L. (1986) Possibilities of disease transmission of embryos. In *Proceedings of the 5th Annual Convention of the American Embryo Transfer Association*, ed. Eldsen, P. R., pp. 55–61. Hastings, Nebraska: American Embryo Transfer Association.

Wright, R. W. & Bondioli, K. R. (1981). Various aspects of embryo culture and *in vitro* fertilization in farm animals. *J. Anim. Sci.*, **53**, 702.

4

Pregnancy Diagnosis and Parturition

RONNIE G. ELMORE

The ability to determine the pregnancy status of each individual animal quickly and accurately is essential to any profitable reproductive herd health program. As the period between breeding and pregnancy diagnosis decreases, the cost/benefit ratio of such a program increases. Early pregnancy diagnosis allows for the rebreeding or culling of non-pregnant animals without undue delay.

Generally, the methods of pregnancy diagnosis in domestic animals can be classified into four categories:

1. Detection of the fetus and its membranes directly by rectal or abdominal palpation, radiography, and ultrasonography.
2. Detection of physical changes in the dam which are associated with pregnancy; for example, increased size of the abdomen, increased size of the uterine arteries, displacement of the uterus, thinning of the vaginal epithelium, and increased size of the mammary glands.
3. Detection of hormonal changes associated with pregnancy, for example, progesterone, estrone, and serum gonadotropins.
4. Detection of maternal behavioral changes secondary to hormonal changes associated with pregnancy, for example, absence of estrus following breeding.

The more direct methods of pregnancy diagnosis are generally less prone to error. Species characteris-

tics often dictate the available methods of pregnancy diagnosis.

COW

Rectal Palpation Techniques

The diagnosis of pregnancy in the cow by rectal palpation of the genital tract is based on the detection of the amniotic vesicle, fetal membrane slip, fetus or placentomes. These are the only rectally palpable positive signs of pregnancy in the cow. The finding of any one of these signs is a sufficient basis for the diagnosis of pregnancy; but it should not be made unless one of these signs has definitely been identified by the palpator. Likewise, no cow should be diagnosed as nonpregnant unless the uterus has been thoroughly palpated throughout its entirety. Even in the most well-managed dairy and beef herds, histories of breeding dates are not always reliable. Therefore every cow examined should be palpated for a possible pregnancy before proceeding with other procedures involving the genital tract.

Palpation of the bovine amniotic vesicle is usually possible beginning around the 29th day of gestation. The vesicle floats freely in the allantoic fluid. To palpate the vesicle, the thumb should be placed on one side of the horn and all four remaining fingers should be placed on the other side of the horn in order to cover large areas of the horn simultaneously. The vesicle can usually be located in the pregnant horn in the vicinity of greatest fluid enlargement and thinnest uterine wall. Early in gestation, the vesicle feels very turgid and is oval in shape. By approximately the 50th day of gestation, the vesicle softens and is less distinct. Generally, palpation of the amniotic vesicle should be avoided unless absolutely necessary to estimate accurately the duration of gestation. This is because of the inherent danger of rupturing either the vesicle or the fetal heartsac. Either of these accidents results in early embryonic death and reabsorption.

The bovine fetal membrane slip can be performed starting at approximately the 30th day of gestation. The tissue recognized as the fetal membrane by rectal palpation is the connective tissue band of the chorioallantoic membrane. A portion of the uterine wall just cranial to the uterine bifurcation is grasped gently and is then allowed to slip between the thumb and forefinger. The chorioallantois and then the uterine wall slip between the thumb and forefinger, in turn, giving a very characteristic sensation if the cow is pregnant, similar to that of slipping a thin, taut string crossways between the fingers. At approximately the 43rd day of gestation the fetal membranes extend into the nongravid uterine horn. By the 60th–70th day of gestation, it is often easier to slip the membranes in the nongravid uterine horn than in the gravid horn.

The bovine fetus can usually be palpated rectally after about the 65th day of gestation. It cannot be palpated until the amnion has softened. A 60 day bovine fetus is approximately mouse size, a 90 day fetus approximately rat size, a 120 day fetus approximately small cat size, and a 150 day fetus approximately large cat size.

Bovine placentomes can be detected by rectal palpation as early as the 75th day of gestation. At this time they can be palpated as ovoid thickened areas in the uterine wall at the level of the intercornual ligament of the horn containing the fetus. The placentomes are larger on the greater curvature of the uterus than near the bifurcation. Palpation of the placentomes is particularly helpful at about 5–6 months of gestation when the fetus is deep in the abdomen and cannot easily be reached. The size of the placentomes located at the base of the pregnant uterine horn can be used for estimation of the stage of gestation. In dairy cows the diameter of the placentomes at the level of the bifurcation is approximately 1.5 cm at 90 days, approximately 2.5 cm at 120 days, approximately 4 cm at 150 days and approximately 5 cm at 180 days of gestation.

Fremitus of the bovine uterine artery is often suggested as an indicator of pregnancy. It can first be palpated at about days 80–120 of gestation. Care should be taken not to confuse the internal iliac artery with the uterine artery. The internal iliac is attached to the shaft of the ilium and is not freely movable. Although most cows with fremitus of the uterine artery are pregnant with a normal fetus, it is possible to find fremitus in pathological conditions in which the uterus is enlarged. Fremitus of the uterine artery is an excellent indicator of pregnancy— but not a *positive* sign.

Errors in conducting pregnancy evaluations are usually the result of inadequate identification of the uterus or failure to palpate the entire uterus. Veterinarians doing routine reproductive herd health work should be able to conduct pregnancy examinations beginning at the 30th–35th day of gestation. Occasionally cows are encountered in which a positive diagnosis is impossible for even an experienced operator. In these situations, they should state frankly that a diagnosis cannot be given and recommend a reexamination. Not all cows pronounced pregnant subsequently calve; there is a 5–10% early embryonic loss due to unknown causes. It is important to remember this figure so that the operator will not lose confidence, and so that this phenomenon can be explained to herd owners. Much practice and review are necessary to develop and maintain the skills required to evaluate bovine internal genital tract structures accurately and quickly by rectal palpation.

Rapid Progesterone Assay Techniques

Rapid progesterone assay techniques can be used to detect nonpregnant cows with nearly 100% accuracy and pregnant cows with approximately 75% accuracy 21–22 days following breeding. High progesterone levels in milk, plasma or serum indicate the presence of a functional corpus luteum. Low circulating levels of progesterone indicate the absence of a functional corpus luteum. If a cow is pregnant 21 days following the last breeding she must have a functional corpus luteum and therefore a high circulating level of progesterone. However if the cow is nonpregnant 21 days following the last breeding, she should be returned to estrus, not have a functional corpus luteum, and have a low circulating level of progesterone.

There are many reasons why 25% of the cows with high progesterone levels at 21–22 days following the last breeding are not subsequently found to be pregnant. Some of these include poor timing in taking samples, breeding at the wrong time, variations in the normal estrous cycle length, early embryonic death, retention of the corpus luteum due to uterine pathology, and ovarian luteal cysts. Improper timing in collecting samples and breeding is probably the most frequent reason for high progesterone levels in nonpregnant cows 21 days following the last breeding. It has been estimated that 5–30% of all cows bred artificially are not in estrus at the time of breeding. If a cow is bred during the diestrual phase of the cycle it will not conceive. A cow bred during diestrus will most likely have a high circulating level of progesterone 21 days following breeding and yet be nonpregnant.

The recent introduction of enzyme immunoassay kits for progesterone has made it possible for virtually every bovine practitioner to assay milk, plasma, and serum samples for progesterone in their clinics. Bovine practitioners can now identify nonpregnant cows at 21–22 days following breeding rather than wait until 35–40 days when accurate pregnancy diagnosis by rectal palpation is possible. Knowing that a cow is nonpregnant at 21 days allows the producer several options for rebreeding. Cows known to be nonpregnant at 21 days following breeding can be injected in 7 days (after the development of a corpus luteum) with prostaglandin and rebred 3–4 days later.

MARE

Rectal Palpation Techniques

Rectal palpation continues to be the most economical and rapid method of early pregnancy diagnosis in the mare. The ovaries serve as suitable landmarks in the mare for beginning an examination of the genital tract for pregnancy. In nonpregnant mares and mares early in pregnancy, the ovaries are usually found in the sublumbar area. They are usually 5–10 cm cranial to the upper third of the shaft of the ilium. The ovaries are drawn medially and ventrally by the enlarging uterus as gestation progresses. Right-handed operators usually find it easiest to first locate the left ovary; those who are left-handed usually locate the right ovary first. After locating either the right or left ovary the hand is passed ventrally down the utero-ovarian ligament onto the uterus. The cupped hand is then slid across the entire cranial border of the uterus with the thumb and fingers extended caudally. In well-relaxed mares the entire palpation can be accomplished without releasing the grasp of the genital tract. The involuted, nonpregnant uterus is usually soft and flat, and measures approximately 4–7 cm across and is about 2–5 cm thick. The position of the nonpregnant uterus in the mare is variable, and may be dorsal or ventral to the level of the anterior brim of the pelvis.

Very early pregnancy diagnosis by rectal palpation in the mare is based upon the detection of increasing uterine and cervical tone. From days 16–21 following ovulation there is a three-fold increase in thickness in the uterine wall in pregnant mares, while in nonpregnant mares the thickness of the uterine wall declines until the onset of the next estrus. Nonpregnant mares usually have soft flaccid uteri 21 days following the last ovulation and pregnant mares usually have tonic, tubular type uteri. An additional finding in early gestation is a tight, firm 'rod-like' cervix. A presumptive diagnosis of pregnancy can be based upon finding uterine and cervical tone 21 days following the last breeding.

The stage of gestation can usually be estimated with accuracy by rectal palpation during the first 3 months of pregnancy. In maiden mares it is often possible to palpate the swelling of a fetal sac, 2.5–3.5 cm in diameter, at 19–21 days, and the uterine wall around the swelling is thinner than the adjacent uterine wall. By days 25–30 the vesicle has expanded to 3–6 cm in diameter. The spherical enlargement bulges ventrally in the lower third of one horn. At this time the nonpregnant horn usually has greater tubularity and tone than the pregnant horn. By days 35–40 of gestation the vesicle is usually 6–10 cm in diameter, is spherical in shape and still has a lot of resilience. By days 50–60 the bulge within the uterus becomes more oval in shape and begins to expand into the uterine body. The vesicle also begins to lose its tenseness by this time. The size of the fetal swelling at 50–60 days is approximately 15–25 cm.

The entire body of the uterus is involved between days 60 and 100. By this time the pregnant uterus begins its descent into the mare's abdomen. Although the uterus cannot be retracted and the ventral bulge cannot be palpated at this time, the conceptus can easily be ballotted in the enlarged uterus. Inexperienced operators often have difficulty diagnosing pregnancy in the mare between 60 and 100 days following breeding. The filled urinary bladder can easily be confused with the uterus. As the gestation progresses the ovaries are drawn forward, medially, and downward. The descent is usually complete by the end of the 7th month of gestation. The fetus can be detected by ballottment in almost all mares even at the time of maximum descent. Ascent of the fetus begins at approximately 7 months of gestation. During this period the fetus can easily be palpated.

Approximately 5–10% of all mares pronounced pregnant on rectal palpation by experienced palpators fail to foal. Early embryonic death and reabsorption of unknown etiology account for many of these failures.

Ultrasound Techniques

Transrectal real time (B-mode) ultrasound is rapidly becoming an important aid in confirming rectal palpation diagnoses in the mare. In some mares the embryonic vesicle can be viewed by transrectal ultrasonography as early as 11–12 days. On the screen the mare's uterus viewed in transverse section appears gray while fluid-filled structures such as the vesicle or endometrial cysts appear dark or black. The uterus usually appears as the circular structure with a granular gray center, the surrounding tissue being more dense and a lighter gray. By days 14–15 the vesicle is 17–22 mm in diameter. Cardiac motion can usually be visualized by days 24–27 in the viable embryo. Ultrasound techniques can be quite helpful in detecting twin pregnancies and in assessing early embryonic death.

The accuracy of detection of the vesicle at days 14–15 using transrectal ultrasound techniques has been estimated to be nearly 99%. Transrectal ultrasound techniques should not be confused with external flank techniques. The equipment that utilizes a sensor probe positioned on the external flank has been demonstrated to be approximately 65% accurate at 35 days of gestation. An experienced operator should be able to detect vesicles at days 21–28 with nearly 90% accuracy.

Pregnant Mare Serum Gonadotropin (PMSG)

Endometrial cups, fetal in origin, form in the pregnant mare at 36–38 days of gestation. These cups secrete pregnant mare serum gonadotropin (PMSG) or equine chorionic gonadotropin (eCG) between days 38 and 120 of gestation. Although early methods to detect eCG involved the use of biological assays, current tests for eCG are immunologic methods. The mare immunological pregnancy test (MIP test, Diamond Laboratories, Des Moines, Iowa, USA) is a passive hemagglutination-inhibition test in kit form, and requires approximately 2 h to perform. Rapid enzyme-linked immunoassay tests for PMSG are currently available.

The accuracy of immunological tests for eCG has been reported to be over 90%. False-positives often occur in mares that have experienced early embryonic death and reabsorption after 38 days of gestation. These mares apparently enter a pseudopregnant state that persists until the endometrial cups regress and eCG has disappeared from the general circulation. These mares are clinically anestrous. The immunological tests for eCG are not accurate in mares carrying a mule fetus where the level of circulating eCG is approximately one-tenth that of a mare carrying a horse fetus. Mares carrying twins usually have higher levels of eCG than those carrying single foals. Ponies tend to have higher levels of eCG than larger breeds of horses. Immunological tests for pregnancy are helpful in mares that are too fractious or too small to palpate rectally or use ultrasound.

Other Methods of Pregnancy Diagnosis

Urinary estrogen concentrations increase markedly after day 80 of gestation in the mare. The Cuboni test for urinary estrogens is approximately 90% accurate after 100 days of gestation and nearly 100% accurate after 150 days. Tests for urinary estrogens for pregnancy are not widely used because of both the complexities of conducting the tests and the length of gestation required before they are efficacious.

Radioimmunoassay (RIA) or enzyme immunoassay (EIA) techniques for detection of circulating progesterone at 17–21 days following breeding or ovulation have been used to make a presumptive diagnosis of pregnancy in the mare. The presumptive diagnosis is based on whether a mare has a functional corpus luteum at the time she should be returning to estrus if not pregnant. These methods are not widely used because other methods such as regular teasing, rectal palpation, and ultrasound techniques are more accurate and less time-consuming.

SOW

Rectal Palpation Techniques

Rectal palpation is an excellent means of pregnancy diagnosis in pluriparous sows and large primiparous gilts. Accuracy of greater than 90% can easily be achieved in animals past the 40th day of gestation. Pregnancy is determined by palpation of the external iliac artery, the uterine artery, the cervix, and the caudal uterine body. Rectal palpation is most easily accomplished while the sow is restrained in a crate. The right hand should be used to palpate the left side of the pelvis and the left hand should be used to palpate the right side. This reduces the risk of injuring the sow's rectum. Starving sows for 12–

24 h before examination is beneficial but not absolutely necessary.

The uterine and external iliac arteries are compared on the basis of size, tone, and the presence of fremitus. The uterine artery is located by first identifying the external iliac artery at the cranial border of the ilium where it is approximately the thickness of a pencil. The external iliac artery has a strong pulse. Tracing along the external iliac artery, the uterine artery is encountered where it crosses over the iliac artery anteroventrally. In the nonpregnant sow the uterine artery is approximately the thickness of a piece of straw and never reaches the thickness of the external iliac artery where the two vessels cross. Uterine arteries of equal or larger size than the external iliacs indicate pregnancy.

The change in character of the pulse of the uterine artery is more diagnostic for pregnancy than the change in diameter. Induction of fremitus by digital pressure can be achieved in practically all pregnant sows in one or both uterine arteries from day 30 of gestation through term. It is extremely important to apply pressure to the correct artery for diagnostic purposes. Spontaneous fremitus of the uterine arteries can be palpated in most pregnant sows after the 37th day of gestation.

Cervical tone is a useful parameter in pregnancy diagnosis by rectal palpation in sows, and is an indicator of estrus; so pregnant sows should not exhibit cervical tone. The fetuses themselves can usually be palpated during the last two weeks of gestation. Rectal palpation is a rapid, accurate, simple, inexpensive method of determining pregnancy in sows and large gilts.

Ultrasound Techniques

Despite the relatively high cost of purchasing an ultrasound machine, these instruments are probably the most common diagnostic tools for pregnancy diagnosis in swine at this time. Two different methods of using ultrasound techniques for pregnancy diagnosis are commonly used in sows. In the first type, ultrasound emitted from a probe is reflected off the walls of blood vessels. The ultrasound is distorted as a result of the Doppler effect in relation to the rate of blood flow through the vessel. The distortion is measured in a sensor contained in the same probe as the emitter, the end result being that pulse rates can be indicated either through audible signals via a stethoscope or loudspeaker or through visual signals on a screen.

Doppler Ultrasound

While conducting a pregnancy examination in a sow with a Doppler ultrasound machine, the sow should be restrained in a crate, and not fed during the procedure as the sounds produced by eating often interfere with interpretation of the sounds from the Doppler machine. The machine probe can be placed externally on the flank of the sow or rectally. Experienced technicians report no difference in the accuracy of the two different sites of placement of the probe. Externally, the probe is placed on the skin of the sow's abdomen lateral to the second to the last teat. A bland coupling medium such as oil is used to exclude air from between the probe and the skin. The probe is rotated on the spot to scan the area of the uterus which in early gestation lies far caudal in the abdominal cavity. The first sound detectable is blood flow in the uterine artery. A strong regular pulse at approximately 80 beats/min is heard, together with characteristic whistling or swooshing. Blood flow in the uterine artery can often be heard as early as 21 days following the last breeding but is not reliably present until 30 days of gestation. Blood flow in the umbilical artery has a similar quality at a slightly higher pitch and a pulse rate that decreases from approximately 240 beats/min at 45 days of gestation to 160 beats/min at term. Blood flow in the umbilical arteries can be detected as early as 32 days of gestation. The fetal heartbeat is at the same rate as the umbilical rate but has more of a clapping or galloping quality, and fetal movements are usually loud, swishing, irregular sounds. The diagnostic key in using Doppler techniques to detect pregnancy in the sow is finding the uterine (fetal) pulse and comparing it to the sow's own pulse. The fetal pulse rate should be approximately twice that of the maternal pulse. Most experienced technicians can diagnose pregnancy by use of Doppler machines in approximately 2–3 min. Doppler methods offer the advantage of detecting not only pregnancy, but also fetal life.

Amplitude Depth or Pulse Echo Machines

The second main method of using ultrasound techniques to diagnose pregnancy in sows is the use of A-mode (amplitude depth/pulse echo) machines. Pulsed ultrasonic sound waves are emitted and received from a transducer held on the skin in the flank of the sow being examined. When the transducer is held against an object, a blip appears on an oscilloscope screen at a point corresponding to the distance between the transducer and the interface of substances with different densities. In examining sows for pregnancy, the amplitude depth ultrasound machine is used to detect the fluid-filled uterus. This method of pregnancy diagnosis in the sow is most accurate between days 30 and 90 of gestation. This is the period when the fluid to fetal tissue ratio is the greatest. Beyond 90 days of gestation, the fetal mass is greater than the fluid volume and cannot easily be differentiated from the sow's own body tissues. False-positives can be caused by erroneously interpreting reflections off the filled urinary bladder as a pregnancy. Also pyometra and other pathological conditions may render a false-positive diagnosis.

Pregnancy diagnosis with an A-mode ultrasound machine is easiest accomplished with the sow restrained in a crate or narrow alleyway. Gentle sows may be examined free of restraint while they are being fed. The transducer head is coated with acoustic coupling gel to provide a positive contact with the skin. The transducer head is placed approximately 5 cm lateral to the teat line cranial to the stifle and caudal to the last rib (usually above the most caudal two teats). The transducer head is directed slightly cranially and dorsally toward the genital tract. Diagnosis can easily be made from either side of the sow. A positive pregnancy diagnosis is made if steady, high amplitude tracings are seen on the right side of the oscilloscope screen. Some machines utilize a series of lights or audible sounds to indicate pregnancy. An experienced technician should be able to diagnose pregnancy in a sow using an A-mode ultrasound machine within approximately 2 min.

Real-time (B-mode) ultrasound scanning gives the clearest indication of pregnancy from about day 25 but the expense of the machines limit their use.

Vaginal Cytology Techniques

Histological evaluation of a cross-section of vaginal tissue collected between days 20 and 25 following the last breeding can be used for pregnancy diagnosis in the sow. Diagnosis of pregnancy by this method has been shown to be 95% accurate. Biopsy specimens for evaluation are taken approximately 5 cm caudal to the cervix using rectal biopsy forceps with a shaft of at least 37 cm. The tissue can be processed by either cryogenic or standard histological techniques.

The thickness of the vaginal mucosa is at a maximum during estrus and then declines with development of the corpus luteum during diestrus or pregnancy. The vaginal epithelium proliferates during the ensuing follicular phase if the sow returns to estrus following breeding but becomes progressively thinner if pregnancy occurs. After the first month of pregnancy the vaginal epithelium comprises only two to three layers, whereas it is five to twenty cells thick in nonpregnant sows, depending on the stage of the cycle.

The greatest advantage of using vaginal biopsies for pregnancy diagnosis in the sow is the early time following breeding that it can be done with accuracy. Accurate diagnosis can be accomplished at 19 or 20 days following the last breeding. The greatest disadvantage of using the procedure is the time and effort required to prepare the vaginal specimens for evaluation. Also accuracy is improved if accurate breeding dates are known; this is not possible on many farms.

Return to Estrus

The return to estrus is still one of the most economical and accurate methods of early detection of pregnancy status on many swine farms. But one of the major disadvantages of such a method is the labor and time required to evaluate each sow at the appropriate time following breeding. Checking for estrus does not detect those sows that have suffered early embryonic death and delayed return to estrus.

Estrone Sulfate Assay

The detection of estrone sulfate in blood is becoming an acceptable method of pregnancy diagnosis in the sow. Estrone sulfate is produced by the placenta and peaks in the plasma between days 23 and 30 in the sow. There is a 10% false-positive rate based on subsequent farrowings, which may reflect the early embryonic death and resorption rates in the herds studied.

Progesterone Assay

Blood progesterone levels can be evaluated at 17–21 days following the last breeding to ascertain pregnancy status in sows. In nonpregnant sows plasma progesterone levels rapidly decline on days 17–19 of the estrous cycle. High levels of progesterone 18–21 days following mating are highly suggestive of nonreturn to estrus and thus a presumptive diagnosis of pregnancy. There are many false-positives for pregnancy in sows when progesterone values at 17–21 days following mating are the method of diagnosis. These false-positives may reflect the high rate of early embryonic death and resorption in sows.

EWE

Pregnancy diagnosis in the ewe has become increasingly important in recent years. There are a variety of methods to detect pregnancy in ewes. The return to estrus as indicated by marker rams wearing marking harnesses has always been used extensively. Careful attention to record-keeping and ewe identification is mandatory if such information is going to be useful. Apparently some flocks experience a fairly high incidence of early embryonic death and reabsorption. These animals are often not identified by using marker rams for pregnancy detection.

Ultrasound Techniques

Pregnancy diagnosis and determination of fetal numbers can be performed using real-time (B-mode) ultrasonic scanners. The most accurate diagnoses are made at about the 80th day of pregnancy but the technique can be used from about the 40th to 100th day. Accuracy depends on the experience and training of the operator. It has been claimed that 99% accuracy can be obtained under the most favorable conditions.

Two types of real-time scanner are available. Formerly, linear array scanners were employed, the scan heads of which measure approximately 3 × 4 × 15 cm. To make good skin contact along the entire scan head the ewes were turned on their backs and, with the fleece about 20 cm anterior to the udder removed, the probe was moved systematically over the abdominal surface in order to view the entire reproductive tract. Acoustic coupling gel is required to maintain an air-tight seal. Recently, sector array scanners have been used. These produce a wedge-shaped image on the screen and require a much reduced area of contact with the subject. The probe is applied to the bald inguinal region and the entire uterus systematically scanned. The ewes need not be turned on their backs nor need any fleece be removed so reducing stress. To achieve maximum throughput the ewes are moved along an elevated race so as to be presented at the eye level of the seated operator. Up to 100 ewes/h can be examined depending on handling facilities.

The ultrasonic fetal pulse detector can also be used. The device makes use of the Doppler phenomenon. Very high frequency sound waves are transmitted and received by a probe. If the rebound is received from a moving object, such as circulating red blood cells, there is a difference in the transmitted and received sound waves. These differences are amplified so that pulse rates can be determined. An experienced technician can decipher maternal and fetal pulse rates with a Doppler ultrasound machine. The most accurate results are obtained when the transducer head is positioned within the emptied rectum. The fetal heart rate is approxim-

ately twice that of the ewe. Therefore sounds thought to be coming from a fetus or the placenta can be compared with those obtained when the transducer is placed over the iliac artery or aorta of the ewe. Accuracy with this method has been reported to be approximately 90% after 65 days of gestation. It is difficult to determine if a multiple pregnancy exists with this detection method.

It has been reported that the use of externally applied A-mode apparatus to detect pregnancy in ewes is about 80–90% accurate following 65 days of pregnancy. By this method different densities of body tissue are detected. Therefore the fluid-filled uterus can be differentiated from the more dense tissues of the ewe. Although this method of pregnancy diagnosis is widely used in sows, it is not of much value in ewes.

Abdominal Palpation

A bimanual rectal probe-abdominal palpation technique has been widely used for pregnancy diagnosis in the ewe. Nearly 100% accuracy at 70–110 days of gestation can be obtained in differentiating pregnant from nonpregnant ewes. The ewe is restrained on her back in a cradle while a lubricated rod (1.5 cm outer diameter by 50 cm length with a rounded tip) is inserted approximately 30 cm into the rectum, and a hand is placed on the external ventral abdomen. Pregnancy diagnosis is based on not being able to palpate the rod, as a pregnant uterus blocks palpating the rod. A nonpregnancy diagnosis is based on being able to palpate it. Thin and relaxed ewes are easier to examine than fat or straining ewes. Fasting for 12 h helps facilitate the evaluations. Approximately 120 ewes/h can be examined by an experienced technician with proper facilities. Care must be taken not to injure the ewes with the rectal probe.

Vaginal Biopsy Techniques

Vaginal biopsy techniques to determine pregnancy in ewes have been reported to be over 90% accurate after 40 days of gestation. It is nearly 100% accurate in detecting pregnancies after 80 days of gestation. However, the technique is only about 80% accurate in detecting nonpregnant ewes at the same time. Vaginal biopsy samples are obtained from the wall just anterior to the urethral orifice. The stratified squamous epithelium of the nonpregnant ewe's vagina is gradually replaced during early pregnancy by layers of cells that tend to be cuboidal in shape. Accompanying changes in the nuclei and cytoplasm are also seen. Multiple fetuses are not detected by vaginal biopsy techniques. Other disadvantages of the technique include the time and laboratory procedures involved in preparing and interpreting the specimens.

Radiographic Techniques

Radiographic techniques for pregnancy diagnosis in ewes is highly accurate after 75 days of gestation. By 80 days of gestation the ovine fetal skeleton is well-calcified. Fetal numbers can usually be easily ascertained from suitable radiographs. Radiographic equipment with a capacity of 100 mA and 90 kV is usually required to produce quality radiographs of the ewe's abdomen, therefore, using radiographic techniques on entire flocks is highly impractical.

Other Methods of Pregnancy Detection

The use of rapid progesterone assays has been demonstrated to be useful in detecting nonpregnancy in ewes at the time of expected return to heat. Since most ewes are not lactating during the breeding season, progesterone assays are conducted on plasma or serum.

A hemagglutination technique for detecting antigens specific for pregnancy in the ewe has been reported. Hemagglutination occurs when rabbit antisheep embryo serum is added to a few drops of blood from ewes between days 6 and 50 of gestation, but not when added to blood from nonpregnant ewes or male sheep. The test does not indicate whether multiple lambs are being carried. The hemagglutination test for pregnancy requires approximately 30 min to conduct.

FEMALE GOAT

There are many valid reasons for conducting pregnancy examinations of goats. Traditionally, owners have observed their goats for the cessation of cycling following breeding as an indicator of pregnancy. Many pregnant goats show false estrus and many nonpregnant or pseudopregnant goats do not demonstrate estrus for the remainder of the breeding season. A teaser male fitted with a marking harness is usually quite helpful in detecting returns to estrus, and rapid progesterone assays can also be utilized. Serum or plasma progesterone concentrations of less than 1 ng/ml on the 21st day following breeding indicates regression of the corpus luteum, return to estrus, and nonpregnancy.

Palpation Techniques

Palpation of the cervix of the goat is a simple field technique for pregnancy diagnosis. One or two gloved and lubricated fingers are inserted into the vagina of the standing animal. The cervix of the nonpregnant, anestrous goat is very firm and conical with distinct folds, and protrudes into the vaginal vault. After 30 days of gestation the cervix becomes softer and more blunt, and after approximately 50 days the soft, blunt cervix is drawn forward over the brim of the pelvis. The cervix will remain out of reach throughout the rest of gestation. A firm, almost cartilaginous cervix palpated in a goat bred more than 50 days ago is indicative of a failure of conception; and a very soft cervix or an unreachable cervix in the same goat indicates pregnancy.

Abdominal palpation for pregnancy diagnosis can be performed by standing behind the animal and attempting to touch both hands together through the abdomen. Fasting the goat for 12–24 h before this procedure is helpful. Usually the fetus cannot be detected by abdominal palpation or ballottement prior to 100 days of gestation. In advanced pregnancy, the kid may be seen to kick in the dam's lower right flank.

A bimanual rectal probe-abdominal palpation technique as described for pregnancy diagnosis in ewes has been used successfully in goats. The animal is placed on its back and a well-lubricated 1.5 × 50 cm rod is inserted about 30 cm into the rectum. The cranial end of the rod is moved from the spine in an arc toward the abdominal wall. If the animal is more than 70 days in gestation, the pregnant uterus can be palpated with a hand on the abdomen. If she is not pregnant or less than 70 days into gestation, the end of the rod can be palpated with the hand on the abdomen. Great care must be taken to not injure the animal while doing this procedure. Some goats are too fractious for this examination.

Radiographic Techniques

By the 65th day of gestation, the fetal caprine skeleton is detectable by radiographic techniques. Enlargement of the uterus can usually be detected by 38 days of gestation, but the pregnancy at this stage cannot usually be differentiated from abnormalities of the uterus. After the 70th day of gestation, nearly 100% accuracy in pregnancy diagnosis can be accomplished, and the number of kids can also be determined.

Ultrasound Techniques

Amplitude depth ultrasonic (A-mode) techniques for pregnancy diagnosis in goats can be done much as it is in sows. The transducer is coated with oil and held firmly in the right lower flank just cranial to the udder. The machine detects differences in tissue densities and can therefore detect the fluid-filled uterus. This method of pregnancy diagnosis seems to be most accurate between days 60 and 90 of gestation.

The Doppler ultrasound technique for detecting fetal circulation is an accurate method of pregnancy diagnosis in goats. The transducer head can be placed either in the rectum or in the flank just cranial to the udder. The fetal pulse can be detected after about the 60th day of gestation in most pregnant animals. The fetal pulse rate is roughly twice that of the dam's pulse rate.

Real-time (B-mode) ultrasound scanning can be used in goats as in sheep with a high degree of accuracy from about day 40.

BITCH

Abdominal Palpation

The ease with which diagnosis can be made and the stage at which it is first possible depends, apart from the skill and experience of the examiner, on the extent to which the animal resists examination, her size and the number of fetuses present. It is impeded in obese animals. These factors, which are more important in the bitch than in any of the other domestic animals, also affect differential diagnosis of pregnancy from pathological conditions simulating it and from physiological pseudopregnancy. Diagnosis before day 30, unless made under the most favorable circumstances must always be guarded. In many cases it may not be possible to make a definite diagnosis until day 40.

Accurate diagnosis depends on identifying the bifurcation of the uterus at the pelvic brim, lying above the bladder and ventral to the colon, and carefully palpating between the fingers each horn as it runs upwards, forwards and outwards to the sublumbar region, ending just posterior to the kidneys. In small lean animals this can sometimes be done with the fingers of one hand; in larger animals and those which are fat, manipulation with both hands is necessary. During the last fortnight of pregnancy, rectal palpation of fetuses placed posteriorly in the uterine horns is possible if the animal is supported on her hind legs.

The sequence of detectable changes is as follows.

Conception to 3 Weeks

No alteration in the configuration of the uterus is detectable until about day 21. At this stage the distended fetal membranes are palpable as discrete, fluid-filled, ovoid swellings in the uterine horns; their size varies with that of the bitch with the approximate average diameter of each swelling being 1–1.5 cm. Between these enlargements the uterus is not detectably larger than when nongravid.

Weeks 3–4

In this period the individual dilations become approximately double in size and tend to a more spherical form, but their consistency does not alter. No appreciable increase in size of the intervening portions of the uterus is palpable.

Weeks 4–7

Between these times a rapid increase in uterine size is detectable. The fetal membranes elongate so that the whole of the uterus becomes enlarged and no individual dilations can be felt. At the same time the position of the uterus alters as it is drawn down by the weight of its contents and each horn forms a shallow arc running from the pelvic brim to the posterior renal sublumbar region.

Up to this stage of pregnancy the fetuses themselves are not palpable, only the uterine enlargement caused by the growth of the fetal membranes.

Week 7 to Term

During this time rapid growth of the uterus is detectable and, as it comes to occupy more of the abdominal cavity, the uterus becomes folded on itself so that each horn runs forward from the cervix, on the abdominal floor, to the liver, then curves upwards and backwards on itself to the sublumbar region behind the kidneys. It is not always possible to palpate the whole length of each horn, particularly in large or fat animals and in the later stages of gestation, but by this time the fetuses or at least some of them are palpable as firm masses, their size varying with the bitch. The landmarks of the pregnant uterus at this time are the fetus in the apex of the horn palpable high up in the flank, and the most posterior fetus, partly in the uterine body and palpable about the mid-line just anterior to the brim of the pelvis.

By about days 50–55 abdominal enlargement is usually evident and movement of the fetuses against the flank may be seen.

Other Diagnostic Methods

Ultrasonic techniques have successfully utilized the Doppler effect to diagnose pregnancy in the bitch from day 30 onwards. Real-time (B-mode) scanning can be used for direct visualization of the pregnant uterus. With experience, pregnancy can be detected from about day 18. Under-estimation of litter size is common because it is impossible to view the whole uterus at one time. In late gestation fetal heartbeats may be detected by a stethoscope. As yet there is no test for maternal endocrinological changes related to pregnancy, although a placental gonadotropin has been suggested as a basis for such a diagnostic test.

Radiography

With careful technique and experience it is possible to obtain radiographic outlines of the swellings in the uterus as early as 30–35 days after estrus if the abdomen is first inflated. Air has been used for abdominal insufflation but, to avoid the possibility of air embolism, human clinicians normally use carbon dioxide. Between 200 and 800 ml of gas are used, depending on the size of the bitch.

Fetal bones do not calcify and become detectable until the last 2 weeks of gestation.

Vaginal Examination

The swelling of the vulva which develops during estrus may persist for a variable part of gestation, but this is usually of little value in diagnosis as the same may happen during pseudopregnancy. It is stated that abundant mucus is present in the first half of pregnancy and that later this disappears and cornified cells can be found in vaginal smears. The cell picture in vaginal smears during pregnancy does not differ sufficiently from that of other periods to provide a means of diagnosis or an aid to it.

Mammary Development

Alterations in the mammary glands are most noticeable in primiparous bitches. A slight, discrete zone of swellings develops around the teats from about the 3rd week onward and becomes progressively greater throughout the gestation period. In the early stages it is more noticeable around the abdominal and inguinal teats. In the case of multiparous bitches no mammary enlargement may be apparent till the last 3 or 4 days of gestation. Early development of the mammary glands can be used only as an aid to diagnosis because of its common occurrence in association with pseudopregnancy.

Hematological Examination

The erythrocyte count, hemoglobin level and packed cell volume all decline from the 3rd week of gestation. There are concomitant increases in sedimentation rates and platelet counts while leukocytes become more numerous between the 3rd and 7th week but then decrease until just before parturition when they again increase. It is suggested that these features may be used diagnostically between days 35 and 50 but the value of using such techniques to arrive at a relatively late diagnosis is open to question. They may be useful in making the sometimes difficult distinction between pregnancy and pseudopregnancy because the blood picture remains normal in the latter condition even in the presence of behavioral signs of pregnancy and lactation. Fibrinogen also increases to two or three times the nonpregnant value during gestation and may provide a method of diagnosis.

Differential Diagnosis

It is necessary to differentiate pregnancy from all conditions causing abdominal distension, such as pyometra, ascites, tumor formation, etc. This can be done only by careful examination and identification of the uterus itself and its contents, and on the basis of other signs and symptoms which may be present and indicate other reasons for enlargement.

Pseudopregnancy may follow estrus in the bitch whether she has mated or not, and be accompanied by signs suspicious in varying degree of pregnancy, such as vulvar swelling, mammary enlargement and milk secretion, and some apparent increase in abdominal size. There is always some uterine enlargement. Differentiation from pregnancy can be made only by careful identification of the uterus by abdominal palpation and determination of the absence of nodular enlargements in the early stages or fetuses in later stages. Repeated examination is often necessary to ensure an accurate diagnosis.

QUEEN

Diagnosis of pregnancy in the cat is usually made by external abdominal palpation which is generally easier than in the bitch because the abdominal wall is thinner and less tense. In difficult cases it may be necessary to anesthetize the cat for thorough palpation. Radiography may be used as in the bitch.

Real-time (B-mode) ultrasound scanning can be used from day 19, as in the bitch, with the same provisos. The hematological changes described for the dog also occur in cats during pregnancy.

PARTURITION

Parturition includes preparation of the pelvic canal, delivery of the fetus, passage of the fetal membranes, and the immediate postpartum reduction of uterine size. Although the various stages of parturition in all animals are somewhat similar, there are some important species differences and a great amount of variation among animals of the same species. Generally, veterinarians should refrain from predicting times of parturition because the predictions frequently will be in error. Just prior to parturition most animals tend to isolate themselves from herd mates and humans if possible. Polytocous animals usually attempt to make nests for their expected newborns.

Very relaxed pelvic ligaments in the *cow* usually indicate that parturition will occur in 24–48 hours. This relaxation of the pelvic ligaments makes the tail head appear to be elevated. The vulva becomes progressively edematous and enlarged. Udder enlargement begins at about the 4th month of gestation. In older, pluriparous cows udder enlargement may not be noticeable until 2–4 weeks prior to parturition. The cow usually exhibits a tenacious, whitish, stringy type of mucus coming from the cranial part of the vagina after 7 months of gestation. During the last few hours before parturition, the cow may exhibit anorexia and restlessness. First calf heifers may show signs of abdominal pain or kicking at the abdomen, treading, switching of the tail excessively, and alternatively lying down and standing.

Udder development in the *mare* usually begins at about 3–6 weeks prior to foaling. In most mares the udder becomes filled and distended with colostrum about 2 days before foaling and oozing of colostrum from the teats, called 'waxing', is observed in 95% of foaling mares 6–48 h before parturition. Within 4 h of foaling, sweating in the flanks is frequently noticed. As foaling nears, many mares show restlessness, slight colic-type signs, excessive tail switching, and repeated lying down and standing. Mares prefer quietness and solitude at foaling and are able to suppress foaling until alone. Approximately 83% of all foals are born during the night.

The signs of approaching parturition in *ewes* and *female goats* are similar to those seen in cows. However the signs are usually not so pronounced. *Sows*, like other polytocous animals, like to build nests before parturition. This behavior may go unnoticed whenever sows are restrained in farrowing crates without bedding materials. During the last portion of gestation, a white vulvar discharge is often noticed in ewes and sows.

Birth Stages

The birth process, labor, can be divided into three stages. Stage I is characterized by active contractions of both the longitudinal and circular muscle fibers of the uterine wall and the dilatation of the cervix. During this stage the cervix is dilated not by pressure of the approaching fetal sacs, but by the contractions of the longitudinal uterine muscles. Oxytocin is seldom released from the posterior pituitary gland prior to the beginning of the second stage of parturition. The cervix of the heifer usually remains tightly closed until 24 h prior to calving. During stage I in the mare, the fetus rotates from its dorsopubic or dorsoilial position into the dorsosacral position. The straining of labor is not seen during the first stage of parturition. The duration of the first stage in cows, ewes, and female goats is usually 2–6 h; in mares 1–4 h; and in sows 2–12 h.

Usually towards the end of the first stage the allantochorion ruptures as it is forced through the dilated cervix into the vagina. Once a portion of the fetus enters the maternal pelvis, reflex stimuli result in straining. This is produced by contractions of the abdominal muscles and diaphragm together with the closing of the glottis. This is the beginning of the stage II of labor.

The second stage is characterized by the entrance of the fetus into the dilated birth canal, rupture of the amniotic sac, strong abdominal contractions, and expulsion of the fetus through the vulva. As the fetal feet pass through the vulva the amniotic sac ruptures. The release of oxytocin is continual throughout most of the second stage of parturition. The normal length of the second stage is ½–4 h in the cow, 5–40 min in the mare, and 1–5 h in the sow.

The third stage of labor is when expulsion of the fetal membranes and initial size-reduction of the uterus occurs. After the fetus is delivered, the uterus continues to contract strongly for 48 h and less vigorously, but more frequently, thereafter. The cow usually expels her fetal membranes within ½–8 h following birth and the mare within ½–3 h. Eating the fetal membranes by the dam has no known benefits as is sometimes suggested and may cause serious after-effects.

INDUCED PARTURITION

Induced parturition is the artificial initiation of the first and subsequent stages of labor to obtain viable, healthy, normal young. In contrast, induced abortion is the termination of gestation without regard to the health or life of the fetus. There are many indications for induced parturition. These include timing the parturition so knowledgeable personnel can be present to assist a dam likely to have difficulty during birth or to aid a high-risk neonate and to terminate abnormal pregnancies such as prolonged gestations and hydrops. Induction of parturition should only be done after the client has been properly instructed regarding all of the advantages and disadvantages of the procedure. Only veterinarians trained and equipped to handle properly any problems encountered should utilize this procedure.

Cow

Induced parturition in cows should only be considered during the last 2 weeks of gestation if the calves are expected to survive. Retained placenta is a common sequela to induced parturition in the cow. The likelihood of retained placenta decreases as the induction time more closely approximates the natural calving time—approximately 75–90% if the calving is 1–2 weeks early and 10–50% if the calving is very near or after the expected calving. Producers should be warned of the possible problems of inducing a large number of cows at the same time. Adequate calving facilities and labor should be available.

Short-acting corticosteroids, prostaglandins, estrogens, and combinations of these drugs are the most common forms of treatment used to induce parturition in cattle. Treatment with corticosteroids stimulates the synthesis and release of estrogens from the placenta which in turn causes the release of prostaglandins and lysis of the corpus luteum of pregnancy.

The short-acting corticosteroids commonly used to induce parturition in cows are dexamethasone (20–30 mg i.m.) and flumethasone (8–10 mg i.m.). Within 2 weeks of the expected parturition, these drugs are 80–90% effective in inducing calving. The period from injection to calving is 24–72 h, with an average of 48 h. With the exception of an increased incidence of retained fetal membranes, calvings following induction with these corticosteroids are normal in all aspects.

The administration of 25 mg of estradiol at the same time as induction of parturition with the short-acting corticosteroids increases the number of cows calving within 72 h and shortens the time between injection and calving by several hours. Field reports vary in regard to whether using estrogens with corticosteroids to induce parturition reduces the incidence of retained placenta. The possibility of milk residues of estrogens needs to be considered when inducing dairy cows.

Induction of parturition with 25 mg prostaglandin $F_{2\alpha}$ (i.m.) or 500 μg cloprostenol (i.m.) in cows is clinically very similar to induction with the shortacting corticosteroids. Approximately 90% of treated cows calve within 24–72 h. Some reports indicate that the incidence of dystocia may be slightly increased and the proportion of live calves may be slightly decreased with prostaglandin-induced parturitions. The incidence of retained fetal membranes is similar to that seen with corticosteroid induction. Although not consistent, some cows induced with prostaglandins exhibit estrous behavior approximately 96 h following injection. The possible advantages of using corticosteroids in combination with prostaglandins for induction of parturition in cows is not well-documented.

Recent studies with the use of relaxin have given encouraging results in the cow. In these experiments, porcine relaxin was administered alone or in combination with prostaglandins and produced a normal parturition with minimal placental retention.

Mare

Although there are many legitimate reasons for inducing parturition in mares, this should not be a routine procedure on most stud farms. In the mare, most procedures used do not induce parturition but are concerned with initiating the second stage of labor. Mares should be selected for labor induction very carefully. The criteria used to determine if a mare is ready for induction of labor include a normal gestation length, mammary gland enlargement with the presence of colostrum, and cervical relaxation. Each of these parameters is equally important. All three should be met before an induction is attempted. Since such a procedure is instituted only when cervical dilatation has occurred, it should be considered induction of labor rather than parturition.

Foals born before 300 days of gestation have little or no chance of survival, even with intensive postpartum care. Although an occasional foal born before 320 days of gestation is clinically mature enough to survive, most foals are not considered mature enough to induce prior to 320 days of gestation. Maintaining the requirement that the gestation be at least 330 days in length assures that the foal will be mature enough to survive. The gestation length should be ascertained by carefully evaluating breeding records. Many owners cannot accurately remember when each of their mares was last bred. Also the possibility of pasture breedings following the last recorded breeding should be determined.

An adequate supply of colostrum in a fully distended udder is probably the best indicator of fetal maturity sufficient for parturition induction. However, since some mares leak colostrum for as long as 2 weeks prior to natural parturition, the decision to induce a mare should not be based solely on the presence of colostrum. Parturition should never be induced in a mare that does not have colostrum present if the foal is expected to survive.

The cervix should be soft and partially relaxed before induction of parturition in the mare. Cervical relaxation can be evaluated by carefully conducting a digital vaginal examination. The mare's vulva and perineal area is scrubbed and then a well-lubricated, sterile, gloved hand is gently introduced into the vaginal vault. The cervix is located and evaluated for softness and dilatation. It should be possible to introduce one to two fingers into the external cervical os. If the mare has colostrum and is at least 330 days into gestation, she will usually have a relaxed, dilated cervix.

Oxytocin is the most commonly used drug to induce labor in the mare. Doses of 20–150 i.u. are given by intramuscular injection. The length of foaling is decreased as the dose of oxytocin is increased. A 20 i.u. dose usually results in a slower, less violent foaling than a 120 i.u. dose; at doses of 50–100 i.u., the mare usually exhibits the preparatory signs of labor within 15 min of injection. Rolling, sweating, nervousness, tail switching, and leaking of milk are usually noticed at this time; 15–20 min following the injection of oxytocin, the veterinarian should do a thorough vaginal examination to determine if the cervix has fully dilated and to determine the position and posture of the foal. At this time it is usually easy to correct malposture or abnormal positions. After the mare proceeds to the second stage of labor, it is extremely difficult to manipulate the fetus. If the red, velvet-like chorioallantois with its cervical star is presented at the vulva, it should be opened to allow the passage of the amnion and foal. Failure to do this may result in the placenta separating from the uterus prematurely and a mild to severely hypoxic foal. The time between the injection of 50–100 i.u. of oxytocin and presentation of the foal at the vulva is usually 25–45 min in normal mares. Following delivery, the mare and foal should be allowed to rest for 20–30 min. During this time care should be taken to assure that the umbilical cord is not prematurely severed. It may be necessary to clear the amnion from the foal's face. The progression of events at an induced foaling is the same as a natural foaling if the mare is near term, has milk in her udder, and has a relaxed cervix.

Although there are no apparent advantages, oxytocin can be administered intravenously to mares to induce parturition; 2.5–10 i.u. can be administered at 15 min intervals until the signs of second stage parturition are evident. An alternative method is to place 100–120 i.u. of oxytocin in 1 liter of sterile saline and administer by slow intravenous drip over the period of approximately 1 h.

Prostaglandins and corticosteroids have been used to induce foaling in mares. However, repeated doses are required and the time from injection to foaling is not very predictable. Therefore, oxytocin is the drug of choice in mares.

Ewe

Induction of parturition in ewes can be accomplished with corticosteroids. However, this procedure is not widely used because the period of effectiveness is quite short and the results are not predictable. Doses of 10–20 mg dexamethasone have been used following 140 days of gestation in the ewe.

Prostaglandins are not good drugs to use for inducing parturition in ewes. The ewe does not depend on a corpus luteum throughout gestation for progesterone. The placental unit is able to provide adequate amounts of progesterone during late pregnancy in the ewe.

Goat

Prostaglandin $F_{2\alpha}$ can be used to induce parturition in goats. A dose of 5–20 mg prostaglandin $F_{2\alpha}$ or 62.5–125 μg cloprostenol given i.m. precipitates parturition within 27–55 h, average 30–35 h. Induction of parturition should not be attempted prior to 140 days of gestation in goats. It is extremely important to have accurate breeding records to calculate injection dates.

Sow

On many swine farms the induction of parturition can improve sow productivity. Having attendants at each farrowing increases the number of live pigs born and improves the survival rate of neonatal pigs. Induced farrowing has apparently decreased the incidence of lactation failure on some farms. The gestation of sows to be induced must be at least 112 days in length if the pigs are expected to survive. In purebred herds where the average gestation length is longer than the usual 114 days, induction should not be done prior to 2 days before the average gestation.

The best drug for induction of parturition in sows is prostaglandin $F_{2\alpha}$ or one of its analogs. Following an i.m. injection of 10 mg prostaglandin $F_{2\alpha}$ or 175 μg cloprostenol, sows farrow an average of 30 h later. Sows injected during the morning hours usually farrow during the daytime hours the next day. To decrease the interval and variability in the interval between treatment and farrowing, 30 i.u. oxytocin can be given 20–24 h following prostaglandin treatment. Typical immediate responses to prostaglandin treatment in sows are attempts to build nests, nervousness, defecation, increased respiratory rate, and increased activity level. The transient side-effects seen following prostaglandin injection are not as pronounced when using the prostaglandin analogs. One must be careful about the timing of prostaglandin induction. If done too early for the given breed or strain of sows, piglets may be weaker and thus more susceptible to effects of cooling and noxious gases from pits (CO) leading to an increased number being crushed by the sow.

OBSTETRICAL OPERATIONS

The primary goals of obstetrical operations are to deliver a viable, healthy fetus that can survive outside the uterus and to prevent injury to the dam during parturition. Both of these goals are extremely important and should be carefully considered whenever obstetrical operations are planned. Obstetrical operations can be divided into four classes: mutation, forced extraction, fetotomy, and laparohysterotomy (Cesarean section).

For the sake of discussion it is necessary to define the orientation of the fetus as it enters the maternal birth canal. The presentation includes the relationship of the spinal axis of the fetus to that of the dam (longitudinal or transverse) and the portion of the fetus that is first entering the birth canal (anterior or posterior in longitudinal presentation and dorsal or ventral in transverse presentation). The position indicates the relationship of the dorsum of the fetus in longitudinal presentation or the head of the fetus in transverse presentation, to the quadrants of the maternal pelvis. These are the sacrum, the right ilium, the left ilium, and the pubis. Therefore a fetus could be dorsosacral, right dorsoilial, left dorsoilial,

dorsopubic, right cephaloilial, or left cephaloilial. The posture signifies the relationship of the extremities, or the head, neck, and limbs to the body of the fetus. The extremities may be flexed or extended. The normal situation in uniparous animals is the anterior longitudinal presentation, dorsosacral position with the head resting on the metacarpal bones and knees of the extended forelimbs. Since the limbs of the multiparous fetus are short and flexible, presentation, position, and posture are of little importance in these species.

Mutation includes the obstetrical operations by which a fetus is returned to normal presentation, position, and posture. These operations include repulsion, rotation, version, and adjustment of the extremities. Repulsion consists of pushing the fetus cranially out of the birth canal within the pelvic inlet into the uterus within the abdominal cavity where space is available to correct abnormal positions or postures. Great care must be taken, particularly in prolonged dystocias in which the uterus is dry and friable, not to push the fetus through the greater curvature of the uterus. Epidural anesthesia is usually helpful in accomplishing repulsion.

Rotation is turning the fetus on its long axis to bring it into a dorsosacral position from a left or right dorsoilial or dorsopubic position. A dorsosacral position is necessary in all but very small fetus in uniparous animals and is the usual position in multiparous animals. In many uniparous animals in which the fetus is in extreme right or left dorsoilial or dorsopubic position at the time of dystocia, there is an accompanying torsion of the uterus. The fetus naturally bends through an arc when being expelled through the maternal birth canal if in dorsosacral position.

Version is the rotation of the fetus on its transverse axis to place it into an anterior or posterior longitudinal presentation. This is most often necessary in the mare. It is extremely rare and anatomically very unlikely for transverse presentations to occur in cows.

Extension and adjustment of the extremities is the correction of abnormal postures, usually due to flexion of one or more limbs. Flexion of the neck and head usually causes dystocia in all species. Flexion of the limbs often causes dystocia in uniparous animals but not in multiparous animals. Care must be taken when repositioning extremities to avoid uterine rupture. Often repulsion is required before abnormally flexed or extended extremities can be repositioned.

Forced extraction is the withdrawal of the fetus from the dam through the birth canal by means of outside force or traction. To apply force, obstetrical (OB) chains must be applied to the limbs and often eyehooks to the head. A loop of OB chain for traction on the limbs should be placed above the fetlock joint and a half-hitch of chain should be applied below the fetlock around the pastern. Chains placed only around the pastern often slip distally causing the hoof to be removed. If excessive force is applied to chains placed only proximal to the fetlock, the epiphysis may be separated. If traction on the bovine head is required, short, blunt eyehooks are recommended, but not when delivering live foals. Chains or devices that go around the head often cause force on the back of the neck and may cause spinal cord and vertebral injury.

Traction, when applied in either anterior or posterior longitudinal presentation, should be applied dorsally and caudally at first to lift the fetus up and over the brim of the pelvis into the birth canal. After the head or the hips pass the vulva, the direction of traction should be more and more ventral until when the back of the fetus is passing through the vulva the direction of traction is perpendicular to the spinal axis of the dam or parallel to her hindlimbs. The direction of traction and that of the fetus as it passes through the birth canal is in the form of an arc. The ventral structures of the fetus are relaxed and concave, and the dorsal structures of the fetus are stretched and convex. The bovine fetus should be rotated approximately 90° when the fetal hips are passing through the maternal pelvis. The reason for this is that the bovine pelvic inlet is not a perfect circle. Its dorsoventral diameter is greater than its horizontal diameter. Rotation of the fetus is not as important in the mare because the mare's pelvic inlet is nearly round.

The force of two to three men (190–360 kg) can safely be applied to most bovine or equine fetuses. No more than the force of one man should be applied to the head of a bovine fetus. Generally, if the head can be pulled into the birth canal while both forelimbs are fully extended into the birth canal the bovine or equine fetus can be delivered by forced extraction. If this cannot be accomplished, some other method of delivery should be considered. If a veterinarian has worked at a mutation or forced extraction for half an hour without making progress, a fetotomy or Cesarean section is strongly considered.

A complete or partial fetotomy should be considered whenever a dead fetus is encountered in those species with a birth canal large enough for the procedure. The reason for doing a fetotomy is to preserve the dam. Recovery following an uncomplicated fetotomy is usually more rapid than with a Cesarean section. During a fetotomy the abdominal cavity is not entered and there are no abdominal incisions to heal following the procedure; so there is less chance of peritonitis or genital tract adhesions following a properly performed fetotomy than with a Cesarean section.

The most common reasons for failures with fetotomy techniques include inadequate training, insufficient experience, and lack of proper equipment. But with all this a veterinarian can do a complete fetotomy in the same amount of time that a Cesarean section would take to complete. An assistant is required to do a fetotomy. The percutaneous fetotomy techniques developed by the veterinarians at Utrecht are the recommended techniques.

Cesarean section is indicated whenever a live fetus cannot be delivered safely by other means, when the dam is a good surgical risk, and when the environment is conducive for major abdominal surgery. Pathological conditions such as uterine rupture and advanced hydrallantois are indications for Cesarean section. There are many approaches for doing Cesarean sections. The dam's characteristics including breed, size, temperament, intended longterm use, etc., and the amount of help available and facilities should be considered when deciding on an operative site. In addition aftercare should be considered before embarking on a Cesarean section. It is more economical in some animals to recommend immediate slaughter.

Dystocia in cows is usually due to disproportion between the size of the fetus and the maternal pelvis, particularly in heifers. Many heifers are bred while too immature, resulting in a normal-sized calf in an undersized dam. Twin dystocia, uterine torsion, fetal monsters, and hydrops are frequently seen in cattle.

In the mare dystocia is usually due to an abnormal presentation, position, or posture, and is often precipitated by the long extremities in the foal. Dystocia due to disproportion of the fetal size and maternal pelvis is rare in the mare.

In the ewe and goat postural abnormalities and twin or triplet dystocias are fairly common. Disproportion of fetal size and maternal pelvis is rare.

In the sow uterine inertia is the main cause of dystocia, but occasionally it is caused by small litters producing relatively large pigs.

Complementary References

Ball, L. (1980) Pregnancy diagnosis in the cow. In *Current Therapy in Theriogenology*, ed. Morrow, D. A., pp. 229–235. Philadelphia: W.B. Saunders.

Barth, A. D. (1986) Induced parturition in cattle. In *Current Therapy in Theriogenology*, 2nd edn, ed. Morrow, D. A., pp. 209–214. Philadelphia: W.B. Saunders.

Bierschwal, C. J. & deBois, C. H. W. (1970) *The Technique*

of Fetotomy in Large Animals, pp. 1–50. Lenexa, Kansas: VM Publishing Inc.

BonDurant, R. H. (1986) Examination of the genital tract of the cow and heifer. In *Current Therapy in Theriogenology*, 2nd edn, ed. Morrow, D. A., pp. 95–97. Philadelphia: W. B. Saunders.

Bundle, J. R. (1986) Pregnancy diagnosis in swine. In *Current Therapy in Theriogenology*, 2nd edn, ed. Morrow, D. A., pp. 918–923. Philadelphia: W. B. Saunders.

Curran, S., Pierson, R. A. & Ginther, O. J. (1986) Ultrasonographic appearance of the bovine conceptus from days 10 through 20. *J. Amer. Vet. Med. Assoc.*, **189**, 1289–1294.

Ginther, O. J. (1986) *Ultrasonic Imaging and Reproductive Events in the Mare*, pp. 195–332. Cross Plains, Wisconsin: Equiservices.

Johnston, S. D., Larsen, R. E. & Olson, P. S. (1982) *Canine Theriogenology*, pp. 33–35. Hastings, Nebraska: Society for Theriogenology.

Hillman, R. B. (1983) Equine parturition. In *Equine Reproduction*, pp. 80–90. Nutley, New Jersey: Hoffman-LaRoche Inc.

Logue, D. N., Hall, J. T., McRobert, S. & Waterhouse A. (1987) Real-time ultrasound scanning: the results of the first year of its application in south-west Scotland. *Vet. Rec.*, **121**, 146.

Neely, D. P. (1983) Pregnancy detection. In *Equine Reproduction*, pp. 65–70. Nutley, New Jersey: Hoffman-LaRoche Inc.

Roberts, S. J. (1986) *Veterinary Obstetrics and Genital Dieases Theriogenology*. Woodstock, Vermont: S. J. Roberts.

West, D. M. (1986) Pregnancy diagnosis in the ewe. In *Current Therapy in Theriogenology*, 2nd edn, ed. Morrow, D. A., pp. 850–851. Philadelphia: W. B. Saunders.

Williams, C. S. F. (1986) Pregnancy diagnosis in the doe. In *Current Therapy in Theriogenology*, 2nd edn, ed. Morrow, D. A., pp. 587–588. Philadelphia: W. B. Saunders.

Zemjanis, R. (1970) *Diagnostic and Therapeutic Techniques in Animal Reproduction*. Baltimore: Williams & Wilkins Co.

5

Male Infertility

B. K. GUSTAFSSON AND D. B. GALLOWAY

'Fertile' can be used in the sense of 'capable of begetting young' or 'reproducing abundantly, prolific'. The latter sense is more appropriate in domestic animals and can be defined quantitatively for males of each species and in particular management systems. Below such performance are degrees of infertility. Slight, moderate, or severe infertility reflects a spectrum of disturbance of reproductive function. Sterility is complete and permanent infertility.

The clinician determines if reproductive function is normal or abnormal. To do this, he selects from a range of techniques including the taking of a clinical history, general clinical examination of the animal, physical examination of the reproductive organs, evaluation of serving behavior, semen examination, tests for specific infectious diseases, and special tests such as endocrine assays, chromosomal examination, and biopsy procedures.

The severity of the disturbance or disturbances should be defined when a diagnosis is made and the implication for fertility stated. A prognosis or the basis on which a prognosis might be made (such as serial examinations) is given. Advice is then given on how the client and veterinarian might best manage the situation to arrive at a satisfactory outcome. A report is given, usually containing a statement of the examinations performed, the results and the conclusions drawn. Legal disputes often arise with respect to male animals, and veterinarians should be meticulous in their examination and in their record keeping. Difficulties in relating the results of examination precisely to fertility and the presence of several unknowns in the field of male infertility can be overcome by the statement that, 'the findings were consistent with high fertility'. Alternatively the findings on examination may be consistent with slightly, moderately, or severely reduced fertility, or with sterility.

In herd and flock preventive medicine programs, the veterinarian must assess the reproductive efficiency of the breeding male or males. Advice is given on how best to achieve the peak efficiency at the time of mating. Advice and assistance may also be needed with respect to mating management and artificial insemination programs. (For a summary of normal semen characteristics see Chapter 2, page 40.)

THE TECHNIQUES OF EXAMINATION

The history should emphasize age, general health and nutritional condition, the dates of transport or illness, and previous reproductive performance. General clinical examination may be limited to a systematic inspection only. Taking the cardinal signs of temperature, pulse, and respiration rate adds objective weight to a statement that the animal 'was in good general health and condition'. Normal conformation and gait are important in male animals. Where abnormalities are noted, particular systems should be examined in detail.

Physical examination of the reproductive organs is done by observation and palpation. Objective measurements should be used whenever possible.

Scrotal circumference measured with a scrotal tape in bulls, rams, and male goats, and scrotal width measured with calipers in the stallion (and also in the dog) are important assessments of testicular size and should always be recorded. Consistency of the testes relates to the structure of the tissues. A firm, resilient testis suggests good spermatogenesis. Fibrous testes feel firm and nonresilient, but degeneration produces a soft testis lacking in resilience.

The tail of the epididymis is a reservoir for spermatozoa and its palpable characteristics reflect the degree to which it is filled out by its contents. Enlargement and increased firmness of any part of the epididymis suggests inflammation or spermiostasis, possibly leading to sperm granuloma formation.

Some of the accessory sex glands can be assessed by rectal palpation in the bull, stallion, and dog. Size, shape and consistency are important in evaluating both normality and abnormality. A smooth muscle relaxant given intravenously to the stallion just before examination allows the veterinarian to palpate the organs much more accurately.

The penis and prepuce are best examined at the time of erection to assess functional normality. Corkscrew deviation of the penis, common in polled bulls, for example, cannot be detected unless the animal is seen attempting to serve. The penis and prepuce can also be examined by palpation and inspection after manually protruding the penis from the prepuce. In bulls, having an assistant insert a gloved hand into the rectum will tend to relax the penis and facilitate manual protrusion. Occasionally in the bull and stallion tranquilizers are given to relax the penis. But since there is some risk of permanent penile paralysis in the stallion, these are only used when necessary and only then with minimal doses and careful handling of the penis to reduce the risk.

The normal sequence of serving behavior involves libido or the desire to serve, courtship activity, erection and protrusion of the penis, mounting, pelvic movements, and in ruminants an ejaculatory thrust. Urethral pulsations are detectable in the stallion, boar, and dog, coincident with ejaculation. Each of these facets may be studied in turn to assess the points at which disturbances of serving behavior are occurring and to help in diagnosing their cause.

Serving capacity as a quantitative measure of behavior has been well-defined in the bull. A practical test has been devised for groups of *Bos taurus* bulls and the result is highly correlated with their serving performance in the field. Essential features of the test include females not in estrus restrained in specially designed service crates, testing a number of animals at the same time from the same age and social group (five bulls; four females), adequate sexual stimulation of bulls before testing and attention to the welfare of the females used.

Serving capacity tests are also available for rams. Each ram is placed with four or five estrous ewes in a small pen (6 m × 6 m) on four occasions. The first two occasions of 20 min duration are to overcome shyness. The following two occasions are of 1 h duration and a ram's serving capacity is taken as the mean number of serves performed by him in these two tests. Modifications from this recommendation have been made to improve economic acceptability of the test. Trials are needed for different flock conditions to verify the efficacy of modified tests.

Semen should be collected from ruminants and the stallion with the artificial vagina whenever possible. The gloved hand method in the boar and manual stimulation of the penis in the dog satisfactorily produce normal ejaculation in most cases. If electroejaculation, or in the bull massage of the pelvic organs, are used in the field, the possible effects of the technique and environmental factors must be taken into consideration. Care should be exercised in ensuring that a representative sample is obtained from the animal.

Semen samples are assessed for volume (gel-free in the stallion and boar), concentration, wave motion (in ruminants), forward progressive motility in per cent, the percentage alive (vital stain), morphology and cells other than spermatozoa. Motility and morphology, concentration, total spermatozoa per ejaculate and the presence of leukocytes are especially important in helping to decide whether or not the reproductive system is functioning normally. The pattern of semen characteristics set out in the form of a spermiogram provides information about the severity, site and cause of the disturbance.

The assessment of wave motion and motility should be made on a warm microscope stage. Immediately after collection air-dried smears can be made for the later assessment of sperm head morphology and a sample preserved in buffered formol saline for assessment of abnormalities of the acrosome, midpiece and tail. These preparations can be sent long distances, even internationally to specialist laboratories.

Specific tests for infectious diseases are dealt with elsewhere (Chapters 2, 11–17).

Luteinizing hormone (LH), follicle stimulating hormone (FSH) and testosterone assays are available so that hormonal parameters in problems of male infertility can be defined. The value of such data, however, are limited because of the difficulty in relating hormonal measurements to potential fertility. Recent work on the response to GnRH injection in bulls shows some promise in this direction. The determination of estrone sulfate in the blood or the testosterone response to human chorionic gonadotropin (hCG) is useful in detecting the presence of a retained testis in sexually aggressive male horses with no palpable organs in the scrotum.

Cytogenetic examination has been useful in detecting the presence of the 1/29 translocation in bulls, associated with reduced fertility in both males and females. Translocations in boars have been associated with low litter size.

Testicular biopsy is not as useful in veterinary medicine as in the human field. The risk of causing degenerative change in the invaded testis and difficulties in obtaining a representative sample are among the disadvantages.

BULL

Both testicular size and serving capacity are highly heritable in the bull. Selection on the basis of testicular size will improve sperm output in future generations and it is associated with some important attributes of female reproduction.

Where large numbers of bulls are being examined, testicular size measured by scrotal circumference and serving capacity are useful objective measurements which can be used to improve herd reproductive efficiency. Both attributes, together with structural soundness, should be emphasized in health and production preventive programs. Breed societies should be encouraged to include a minimum scrotal circumference at a given age as part of breed descriptions.

Good nutrition is essential during the rearing period for a bull to manifest his potential testicular size. In the adult, diets that maintain good health and body condition are adequate also for good testicular function and other aspects of reproductive efficiency.

Testicular Dysfunction

Testicular dysfunction can be divided into three broad categories. *In the first* are disturbances of the spermatogenic epithelium where there is an intrinsic fault in the cellular production lines. This includes the testicular hypoplasia complex. Generally, bulls with testicular hypoplasia have nothing in the history or in the results of general clinical examination that could account for failure of testicular development. There appears to be a range of severity from

the aspermic bull to animals that are close to normal. The testes may both be small with a scrotal circumference of 24–30 cm at the time of diagnosis which is generally at 1–3 years of age. The condition can also be unilateral. Epididymal tails are firm and lack resilience. Serving behavior is not affected. Semen is of low concentration and motility. In some cases, sperm head morphology is within normal limits, but in other cases severely disturbed head morphology is found along with giant cells indicating severe dysfunction of the spermatogenic epithelium. Morphologic abnormalities of the head may represent degenerative change superimposed on the basic testicular problem or a more severe degree of the intrinsic disturbance. Abnormalities of the midpiece and tail are generally increased with various combinations of spermatozoa with attached proximal cytoplasmic droplets, single bent and coiled tails, and detached heads.

In some bulls a proportion of the spermatogenic epithelium appears to be coded to produce a specific type of abnormal spermatozoa. Again there can be a wide range of severity, from bulls in which most of the spermatozoa are abnormal and fertility is normal or severely affected. Sticky chromosomes is an uncommon defect in the spermatogenic epithelium which results in the production of pyknotic nuclei and hyperchromatic spermatozoa-like bodies which are evident in stained semen smears. Specific defects include abaxial midpiece attachments, acrosome abnormalities, and defects of development of the midpiece and tail. Tailless heads, when they are consistently present in the ejaculate in large numbers without other signs of testicular dysfunction appear to be another form of defect. Genetic factors are very important in the occurrence of these primary disturbances of differentiation of the spermatogenic epithelium.

The second category of dysfunction involves abnormalities of the nutritional or hormonal support for the growing testes. Small testes arising from poor nutrition in the rearing period or the improper use of estrogenic growth promotants are examples.

The third category involves degeneration of the spermatogenic epithelium due to damaging external influences. Testicular degeneration is common in bulls. Disturbances in general health, especially when accompanied by fever or toxemia are likely to cause degeneration. Local inflammation of the scrotal area results in heat degeneration of the testis. Beef bulls that are prepared intensively for exhibition and sale may be unable to maintain low testicular temperature. Fat in the scrotal neck region, tropical or subtropical environmental temperatures, housing and bedding leading to a warm moist environment for the scrotum and high nutritional plane are the main contributing factors.

Testes affected by degeneration are often reduced in size and are softer and less resilient than normal. Initial changes in the semen picture occur between 10 and 50 days after the cause begins to act depending on the severity of the cause and the cell populations affected. Low concentration and motility of spermatozoa, increased sperm head abnormalities and varying combinations of spermatozoa with attached cytoplasmic droplets, tailless heads, and bent and coiled tails are typical semen characteristics. The degeneration can be mild to very severe. If the spermatogonial population is severely damaged then regeneration cannot occur. Where regeneration is possible it may take several months. Most clinically obvious degenerations cause reduced fertility and take at least 2 months to recover after the damaging incident.

Epididymal Dysfunction

Epididymal dysfunction with abnormal composition of the epididymal plasma in the tail is not associated with any palpable changes. The semen picture is characterized by low motility and high numbers of spermatozoa with singly bent tails. Exhaustive ejaculation helps to define the condition, since the motility increases after five or more ejaculates and the percentage of spermatozoa with singly bent tails decreases. The potential for this type of epididymal dysfunction appears to be congenital.

Abnormal Development of the Mesonephric Duct

This can give rise to several clinical pictures. Where the seminal vesicles have failed to develop, the defective organs can be felt per rectum. There are no other clinical signs. If a segment of the vas deferens or the epididymis is missing, the testis on that side cannot contribute to the ejaculate. The head of the epididymis may appear normal on palpation for a considerable time due to resorption of spermatozoa. However, at some stage a spermatic granuloma usually forms causing enlargement and increased firmness. An apparent fusion of the mesonephric ducts to form a cyst into which the vasa deferentia and vestigial seminal vesicles empty and which connects with the pelvic urethra has been found in some bulls. Low sperm concentration, low motility, and a high percentage of tailless heads are features of the semen picture.

Spermiostasis

Spermiostasis occurs in bulls and is usually manifest by a firm enlargement of the epididymal head. The origin is a disturbance of efferent tubule development. The condition is described further in the section on the ram (page 85).

Serving Inability

Serving inability and lowered serving capacity can be purely behavioral. The fault appears to be in the central nervous system since hormonal levels and the function of the reproductive organs are generally within normal limits. Other disturbances of normal serving behavior can be related to abnormalities of the back, legs, feet or the penis and prepuce. Genetic factors which are important for libido and serving capacity in Hereford and Angus bulls in southern Australia were found to have a heritability of 0.59 ± 0.15. Structural abnormalities of the back, legs, and feet and corkscrew deviation of the penis should be considered heritable problems affecting serving efficiency.

Prolapsed Prepuce

Prolapsed prepuce is seen commonly in some *Bos indicus* cattle and in polled *Bos taurus* breeds. A deficiency of the preputial musculature is responsible and selection against bulls that tend to prolapse the prepuce is recommended.

RAM

Testicular size is affected by genetic factors, age, nutrition and season. Since each gram of normal testicular tissue produces approximately 20×10^6 spermatozoa/day, large testes produce more spermatozoa/day than small testes. In western Australia Merino flocks, 400 g of testis tissue per 100 ewes has been found to be adequate for normal fertility. Individual rams varied markedly in paired testicular weight (100–800 g).

Selection of rams should be made on measured productive characteristics (for example, wool fiber diameter) and on reproductive efficiency. Adaptation to the particular environment in terms of maintaining high reproductive efficiency is important.

Good general health and condition, normal reproductive organs, large testicular size and excellent semen quality form a good basis for assessing reproductive efficiency. Serving capacity testing may be considered if economically applicable.

Group Assessment

In flock health and production programs the ram team may be examined and divided into three groups on the basis of general health and condition, testicular size and consistency and the presence or absence of abnormalities of the reproductive organs. *Group A rams* are in excellent condition for joining with the ewes. Their testes are large, firm and resilient, and the epididymal tails are filled out with stored spermatozoa. Semen may be collected from a sample of these rams to verify that they are producing ejaculates of high quality. *Group B rams* are less than optimum with respect to body condition and the size and condition of the testes, but they show no evidence of serious pathological processes. Semen from a sample of these rams will usually be of lower quality than that in group A, and the extent will depend on the severity of the disturbances of testicular function. Advice is given as necessary on management, nutrition, and disease control in these rams to bring them to the peak of reproductive efficiency at the point of joining with the ewes. *Group C rams* have abnormalities which have serious implications for reproductive efficiency. Diagnostic examinations of these rams, including semen examination and tests for infectious disease (such as *Brucella ovis*, see page 215), assist in defining the factors involved in ram wastage in the flock. Group C rams are not used for mating.

Testicular Dysfunction

Small testes occur in rams associated with disturbances of descent, abnormal chromosome constitution, and poor nutrition and parasitism during the rearing period. Genetic factors should be considered as a reason for testicular hypoplasia, particularly in inbred strains of sheep. Cryptorchidism is inherited and affected rams should not be used for breeding.

Some flock problems of developmental failure of testicles appear not to be genetic. A 'Sertoli cell only' histological picture is typical. In one case the ovaries of some ewes born at the same time as affected rams were hypoplastic. There appeared to be germ cell destruction at an early stage of embryonic development. Further work is needed to characterize possible toxic agents (such as fungal toxins) that could be responsible for underdeveloped testes.

Testicular degeneration is common in rams, particularly when management and environmental factors militate against the normal processes of testicular cooling. Sheep that are heavily fed, maintained in full wool, and with a thick wool covering of the scrotum, and housed in warm, humid or hot weather are especially at risk. Thickening of the scrotal skin from scrotal mange leads to testicular degeneration. Blowfly strike, with its attendant stress, fever and toxemia, and arsenic absorbed from dipping fluids or ingested are other causes of testicular degeneration in the ram. The clinical signs and seminal changes are similar to those described for the bull (page 83).

Spermiostasis

Spermiostasis is the result of abnormal development in the embryo of the efferent tubules from the mesonephric structures. Blind-ended tubules fill with spermatozoa after puberty. The wall breaks down and spermatozoa gain access to the interstitial tissue causing a granuloma. The affected epididymal head is enlarged and very firm in consistency, and the tail on that side feels small and empty. While the duct system is still patent the semen contains increased abnormalities of the midpiece and tail. The lack of polymorphonuclear leukocytes in the semen and in the lesion on postmortem examination helps to distinguish spermiostasis from infectious epididymitis. Genetic factors are considered to be the primary cause of spermiostasis, the prevalence varying among breeds. Some environmental factors such as plane of nutrition may influence prevalence. In some flocks both spermiostasis and infectious epididymitis, often due to *Actinobacillus seminis*, occur simultaneously. Some lesions in the head of the epididymis appear to have started as spermiostasis with later invasion of the lesion by the infectious organism. Control of both genetic and infectious factors is indicated.

Diseases

Diseases such as pneumonia, parasitism in young rams, footrot and foot abscess, and *Corynebacterium renale* infection of the prepuce will adversely influence serving ability and reduce serving capacity. Some young rams may show inhibition of mating behavior when first put in with a flock of ewes. The majority start mating within 2–3 weeks, and a normal mating behavior follows. Sexual inhibition of young rams during their first mating season can also contribute to low fertility.

GOAT

General principles apply as for the ram. The male has not been studied in as much detail as the ram and the bull. Testicular hypoplasia, which appears to be familial, occurs. Testicular degenerations are not as common as in the ram possibly because of the more open hair covering of the scrotum and the different conditions under which goats are kept.

Spermiostasis is a serious problem in some breeding lines of milking goats with bilateral aspermic cases being more common than unilaterally affected animals. The symptoms are similar to those seen in rams (see above). Genetic factors again appear to be important. Angora goats seem to be relatively free from the problem.

BOAR

In order to minimize repeat breeding, emphasis must be placed on boar selection, a procedure which should emphasize the purchase of boars from herds free from disease. Also, purchase should not be made from herds suspected to have a high incidence of unfavorable genetic traits. A thorough examination of the locomotor function is an important part of a prepurchase procedure. A breeding soundness examination should be considered an essential safety measure. A boar usually needs an acclimatization period to adjust to the new herd, which may be from 6 weeks to 2 months. During this time appropriate preventive medicine (such as vaccinations) can be applied. An evaluation for breeding soundness including semen evaluation with or without test mating can preferably be conducted during this period if this had not been done as a prepurchase procedure. The mating system (for example, hand mating, group mating, pasture mating, double mating, artificial insemination) must be considered when evaluating the role of the boar with infertility problems in a herd. The age of the boar at the start of routine usage and the service frequency are also factors that need to be considered.

Reviewing Records

If the mating system permits, an examination of boar infertility should be preceded by a thorough review of records: nonreturn rate to first service, farrowing rate, litter size, postbreeding estrus intervals, vaginal discharge, etc. A semen evaluation should always be included. If the examiner is not quite proficient in semen evaluation (especially the morphologic part) it is important that an appropriate sample be sent to a recognized semen laboratory. Spermatozoa fixed in buffered formol saline solution can be stored and mailed long distances for morphologic examination. It is important to realize that what happens in a herd at a given time is a re-

flection of what happened some time ago in the testes or in the excurrent duct system. Thus, young boars that have been used before they were sexually mature might very well be normal at the examination but still be responsible for the problem. The causes of noninfectious infertility in the boar can generally be listed under three broad categories: (1) disturbances of the mating ability; (2) testicular dysfunction; (3) epididymal dysfunction.

Disturbances of the Mating Ability

The serving capacity can be impaired by poor libido, which may have a genetic background, or by weakness of the locomotor system. However, information on past illness or injuries, the age at the onset of the condition, the exact nature of the dysfunction, and the social, physical, and climatic environments must be obtained to rule out any acquired causes. The clinical examination of the boar should focus on its behavioral response to a highly receptive female in a normal mating arena. If abnormalities of the penis are suspected it might be necessary for the boar to be examined under anesthesia.

The most common cause of dysfunction of serving behavior is locomotor dysfunction. In several countries locomotor dysfunctions are the most common single reason for culling boars and have been listed as one of the four common causes of reproductive inefficiency in boars. These locomotor dysfunctions are generally referred to as leg weakness. Although it is a fairly well-documented clinical entity known to be associated with rapid growth rate, the exact etiology has not been determined. The disease is often related to osteochondrosis and arthrosis with localization in the hindlimbs causing a swaying action of the hindquarters, a stiff gait or an arched back with all four legs bunched together under the body. The serving behavior is characterized by difficulties in both mounting and completing the copulation. A tendency to fall off the sow and the adoption of a dog-sitting posture is common. Treatment is of questionable value. Boars should be selected from an adequate genetic pool of boars who have the ability to withstand a high intensity of feeding and the life under restricted exercise. Good conformational constitution and good movements are other criteria upon which to select. The physical environment of the mating pen is important and floors should provide good footing.

Testicular Dysfunction

Among testicular dysfunction problems resulting in

quantitatively or qualitatively insufficient sperm output and infertility, two conditions, testicular hypoplasia and testicular degeneration, are of major interest.

Testicular Hypoplasia

Testicular hypoplasia is an inherited congenital underdevelopment of the testes, which can be unilateral or bilateral, total or partial. In total bilateral hypoplasia the seminiferous tubules lack germinal epithelium and sperm production does not occur. These boars are sterile. Other types of hypoplasia (partial bilateral or unilateral or total unilateral) may result in a reduced sperm output with subnormal fertility. The fertility can occasionally be within normal range especially at low service frequency. Such cases may lead to a spread of this heritable defect. Clinically, testicular hypoplasia is characterized by small testis size and small and flaccid epididymal tails on the affected side or sides. The ejaculate is characterized by various degrees of oligospermia from virtual aspermia to a slightly lowered concentration. The sperm motility is usually reduced and the incidence of pathological spermatozoa is frequently increased. A striking feature in partial hypoplasia seems to be an increased incidence of spermatozoa with proximal cytoplasmic droplets (immature spermatozoa). An increased frequency of abnormal sperm heads is another common sign. The clinical diagnosis is based on breeding history, palpation of the testes and epididymides and semen evaluation. Affected boars usually have normal libido and mating behavior. There is no treatment for testicular hypoplasia and because the condition is suspected to be hereditary, affected boars should be culled.

Testicular Degeneration

Testicular degeneration is probably the most common cause of infertility in the boar. It is an acquired disorder, the cause of which is often complex and difficult to establish in the individual animal. Causative factors include systemic disease, fever, chronic diseases, traumatic injury, toxins, nutritional imbalance, high ambient temperature, hormonal imbalance and stress. Local irritation or inflammation caused by insect bites, disinfectants or insecticides can also result in testicular degeneration. Many parts of the world that raise pigs are seasonally very hot and the boar may play a role in the so-called seasonal infertility syndrome (summer infertility). Periods of extremely hot weather are frequently followed by increased incidence of abnor-

mal spermatozoa. Even extremely cold weather can cause testicular degeneration as has been noticed in the midwestern states of the United States. Frostbite can sometimes be seen on the scrotum but frequently there is no physical evidence of injury. Other environmental factors that are increasingly important are toxic agents like cadmium. Even feed additives, rodenticides and mycotoxins may cause testicular degeneration. Clinically, there is usually no sign of systemic disease. Sexual behavior is usually normal. The size of one or both testes may be somewhat smaller or larger than normal. Testicular consistency may be increased and localized indurations may be palpated. In advanced cases, testicular atrophy develops. Affected boars usually produce a normal semen volume and sperm concentration may be normal or reduced. Different degrees of reduced sperm motility is a major finding. A variety of morphological alterations of the sperm head, acrosome, midpiece or sperm tail may occur. A high incidence of proximal cytoplasmic droplets and midpiece defects seem to be a characteristic feature. An excessive degeneration of the germinal epithelium often results in a clinical picture similar to that of testicular hypoplasia. However, boars with testicular degeneration have usually had prior normal fertility and semen quality. If the causative agent is eliminated, a regeneration of the germinal epithelium may occur. Complete recovery depends on the cause and the duration of the disease. Reevaluation of boars in about 2 months will aid in establishing a definite diagnosis.

Effective medical treatment for testicular degeneration is unknown. It should be noticed that semen produced at early stages of puberty, for example, at 6–8 months of age, and in some boars with delayed puberty (8–10 months old) is characterized by a high incidence of abnormal spermatozoa, particularly abnormal head shapes and proximal cytoplasmic droplets. This picture is similar to the one seen in cases of testicular degeneration but is normal before the boar has reached full maturity.

Epididymal Dysfunction

Apart from epididymitis associated with orchitis (see page 217) epididymal disorders are not common in the boar. Occasionally, aplasia of the tail of the epididymis may be diagnosed by palpation. If other parts are involved the diagnosis is more difficult. In some cases of segmental aplasia, spermiostasis (sperm granuloma, spermatocele) develops and can be palpated. Unilateral segmental aplasia results in lowered sperm concentration in the ejaculate.

Functional disturbances of the epididymis may result in abnormal composition of the epididymal plasma. The clinical picture is characterized by lowered sperm motility and increased frequency of single bent or coiled sperm tails. The incidence of proximal cytoplasmic droplets may be increased but the sperm head is normal. Repeated ejaculations within a short time period may result in improved sperm motility and sperm morphology. These exhaustion tests are used to differentiate between disorders of epididymal and testicular origin. The cause of the epididymal dysfunctions is not entirely known. Varying degrees of infertility have been found in bulls. In boars the relationship between epididymal dysfunction and fertility is not well established but lowered fertility has been found in such boars at artificial insemination with liquid semen stored for more than 30 h. There is no medical treatment for this condition but a high ejaculation frequency may increase the fertility of some boars.

STALLION

It is often difficult to evaluate a stallion's reproductive efficiency. Breeding practices, the quality of the mares, the distribution between maiden, barren and foaling mares, the total number of mares assigned to a stallion are factors that make breeding records difficult to interpret. The best, although retrospective, measure of stallion fertility is the foaling rate achieved with mares of normal fertility under optimal management conditions. A normally fertile stallion is one which is capable of efficiently rendering at least 75% of 40 or more mares pregnant when bred naturally, or 120 mares when bred artificially in one breeding season provided that the mares have a reasonably good fertility and are under reasonably good management.

In problem stallions, breeding records must be carefully studied. Of particular importance is a measure of previous fertility in each of three groups of mares—the maiden, barren, and foaling mares. Services per foaling, services per pregnancy, estrous periods per foaling or pregnancy are valuable indices. When the apparent fertility measures are low, the management and veterinary programs under which the stallion has performed should be evaluated.

This includes nutrition and parasite control programs, use of artificial light, teasing and palpation program as well as immunization, diagnostic and therapeutic procedures. Especially for race and performance horses it is desirable to obtain as much information as possible concerning medications given in the past. Physical examination of the genital organs and semen evaluation should always be included in problem stallions. Abnormal mating behavior and testicular and epididymal problems are major categories of noninfectious infertility.

A normal stallion should be interested in the estrual mare and be anxious and able to mount, be able to seek and find the vulva or be willing to insert in the artificial vagina, be able to thrust and to ejaculate promptly. Abnormal mating behavior is seen in inexperienced stallions or in stallions with a negative experience of sexual activity. For example, race and performance horses have frequently been exposed to punishment for showing sexual arousal at inappropriate times. This may result in difficulties to express normal behavior toward an estrual mare. It has been convincingly demonstrated experimentally that the sexual behavior of a stallion can be rapidly modified by negative experience.

Various forms of abnormal behavior occur including failure to obtain an erection, prolonged reaction time, mounting without erection, multiple mounts before intromission, multiple intromissions before ejaculation, lack of ejaculation and abusing the mare. These disorders require retraining of the stallion under the best possible conditions. The retraining may be accomplished by presenting a variety of estrous mares to the stallion twice a day in quiet undisturbed surroundings until normal behavior patterns are established. Quiet, older mares may be useful for that purpose. The time it takes to attain normal breeding behavior depends on the magnitude and duration of the altered behavior and also on the stallion's innate sex drive.

Genetic Predisposition

It is always a possibility that an abnormal behavior can depend on a genetic predisposition. Training of such stallions does not usually result in any improvement. Unfortunately, there is no test by which one could determine genetic influence. The steroid concentrations in blood are usually normal in all of these cases. Hormonal treatments (hCG i.v.) have been tried to increase the circulating testosterone levels but without much success. Ejaculation difficulties have been treated with beta-blockers, oxytocin or prostaglandin $F_{2\alpha}$ with some success. In stallions in which the dysfunction is clearly acquired or related to age such treatments might be justified. Prostaglandin $F_{2\alpha}$, 5–10 min before mating or semen collection, might stimulate erection and ejaculation.

Also, 10–20 USP units of oxytocin i.v. or i.m. 1–3 min before mating have shown a good effect on the sex drive and ejaculation in some stallions. Experiments involving experience-related sexual behavior dysfunctions have shown a positive effect of treatment with benzodiazepine derivatives. Diazepam (Valium) treatment (slow intravenous injection of 0.05 mg/kg diazepam, 5–10 min before breeding) has been used successfully in spontaneously inhibited stallions.

Testicular and Epididymal Dysfunctions

The testicular and epididymal problems do not deviate clinically from what is seen in other species (for example, bull and boar). A number of external and internal factors can cause a disturbance of the testicular function. Since testicular hypoplasia is congenital and probably genetically based it is important to differentiate between this condition and testicular degeneration which is an acquired condition. If a stallion has had normal testes which have now become abnormally small, it is obvious that the condition is acquired and should be classified as testicular degeneration or atrophy. However, in many cases there is insufficient evidence to determine the course by which the testes reached their present subnormal size. Nevertheless such stallions are poor prospective breeders if they produce an abnormal semen picture. To rule out the possibility that an improvement might occur, the examination should be repeated again in about 2 months followed by an examination before the next breeding season. The examinations should include a semen analysis (sperm motility, morphology, presence of other cells than spermatozoa). Since many stallions have had a racing career and were probably exposed to steroid treatment one must realize that steroids may have had a suppressive effect on spermatogenesis and epididymal function. Whether or not a steroid results in permanent damage may be dependent on the amount and duration of treatment and on the age of the stallion at steroid administration. The increased use of such agents should be of concern to the horse industry until more is known about their potential effect on future reproductive performance.

DOG

Reproductive efficiency in the male dog has not been well defined. This is due to many factors. For example, unlike the situation in the food animal species the economic justification for high reproductive efficiency has existed only to a limited extent. Under regular household conditions a particular male is bred only to a limited number of females in a lifetime. Furthermore, artificial insemination has not been widely used. The importance of semen examinations is just beginning to be generally recognized.

Primary Infertility

Male dog infertility is commonly classified as primary infertility or acquired infertility. Among causes of primary infertility, testicular hypoplasia should be considered in the first place since a hereditary predisposition might exist. As in other species (for example, bull, boar) the underdevelopment of the testes may occur in varying degrees resulting in a variable decrease in sperm production. Bilateral total hypoplasia results in total aspermia. The testes are small and may be either hard or soft in consistency. The epididymines are easily palpated but the tail appears flaccid and empty. The libido is not affected. The differential diagnosis between testicular hypoplasia and a segmental aplasia of the epididymis is obtained by careful palpation of the scrotal contents. Differentiation between hypoplasia and excessive testicular degeneration (testicular atrophy) may present certain difficulties especially in cases where sperm are present but in low concentration (oligospermia). In the absence of historical evidence, there is no recourse except to repeat the examination in 2–6 months. If there is no change in the physical appearance of the genital organs or in the semen picture it is most likely a case of hypoplasia. A biopsy may help at this stage at least to verify the severity of the condition.

Other cases of primary infertility may involve lowered sperm motility with or without an increased frequency of sperm morphological defects (acrosome defects, abnormal head shape, abnormal sperm tails, abnormal midpieces) without affecting the size of the testes or epididymides. This might be associated with a functional disturbance of the epididymis or a disturbance of certain phases of spermatogenesis. The background may be an inborn hormonal dysfunction. To rule out an acquired condition it is important to repeat the examination at least twice at an interval of about 4 months between the examinations.

Acquired Infertility

Among the causes of acquired infertility, testicular degeneration is most common. As in other species a variety of causative factors are involved, such as hormonal disturbances, heat, stress, toxins, scrotal irritation or dermatitis, autoimmune disorders, etc. The clinical picture is similar to that in other species: low sperm motility, a high incidence of sperm defects, and palpable changes of the testicles. To differentiate from primary infertility it is necessary to have access to a reliable history.

Epididymal Disorders

These are not well known in the dog. Functional disturbances are characterized by low sperm motility and a high number of spermatozoa with sperm tail defects (single bent or coiled tails). Frequent ejaculations may result in an improvement which can serve as a differential diagnosis.

In general, there are no effective medical treatments for non-infectious infertility problems in the dog. If the causative agent or condition can be removed a testicular degeneration can be reversed. Mating problems (poor libido) might sometimes be remedied by changing the dog's environment and management. In cases of unilateral testicular pathology (for example, tumor or inflammation) removal of that testis eliminates an adverse influence on the intact testis. A dog with an epididymal dysfunction may benefit from frequent ejaculations before a particular mating. If a very young dog shows inadequate reproductive function including a pathological semen picture it is wise to wait with a definite diagnosis until a condition of delayed puberty can be ruled out.

Complementary References

Blockey, M. A. de B. (1981a) Development of a serving capacity test for beef bulls. *Appl. Anim. Ethol.*, **7,** 307–319.

Blockey, M. A. de B. (1981b) Modification of a serving capacity test for beef bulls. *Appl. Anim. Ethol.*, **7,** 321–336.

Blockey, M. A. de B. (1981c) Further studies on the serving capacity test for beef bulls. *Appl. Anim. Ethol.*, **7,** 337–350.

Blockey, M. A. de B., Straw, W. M. & Jones, L. P. (1980) Heritability of serving capacity and scrotal circumference in beef bulls. *J. Anim. Sci.*, **47:** Suppl. 1, 253.

Blockey, M. A. de B. & Wilkins, J. F. (1984) Field application of the ram serving capacity test. In: *Reproduction in Sheep*, pp. 53–58, eds Lindsay, D. R. & Pearce, D. T. Canberra: Australian Academy of Science.

Bonte, P., Vandeplassche, M. & Lagasse, A. (1978) Functional epididymal disorders in boars. *Zuchthygiene*, **13,** 161.

Cox, J. E. (1987) Cryptorchidism. In: *Current Therapy in Equine Medicine*, 2nd edn, ed. Robinson, N. E. Philadelphia: WB Saunders Co.

Deschamps, J. C., Ott, R. S., McEntee, K., Heath, E. H., Heinrichs, R. R., Shanks, R. D. & Hixon, J. E. Effects of zeranol on reproduction in beef bulls. Scrotal circumference, serving ability, semen characteristics, and pathological changes of the reproductive organs. *Amer. J. Vet. Res.*, **48,** 137–147.

Einarsson, S. & Gustafsson, B. (1973) A case of epididymal dysfunction in boar. *Andrologie*, **5(4),** 273–279.

Gherardi, P. B., Lindsay, D. R. & Oldham, C. M. (1980) Testicle size in rams and flock fertility. *Proc. Aust. Soc. Anim. Prod.*, **13,** 48–50.

Gustafsson, B., Einarsson, S., Nicander, L., Holtman, M. & Soosalu, O. (1974) Morphological, physical, and chemical examination of epididymal contents and semen in a bull with epididymal dysfunction. *Andrologia* **6(4),** 321–331.

Gustavsson, I. (1979) Distribution and effects of the 1/29 Robertsonian translocation in cattle. *J. Dairy Sci.*, **62,** 825–835.

Gustavsson, I. (1984) Chromosome evaluation and fertility. *Proc. 10th Int. Congr. Anim. Reprod. AI.*, **4,** VI-1–VI-8.

Hancock, J. L. (1957) The morphology of boar spermatozoa. *J. Roy. Microscop. Soc.*, **76,** 84–97.

Holst, S. J. (1949) Sterility in boars. *Nord. Vet. Med.*, **1,** 87–120.

Kilgour, R. J. (1984) Sexual behavior in male farm animals. In: *The Male in Farm Animal Reproduction*, ed. Courot, M. Boston: Martinus Nijhoff.

Larsen, R. E. (1980) Infertility in the male dog. In: *Current Therapy in Theriogenology*, pp. 646–654. Philadelphia: WB Saunders Co.

Larsson, K. (1986) Evaluation of boar semen. In: *Current Therapy in Theriogenology*, 2nd edn, pp. 972–975. Philadelphia: WB Saunders Co.

McDonnell, S. M. (1986) Stallion sexual behaviour dysfunction: Experimental models and clinical considerations. *Proc. Ann. Meeting. Soc. Theriogenology, Rochester, NY*, 1–12.

McDonnell, S. M., Kenney, R. M., Meckley, P. M. & Garcia, M. C. (1985) Condition suppression of sexual behavior in stallions and reversal with diazepam. *J. Physiol. Behav.*, **34,** 951–956.

McDonnell, S. M., Kenney, R. M., Meckley, P. M. & Garcia, M. C. (1986) Novel environment suppression of sexual behavior in stallions and effects of diazepam. *J. Physiol. Behav.*, **37,** 503–505.

Post, T. B., Christensen, H. R. & Seifert, G. W. (1987) Reproductive performance and productive traits of beef bulls selected for different levels of testosterone response to GnRH. *Theriogenology*, **27(2),** 317–328.

Sekoni, V. O., Gustafsson, B. K. & Mather, E. C. (1981) Influence of wet fixation, staining techniques, and storage time on bull sperm morphology. *Nord. Vet. Med.*, **33,** 161–166.

Swierstra, E. E. & Dyck, G. W. (1976) Influence of the boar and ejaculation frequency on pregnancy rate and embryonic survival in swine. *J. Anim. Sci.*, **42,** 455–460.

Toelle, V. D. & Robison, O. W. (1985) Estimates of genetic correlations between testicular measurements and female reproductive traits in cattle. *J. Anim. Sci.*, **60(1),** 89–100.

6

Anestrus and Infertility in the Cow

R. S. YOUNGQUIST

with a section on Postpartum Uterine Infections with T. W. A. LITTLE

CONGENITAL DEFECTS OF THE GONADS

Ovarian Hypoplasia

Ovarian hypoplasia has occurred in Swedish Highland cattle as an autosomal recessive trait with incomplete penetrance but may occur sporadically in other breeds. The condition may be partial or complete, unilateral or bilateral. When unilateral, the left ovary is more likely to be hypoplastic than the right. The affected ovary may vary from a small cordlike thickening in the cranial edge of the mesovarium to a bean-sized structure. The tubular portion of the genital tract may remain infantile in animals with complete bilateral hypoplasia or may develop to normal or near-normal size in heifers with unilateral or partial ovarian hypoplasia. Animals with complete bilateral ovarian hypoplasia are sterile while those with partial or unilateral ovarian hypoplasia may be subfertile. Females with an abnormal karyotype such as XXX or XO are also affected by ovarian hypoplasia. Ovarian hypoplasia should be differentiated from nonfunctional ovaries associated with malnutrition or debilitating diseases. Treatment of ovarian hypoplasia with exogenous hormones is not likely to be successful and affected animals should be salvaged by slaughter.

Ovarian Agenesis

Occasionally, agenesis of one or both ovaries may be encountered. The tubular genital tract may be absent or infantile in cases of bilateral ovarian agenesis.

CONGENITAL DEFECTS OF THE TUBULAR TRACT

Segmental Defects

Segmental defects in the development of the paramesonephric (Müllerian) duct system, which normally gives rise to the cranial vagina, cervix and uterus, are not uncommon in cattle. The defect is associated with the white coat color in Shorthorn cattle, hence the name 'white heifer disease', but segmental aplasia is not confined to that breed and occurs sporadically in other breeds. Usually the cranial portions of the tract (the ovaries, uterine tubes and cranial portion of the uterine horns) are normal and secretions from the endometrium accumulate in the portions of the uterine horns that are present. A wide range of defects may occur. The hymen may be imperforate and block the drainage of secretions from a normal tract, distending the vagina and cervix. If the condition is allowed to persist, the dilatation may lead to atrophy of the tubular organs. Early treatment by incision of the hymen may allow the tract to function normally. Pyometra may develop if bacteria gain access to the accumulated fluid.

Aplasia of the Paramesonephric Ducts

Aplasia of one paramesonephric duct leads to the development of only one uterine horn (uterus unicornis). Affected animals may have normal fertility but are more likely to be subfertile.

Incomplete Fusion of the Paramesonephric Ducts

The caudal portions of the paramesonephric ducts may fail to fuse properly resulting in duplication of various portions of the caudal tubular tract. Most frequently, abnormalities of fusion occur in or around the area of the cervix. In some cases, the entire cervix may be duplicated and the cranial vagina divided by a dorsoventral band of tissue, while in others the cervix and vagina may be normal with the exception of a band of tissue extending from dorsal to ventral across the external os of the cervix. Partial failure of fusion may involve only a portion of the cervix resulting in a single uterine body and internal cervical os, duplication of a portion of the cervical canal and a double external cervical os. Uterus didelphys results when the cervix and uterine body are completely divided. Affected cows may conceive from natural service or if artificially inseminated into the cervix and uterine horn ipsilateral to the ovary that ovulates. The resulting pregnancy may not continue to term due to lack of placental attachment in the nongravid uterine horn.

Freemartinism

A freemartin is a genetic female born co-twin to a bull. While the effect on the male may be minimal, the reproductive organs of the female are severely altered. The condition arises due to anastomoses between the placental circulations of the twins. Blood is exchanged between the fetuses and each is colonized by cells from the other. Since sexual differentiation of the male embryo occurs earlier than that of the female, the male twin may sterilize the female by transfer of the H-Y antigen which inhibits development of the female gonad. The ovaries of freemartins are underdeveloped and contain seminiferous tubules. Defects of the tubular genital tract vary in severity and the structures present range from cordlike bands in the broad ligaments to near-normal uterine horns. In most cases, there is no communication between the uterus and vagina. Vesicular glands of varying size are nearly always present and an imperforate hymen occludes the hypoplastic vagina.

Over 90% of the female calves born co-twins to males are freemartins, thus the history would suggest a diagnosis in most cases. Single-born freemartins are possible if heterozygous twins of unlike sex are conceived and the male twin is lost after day 30 of gestation. In breeding age heifers, rectal examination will reveal segmental aplasia of the tubular genital tract and hypoplastic ovaries. Animals that are too small for palpation per rectum may be examined with a small glass vaginal speculum. The vagina of a freemartin is usually shorter than normal. Comparison with heifers of a similar age known to be singletons may be helpful. A definitive diagnosis may be made by karyotyping the suspected individual. Varying percentages of male cells are found in freemartins.

Testicular Feminization

Insensitivity of embryonic tissue to androgens caused by a lack of receptor sites results in birth of an animal that is a phenotypic female with an XY genotype, inguinal or abdominal testes that secrete testosterone, and aplasia of the tubular portion of the genital tract. The fetal testes secret normal amounts of testosterone resulting in degeneration of the derivatives of the paramesonephric duct system while the mesonephric duct system degenerates because of its insensitivity to androgens. The gene controlling androgen insensitivity is thought to be X-linked.

Parovarian Cysts

Remnants of the mesonephric or paramesonephric duct systems may persist and develop into cystic structures of varying size near the ovaries. These cysts rarely exceed more than a few centimeters in diameter and have little effect on fertility unless they reach a size sufficient to interfere with ovulation or function of the fimbriated end of the uterine tube. Parovarian cysts may cause confusion in the diagnosis of cystic ovarian disease.

ACQUIRED DEFECTS OF THE GONADS

Ovulation Tags

Ovulation tags develop following ovulation due to hemorrhage associated with rupture of the follicle and may result in fine adhesions between the ovarian surface and the uterine tube. Most resolve spontaneously and have little effect on subsequent function of the ovaries or uterine tubes.

Ovarian Hemorrhage

Ovarian hemorrhage may follow traumatic manipulation of the ovaries. Hemorrhage following enucleation of corpora lutea of pregnancy or those associated with pyometra is more severe than that following enucleation of corpora lutea in cycling cows. One half to several liters of blood are usually lost and fatal hemorrhage may occur. Organization of the resulting blood clot leads to adhesions between the ovary and ovarian bursa which may interfere with their normal function. In cases of pyometra, release of infective exudate results in severe adhesions leading to infertility. Enucleation of corpora lutea is an archaic practice and has been supplanted by judicious use of prostaglandin $F_{2\alpha}$ or its synthetic analogs (PGF).

Oophoritis

Inflammation of the ovary may follow traumatic manipulations, enucleation of corpora lutea associated with pyometra, and attempts to drain ovarian cysts via a needle inserted through the vagina. Ascending infections from the uterus may also affect the ovary.

ACQUIRED DEFECTS OF THE TUBULAR GENITAL TRACT

Uterine Tube Disease

Hydrosalpinx

Hydrosalpinx is characterized by the accumulation of a clear to slightly cloudy mucus within the lumen of the uterine tube following obstruction of either the ovarian or uterine extremity. Hydrosalpinx may be secondary to stenosis caused by chronic irritation of the uterine tube. Distension of the tube may be uniform or segmental and may reach 1.5 cm in diameter. Traumatic manipulations of the ovaries and intrauterine irrigation may cause inflammation of the uterine tube leading to bursal adhesions and secondary hydrosalpinx.

Salpingitis

Salpingitis is characterized by inflammation of the uterine tube without obvious enlargement of the organ. The lesion may not be detectable by palpation per rectum. Infections causing salpingitis commonly ascend from the uterus. Histological changes in the tubal epithelial cells are a significant cause of infertility since the functional integrity of the mucosa is necessary for transport of both male and female gametes, fertilization, and nourishment of the fertilized ovum. The surface epithelium of the uterine tubes may be more easily damaged than that of the uterus.

Pyosalpinx

Pyosalpinx is not as common as hydrosalpinx and is characterized by accumulation of purulent exudate within the uterine tube. The tube is not usually affected over its entire length. Pyosalpinx frequently follows severe cases of uterine infection and may be complicated by perimetritis and localized peritonitis.

Diagnosis of Tubal Obstructions

Examination of the uterine tubes by palpation per rectum may or may not be adequate to diagnose lesions of the tubes. In some cases, the lesions may not be grossly obvious but have a severe effect on fertility; while in others, apparently severe adhesions do not prevent gamete transport and fertilization.

Tests for Tubal Patency Several tests for determining the patency of the uterine tubes have been described:

Starch Test For this test 1 g of starch suspended in 10 ml water is injected through an 18 gauge × 30 cm needle inserted through the sacrosciatic ligament onto the surface of the ovary ipsilateral to the uterine tube in question. The test should be performed during the luteal phase of the estrous cycle. Cervicovaginal mucus or washings are collected 24–48 h after injection. The mucus is placed on a microscope slide, stained with Lugol's iodine, and examined microscopically for purple-stained starch granules. Starch grains are not thought to traverse the pelvis frequently, thus the test might be used to demonstrate unilateral tubal blockage but may be more suited to demonstrate bilateral blockage. While normal fertility has been reported to follow application of the starch test, the clinician should be aware that foreign body granulomas on or near the ovaries may be a sequel to the injection of starch into the peritoneal cavity.

Phenosulfonphthalein Dye Test The phenosulfonphthalein (PSP) dye test is based on the fact that PSP dye is not absorbed rapidly by the endometrium but is absorbed rapidly by the peritoneum and excreted by the kidneys. Dye infused into the uterus of a cow with normal uterine tubes passes through the tubes into the peritoneal cavity and imparts a red or pink color to alkaline urine shortly after infusion. In cases of bilateral tubal occlusion, the dye does not appear in the urine until more than 1 h after infusion. The urinary bladder of the cow is catheterized with a retention catheter and emptied of urine; 20 ml of dye solution (0.1 g PSP/100 ml water) is infused into the uterus and urine is collected every 15 min and alkalinized. Appearance of the dye in the urine at 15 min after infusion is interpreted to mean that both tubes are patent. Unilateral occlusion is suspected when the dye appears between 15 min and 1 h after infusion, while bilateral occlusion is suspected when the dye is not present by 1 h. The PSP dye test may be more accurate in identifying cases of bilateral occlusion than unilateral occlusion, but some investigators have found that the results of the PSP test are variable and do not correlate well with recovery of embryos.

Pollen Grains   Pollen grains (80 μm in diameter) have been used to assess the patency of the uterine tubes in slaughterhouse specimens. In some cases, uterine tubes that appeared to be patent based on the PSP dye test did not permit passage of the pollen grains, suggesting that some lesions may permit the passage of fluid but not the passage of ova. None of the above tests for uterine tubal patency are capable of identifying specific abnormalities of tubal function that may affect the passage of gametes or fertilized ova.

Embryo Recovery   Embryo recovery after either a single ovulation or superovulation is evidence that one or both uterine tubes are patent and functional. Flushing of the uterus for recovery of embryos has the additional advantage that it may be of some therapeutic benefit. If normal embryos are recovered, they may be transferred to synchronized recipients, frozen for future use, or a single embryo may be replaced in the uterus of the donor. Attempts to recover embryos should be repeated several times since there is some variation in recovery rates.

Control and Treatment of Uterine Tube Disease

Treatment of diseases of the uterine tube is usually not possible. Concurrent uterine infections should be treated as indicated and a period of sexual rest may be of some benefit in valuable animals to per-

mit resolution of the lesions. Systemic antibiotics may be indicated in some cases. Some authors recommend removal of the ovary on the affected side in unilateral cases to ensure that ovulation occurs only ipsilateral to the patent uterine tube, but others suggest that surgical removal may not be of benefit. *In vitro* fertilization of ova harvested from affected cows may be a therapeutic possibility. The prognosis for reproduction in cases of bilateral occlusion of the uterine tubes is poor.

Because many of the causes of uterine tube disease are iatrogenic, the clinician should refrain from any of the treatments or practices that contribute to the problem. These include: traumatic manipulation of the ovaries (enucleation of corpora lutea and intentional rupture of ovarian cysts); infusion of large volumes of fluid or irritating chemicals into the uterus; and the administration of large doses of exogenous estrogens that may cause violent uterine contractions and force infected exudate into the uterine tubes.

Retained Placenta

Cows that retain the placenta for more than 12 h after calving are more likely to develop uterine disease than are cows that do not retain their placenta. However, those cows that rapidly return to normal following a retained placenta are as fertile as their herdmates indicating that, in the absence of a subsequent reproductive tract abnormality, retained placenta has a minimal effect on reproductive performance.

Prevalence

Retained placenta is more common in dairy than in beef breeds and the prevalence ranges from 8 to 12% following spontaneous delivery of single calves. The prevalence of retained placenta is higher following delivery of male calves and twins and following deliveries complicated by dystocia. Delivery of a calf outside the normal gestation length (shortened or prolonged) is accompanied by an increase in the prevalence of retained placenta.

Etiology

The cause of retained placenta is failure of the villi of the fetal cotyledon to detach from the crypts of the maternal caruncle. The loosening process normally begins during the last months of pregnancy. At term, rupture of the umbilical vessels interrupts the blood flow through the fetal placenta resulting in shrinkage of the villi. Strong uterine contractions during the third stage of labor and changes in shape of the maternal caruncles contribute to final separation of the placenta. The precise reason for failure of this separation process in apparently normal cows is not known. European workers have implicated lack of normal neutrophil invasion as a possible factor.

Clinical Signs

The clinical signs of retained placenta are usually obvious to the herder, but in some cases the placenta may be entirely within the genital tract. The majority of affected cows show no serious clinical signs other than a transient decrease in appetite and milk production. Some cows (20–25%) affected by retained placenta develop moderate to severe metritis (see page 98). The most objectionable clinical signs are the malodorous discharge and the unsightly mass of tissue hanging from the genital tract. Retained placentas are usually expelled by 7–10 days after calving when the caruncular tissue has become necrotic and sloughed.

Treatment of Retained Placenta

A variety of treatments has been advocated for retained placenta including aggressive attempts at manual removal, myometrial stimulants, intra-uterine and/or systemic antibiotics (alone or combined with manual removal), and no therapy whatsoever.

Manual Removal Most contemporary authors agree that manual removal of the placenta is indicated only when it may be accomplished by gentle traction, signifying that most or all of the placentomes have separated. Manual removal is specifically contraindicated when the patient shows any sign of toxemia or septicemia. Complete removal of the fetal membranes is nearly impossible and the trauma associated with the procedure inhibits phagocytosis by uterine neutrophils. Unfortunately, many herders are accustomed by tradition to manual removal and may insist on attempting the procedure to the detriment of the patient's health and future fertility.

Myometrial Stimulants Administration of oxytocin within the first 24–48 h after calving has been suggested to be of benefit in prompting expulsion of the placenta. However, treatment with a single dose of oxytocin does not reduce the prevalence of retained placenta in cows that calve normally nor in cows that require assistance at calving. Treatment with an estrogenic hormone immediately after calving may decrease fertility in cows with retained placenta. Furthermore, cows with a retained placenta have an elevated plasma concentration of estrogens during the period of retention. Treatment with estradiol benzoate after day 6 postpartum increases phagocytosis by uterine neutrophils and is not accompanied by undesirable side-effects. Retained placenta may be secondary to hypocalcemia in dairy cows and treatment with intravenous calcium solutions is indicated in those cases.

Antibiotics The results of treating cows affected by retained placenta with antibiotics are difficult to evaluate. The reproductive performance of cows with retained placenta treated with intrauterine tetracycline may be similar to unaffected herdmates or may be reduced by treatment. The prevalence of metritis associated with retained placenta may not be reduced by antibiotic therapy and pyometra may develop even in treated cows. Intrauterine antibiotics can reduce bacterial putrefaction and lysis of the villi, thereby reducing the disagreeable odor. The placenta will be freed upon necrosis of the caruncle which is unaffected by antibiotic treatment. A further complication of antibiotic therapy is the potential for depression of normal phagocytic activity by leukocytes.

Control and Prevention of Retained Placenta The prevalence of retained placenta can be reduced by providing an adequate dry period (6–8 weeks), a properly balanced ration (with special attention given to calcium, phosphorous, vitamins A and E, and selenium), exercise, reduction of stress, immunization when possible against infectious diseases that cause abortion, and a sanitary environment at parturition. Those cows that require treatment should be treated appropriately, and those that do not should be observed for any change in their condition.

POSTPARTUM UTERINE INFECTIONS

Infections of the uterus are more common in dairy than in beef cows, vary in severity from mild endometritis to toxic metritis, and may delay conception or lead to death of the affected animal. A number of factors influence the severity and prevalence of uterine infections including the species and pathogenicity of the causative organism, the cellular and immunological defenses and dietary management of the affected animal, and environmental sanitation.

They are particularly common if the placenta is retained and although a variety of bacteria has been implicated, *Actinomyces pyogenes* (formerly *Corynebacterium pyogenes*) is the organism most frequently involved.

A number of prospective studies have shed considerable light on the etiology and control of this condition. There is a high correlation between placental retention and metritis; some studies have indicated that only 16% of cows with metritis have not retained their placenta. The total incidence of metritis ranged from 8 to 20% in these studies. The retained placenta delays involution, thus facilitating uterine infection. However, the defect in neutrophil function reported to be associated with placental retention, also may be an important predisposing factor for metritis.

A number of specific diseases such as brucellosis and campylobacteriosis, which result in embryonic death, may cause metritis but these conditions are largely controlled.

Microbiology

The uterus of all cows is contaminated during parturition by microorganisms from the environment. A variety of bacteria can be isolated from the uterus of the cow during the 3 weeks after calving. Most of them are merely transient residents of the reproductive tract, soon eliminated from the involuting uterus in normal fertile cows, and any endometritis resolves prior to the time the cow is served. The flora often is composed of potentially pathogenic organisms including *Staphylococcus aureus* and α and β hemolytic streptococci as well as coagulase-negative staphylococci and nonhemolytic streptococci, but these organisms are usually rapidly eliminated after 10 days postpartum although some will progress to produce metritis.

In cows that develop uterine disease, *A. pyogenes* persists in the uterus and is a significant pathogen. A direct correlation has been found between the presence of *A. pyogenes* infection and metritis and it is found in over 40% of cases. Initially there is often a mixed infection but subsequently *A. pyogenes* is often isolated in pure culture. This organism is the predominant isolate from cows which fail to conceive to their first service after parturition.

In the early stages of *A. pyogenes* infection the endometritis is usually mild but if it persists for more than a week, a severe endometritis follows which may gradually clear after a month. In this case the uterine lesions progressively decline 3–4 weeks after the clearance of *A. pyogenes*. Many of these cows are subsequently fertile. When the infection is very persistent the endometritis progresses to metritis and

pyometra. Such cows may show prolonged infertility or even sterility.

In addition, gram-negative anaerobic bacteria are frequently isolated from cases of severe uterine disease. There appears to be synergism between *A. pyogenes* and *Fusobacterium* and *Bacteroides*, each enhancing the other's ability to cause uterine infections. *Clostridium* spp. occasionally colonize the anaerobic postpartum uterus causing severe toxic metritis. Other species of bacteria may be found in the uterus but they have little effect on fertility. These organisms may, however, produce penicillinase and influence the selection and route of administration of drugs used in treating uterine infections.

There is no evidence that cows with ovarian abnormalities are more susceptible, although there is often a persistent corpus luteum in cases of endometritis and pyometra. This is due to failure of the normal regression of a newly formed corpus luteum subsequent to the uterine infection. Endometritis has been associated with prolonged luteal activity and high concentrations of progesterone. In contrast, the high concentration of estrogen associated with estrus appears to increase the rate at which infections are eliminated and to accelerate the rate of repair. This may explain why conception rates are higher if the time of first service is delayed beyond 40 days postpartum.

Defenses

Bacteria are normally removed from the uterus through phagocytosis by neutrophils. Phagocytosis is depressed by an abnormal delivery (dead fetus and/or dystocia), by trauma to the uterus through obstetric manipulations or attempts to remove retained placentas, and by antiseptics and antibiotics.

The endogenous ovarian steroid hormones also affect the defense mechanism of the uterus. Leukocytosis is stimulated by estrogen and inhibited by progesterone. Cows that ovulate early in the postpartum period are more likely to develop pyometra because the endometrium is brought under the influence of progesterone before the infecting microorganisms are eliminated from the uterus.

Dietary Management

Uterine infections are more common in cows that are overfed during the dry period (fat cow syndrome), and in cows fed rations improperly balanced for calcium and phosphorous. Retained placenta (and subsequent metritis) is associated in some areas with deficiencies of selenium, and vitamins E and A.

Sanitation

The cleanliness of the calving environment has a major influence on the prevalence and outcome of cases of uterine infection. Dairy cows are often placed in maternity stalls when parturition is imminent. These areas are frequently heavily contaminated by pathogenic bacteria that gain access to the uterus during calving. Intervention in dystocia without strict attention to sanitation increases the probability of infection. Beef cows are less likely to develop uterine infections than are dairy cows because beef cows usually calve on uncontaminated pastures and less frequently suffer dystocia.

Normal Involution of the Uterus

The uterus of the cow continues to contract strongly for 48 h following delivery of the fetus. During this time (the third stage of labor), the placenta is usually shed and the majority of uterine fluid (lochia) is evacuated. Abnormalities of involution cannot be diagnosed by palpation per rectum during the first several days after calving when both normal and abnormal uteruses are out of the examiner's reach and cannot be safely retracted. By 10–15 days after calving, the entire uterus can be palpated if involution is normal. The previously gravid horn never returns to its original size but continues to be larger than the nongravid horn after involution is complete. The cervix involutes more slowly than does the uterus and is the last part of the tubular genital tract to undergo complete involution. Fluid should not be palpable within the lumen of the uterus by 14–18 days after calving if involution is normal. Gross reduction in size and histological repair of the endometrium are complete in dairy cows by 40–50 days after calving.

Lochia is normally expelled during the first 2 weeks after calving and may range in color from dark red or brown to white. If involution is delayed, discharge of lochia may continue until 30 days postpartum. The discharge of lochia should not be considered abnormal unless the fluid is fetid, continues to be discharged for longer than 30 days, or the cow develops other clinical signs. Reexamination of cows with a prolonged discharge of lochia at a later date will frequently reveal that involution has occurred and was simply delayed.

Types of Uterine Infection

Uterine infections range from mild to severe and may progress rapidly from less to more severe in naturally occurring cases and should progress from more to less severe during recovery. For purposes of discussion, infections of the uterus are divided into the following categories: endometritis, metritis and pyometra.

Endometritis

Endometritis is the least severe form of uterine disease and is characterized by inflammation of the uterine mucosa. Endometritis may be the primary lesion or the condition may progress rapidly to more severe forms of uterine disease. The bovine uterus is normally contaminated by a wide variety of microorganisms during the puerperium. Bacteria are removed from the endometrial cavity during the first few weeks after calving by phagocytosis which is enhanced by estrogen and inhibited by progesterone.

Clinical Signs   The first symptoms noticed in endometritis are usually the discharge of an excess of clear or white mucus. With *Actinomyces pyogenes* infection this tends to be purulent and has a characteristically foul odor. A clinical evaluation of the state of the uterus can be made by rectal examination. The size of the uterus, the thickness of the uterine wall and fluid content of the uterus are judged in relation to the number of days postpartum.

The clinical signs of endometritis range from slight opacity of the estrual mucus to slight enlargement of the uterus which may contain varying amounts of lochia. Purulent exudate may be observed in the cranial vagina and cervical canal by examination with a vaginal speculum. The history may indicate that the cow has failed to conceive after several services. The patient is otherwise healthy but may display a purulent vaginal discharge and the uterus may contain palpable fluid. Endometritis is usually diagnosed between 2 and 8 weeks after calving. Acute endometritis is characterized by infiltration of inflammatory cells while chronic lesions of endometritis include periglandular fibrosis and cystic dilatation of the endometrial glands. The prognosis for recovery from endometritis is usually good if the condition does not progress to more severe forms of uterine disease.

Metritis

Metritis is characterized by inflammation of all layers of the uterine wall. Retained placenta may or may not be associated with metritis. Metritis usually develops within a few days to 2 weeks after calving and may be accompanied by severe septicemia or toxemia (septic metritis). Metritis is usually a sequel to uterine inertia and delayed involution caused by prolonged dystocia, traumatic obstetric operations, uterine torsion or uterine eversion. A wide variety of bacteria have been isolated from cases of metritis, the most common being coliforms, *A. pyogenes*, *Pseudomonas aeruginosa*, hemolytic streptococci and staphylococci, and clostridia.

Clinical Signs The clinical signs of metritis vary with the number and virulence of the invading microorganisms. The affected cow may show signs of septicemia including depression, anorexia, inability to rise, and decreased milk yield. Early in the disease, the rectal temperature may be elevated but may be normal to subnormal if the case is neglected. Some cases may be complicated by tenesmus. Vaginal discharges vary from scanty white mucus to copious amounts of red to red-black watery material with a foul odor. Palpation per rectum will reveal the uterus to be enlarged and atonic. In some cases, the inflammation may spread through the uterine wall and cause peritonitis. Septic metritis should be differentiated from other conditions that cause involuntary recumbency during the postcalving period such as hypocalcemia, traumatic gastritis, and septic mastitis.

Treatment Initial treatment should be directed toward controlling the septicemia. Large systemic doses of broad-spectrum antibiotics are indicated along with fluids and supportive therapy. Attempts to remove a retained placenta or irrigate the uterus are contraindicated during the acute phase of the disease. After the patient has recovered from the acute septicemia, appropriate intrauterine therapy may be considered.

The course of septic metritis is usually short with recovery or death of the patient in 2–6 days. Sequels to the disease include laminitis, perimetritis, salpingitis, chronic endometritis and pyometra.

The prognosis for the life of the animal in cases of septic metritis is fair to poor and fatalities are frequent in spite of aggressive therapy. Future fertility may be compromised.

Pyometra

Pyometra in the cow is defined as the accumulation of a variable amount of purulent exudate within the lumen of the uterus and the persistence of a corpus luteum in one of the ovaries. Pyometra develops in cows that ovulate before the organisms infecting the uterus during the postpartum period are eliminated

by the normal defense mechanisms. The corpus luteum persists possibly because the abnormal uterine contents suspend the release of prostaglandin from the endometrium or sequester it within the uterine lumen. Thus, the uterus is brought under the prolonged influence of progesterone which, in turn, further depresses phagocytic activity of uterine neutrophils allowing the bacterial infection to persist. Cows affected with pyometra seldom display any clinical signs; however, a purulent vaginal discharge may be observed in a few cases. Usually the presenting complaint in cases of pyometra is anestrus caused by persistence of the corpus luteum. The uterine enlargement is differentiated from that caused by pregnancy by the character of the fluid within the uterus and the thickness of the uterine wall. Fetal fluids are not as viscous as those associated with pyometra and the wall of the pregnant uterus is thinner and more resilient than that in a case of pyometra. In addition, the examiner must determine that the positive signs of pregnancy (fetal membrane slip, amniotic vesicle, placentomes, and fetus) are not present. Cases of pyometra that occur during the postbreeding period may be caused by *Tritrichomonas fetus*, a protozoan transmitted venereally among cattle. The prognosis for recovery from pyometra is fair to good, especially if diagnosed early in the course of the disease.

Treatment of Uterine Infections

A number of hormones, antibiotics, and antiseptics have been advocated for treatment of uterine infections in cows. Unfortunately, many of the recommendations have been based on uncontrolled observations, leading one author to conclude that '... many cows become pregnant in spite of rather than because of treatment'.

There is still much dispute over the value of the treatment available for chronic endometritis as many cases will recover spontaneously with the reestablishment of estrous cycles.

Antibacterial Drugs

The use of intrauterine antibiotics is advocated by some, but evidence for their efficacy is difficult to find. A very wide range of antibiotics has been used often in insufficient amounts. Parenteral administration of antibiotics for several days may be better but is not popular with farmers as cattle are usually in peak production when treatment is required.

Examination of uterine swabs for the presence of *A. pyogenes* or other pathogens might assist in better selection of antibiotics to be used and an improvement in the outcome in treatment. Interpretation of culture results is difficult, however, due to frequent contamination from the vaginal or cervical bacterial flora.

To be useful in treating uterine infections, an antibacterial drug must be active against the primary uterine pathogens (*A. pyogenes* and gram-negative anaerobes); it must reach concentrations at the site of infection above the minimum inhibitory concentration (MIC) for the infecting organism; it must be active in the presence of organic debris, and in the anaerobic environment of the postpartum bovine uterus.

The organisms infecting the uterus are usually sensitive to penicillin but during the first 4 weeks after calving, contaminating microorganisms produce penicillinase. Thus, *penicillin* would not likely be effective if given locally during the early postpartum period but would be useful if given systematically. By 30 days after calving, the organisms that produce penicillinase are usually eliminated from the uterus and intrauterine treatment with penicillin is beneficial. Daily doses of penicillin that have been recommended to reach the MIC are 5000–10 000 i.u./kg systematically, and 1 000 000 i.u. by intrauterine infusion.

Oxytetracycline is a broad spectrum antibiotic active against many of the microorganisms that infect the bovine uterus. The activity of oxytetracycline is only slightly reduced by organic debris and the absence of oxygen. The MIC of oxytetracycline for *A. pyogenes* is usually higher than the concentration that can be achieved by systemic administration of the drug. Thus, intrauterine infusion of oxytetracycline might be considered in treating uterine infections but systemic administration of the drug is not indicated. Some preparations of oxytetracycline irritate the endometrium, cervix, and vagina and should be used with care or avoided.

Sulfonamides are inactivated by organic debris and are a poor choice for intrauterine therapy. Systemic administration of sulfonamides might be indicated in some cases.

The *aminoglycoside antibiotics* are not active in an aerobic environment and are thus not indicated in the treatment of uterine disease. *Nitrofurazone* has been recommended for use in treating uterine infections, but it is nearly impossible to achieve MIC for the infecting microorganisms at the site of infection, the chemical is irritating, and it has been shown to reduce fertility in treated cows.

Many antibiotics and antiseptic chemicals interfere with the normal uterine defense mechanism by reducing phagocytosis; thus, the potential benefits of intrauterine therapy must be weighed against the potential for adverse effects. Based on the usual antibiotic sensitivity of the microorganisms commonly isolated from cases of uterine disease, the characteristics of the antibiotics, and the environment of the uterus, the most reasonable therapy (when treatment with antibiotics is indicated) for uterine infections in cows is intrauterine administration of a nonirritating preparation of oxytetracycline and/or systemic administration of penicillin during the early postcalving period and intrauterine and/or systemic administration of penicillin after 30 days postpartum. Treatment of dairy cows results in residues in the milk from treated animals and appropriate withdrawal times must be observed.

Hormones

Various hormone preparations have been used to treat uterine infections both alone and in combination with antibacterial drugs. Much treatment is aimed at providing luteal regression and estrus; the use of exogenous prostaglandin to achieve this may have a valuable effect on the clinical condition.

Endogenous estrogen associated with the follicular phase of the estrous cycle has a beneficial effect on phagocytosis by uterine neutrophils. The common practices of allowing a period of sexual rest or shortening the estrous cycle with serial administration of PGF prior to attempts at breeding as methods of treating uterine infections are based on this effect. Exogenous estrogens, however, are of limited benefit in treating uterine infections and may, in some cases, be harmful, although it has been claimed that where no corpus luteum is present, the use of exogenous estrogen to mimic natural estrus can be successful, and the use of estradiol benzoate (10 mg) gives results at least as good as those of prostaglandin if given in the first 40 days after calving.

Treatment of cows with gonadotropin releasing hormone (GnRH) at 2 weeks after calving has been shown to improve fertility in some, but not all, trials. In herds with a high prevalence of postpartum uterine disease, treatment with GnRH may decrease fertility by increasing the prevalence of pyometra.

Prostaglandin $F_{2\alpha}$ (or its synthetic analogs) is the treatment of choice for bovine pyometra. Treatment with PGF is followed in 3–9 days by uterine evacuation in 85–90% of treated cows. After endometrial lesions are allowed 30 days to heal, fertility is restored in most patients. In cases of chronic metritis, treatment with PGF one or two times at 10–14 day intervals decreases the number of days open.

The use of Lugol's solution of iodine (one part of

Lugol's solution in 400 of water), to irrigate the uterus in cases of endometritis has in the past been a favorite method of treatment. Up to 150 ml of solution can be safely injected. The beneficial efffect has been attributed to the ability of Lugol's iodine to stimulate the endometrial stroma by increasing the blood supply leading to increased neutrophil infiltration and production of macrophages. However, this has never been shown to be true and there is no good reason to continue using this irrational method of treatment.

The spontaneous recovery of many cows makes evaluation of all methods of treatment difficult.

Control and Prevention of Uterine Infections

Cows that suffer from abnormalities around the time of calving such as hypocalcemia, dystocia, and retained placenta are more likely to suffer from uterine diseases than are cows that calve normally. Affected cows should be observed closely for abnormal clinical signs and treated appropriately. Routine treatment of cows with antibacterial drugs and chemicals has not been shown to be beneficial and in some cases has reduced fertility. Single intrauterine treatments with antibiotics do not shorten the time required for recovery from the uterine disease. Postpartum uterine infections may be prevented or the number of such infections reduced by strict sanitation in the calving environment and during assistance with delivery along with proper management during the dry period. This approach will probably be more successful than attempts to treat uterine disease with antibacterial drugs.

Perimetritis

Perimetritis may be a sequel to severe metritis, uterine rupture, perforation of the vagina by the penis of a bull, traumatic obstetric procedures, and Cesarean section. Perimetritis is characterized by inflammation of the peritoneal surface of the uterus and may be accompanied by local or diffuse peritonitis followed by development of adhesions between the uterus and the broad ligaments or other abdominal organs. The condition should be differentiated from abdominal fat necrosis and traumatic gastritis. Lesions range from a few minor strands of connective tissue to severe and extensive adhesions. Signs of peritonitis early in the course of the disease should be treated aggressively with systemic antibacterial drugs. The prognosis depends upon the extent of the lesions. Fatalities can occur in cases of vaginal rupture because the affected animals may not be presented for treatment until peritonitis is advanced.

Severely affected animals are frequently rendered sterile.

Abscess of the Uterine Wall

Abscesses of the uterine wall may follow severe metritis or traumatic manipulations such as artificial insemination, embryo recovery, or embryo transfer. Abscesses of various sizes are detected by palpation per rectum and must be differentiated from uterine neoplasms. This condition is frequently accompanied by infertility. Treatment is usually unrewarding but systemic antibiotics may be indicated in some cases. Spontaneous drainage may lead to recovery if the abscess ruptures into the lumen of the uterus or rectum, but may lead to peritonitis if it ruptures into the peritoneal cavity.

Cervicitis

Inflammation of the cervix commonly accompanies metritis or may be due to chronic irritation associated with pneumovagina and urovagina. Cervicitis may also be induced by injudicious attempts to pass instruments through the cervical canal. The clinical signs of cervicitis observed through a vaginal speculum include swelling and edema of the external cervical os, hyperemia of the mucosa, and the presence of mucopurulent exudate within the cervical canal and cranial vagina. Prolapse of the caudal one or two cervical rings is common in pluriparous animals and is not thought to contribute substantially to infertility, although some authors have suggested that prolapsed cervical rings be amputated. Hypertrophy of the cervix is a normal consequence of parturition in *Bos indicus* cows and their crosses. Chronic and severe irritation of the cervix by caustic chemicals or pathogenic bacteria may lead to fibrosis and stenosis of the cervix and cause infertility in nonpregnant cows and severe obstructive dystocia in cows pregnant at the time of the insult.

Treatment of cervicitis should be directed towards removal of the cause of the irritation. Spontaneous recovery may occur after a period of sexual rest. Cases of cervicitis associated with metritis usually respond to the treatments indicated for the primary disease while those caused by pneumovagina and urovagina are treated with the appropriate surgical procedure, episioplasty or urethroplasty, respectively. Caustic chemicals should never be placed in contact with the cervical mucosa.

Cervical (Nabothian) Cysts

Retention cysts may develop when the duct of a cervical gland is occluded. These fluid-filled cysts may reach several centimeters in diameter, are usually benign, and may be easily treated by surgical drainage.

Vaginitis

Inflammation of the vagina may be secondary to metritis and pneumovagina or may be caused by traumatic obstetric operations such as forced extraction or fetotomy. Other causes of vaginitis include the infectious bovine rhinotracheitis–infectious pustular vulvovaginitis (IBR–IPV) virus and the bovine venereal diseases which are discussed in Chapters 11, 13 and 16. The clinical signs of vaginitis vary with the severity of the insult, and range from a cloudy mucus discharge and hyperemia of the vaginal mucosa to necrosis of the vaginal mucosa accompanied by tenesmus, cellulitis, and septicemia. In severe cases, the animal's life may be threatened.

Treatment should be directed toward removal of the cause of irritation, control of tenesmus with epidural anesthesia, appropriate surgical correction of vulvar defects and urovagina, and systemic antibiotics and other supportive treatment as indicated in cases of septicemia. Fibrosis may follow severe vaginitis, necessitating delivery by Cesarean section should the animal conceive again.

Perineal Lacerations

Lacerations of the perineal tissue are classified by their depth and the degree of tissue destruction. Superficial lacerations of the vaginal and vulvar mucosa are first-degree lacerations while those that involve the entire wall of the vagina and vulva are second-degree lacerations. Lacerations that involve the entire thickness of the vagina, rectum, perineal body, and anal sphincter resulting in a common opening of the genital and digestive tracts are third-degree lacerations. Rectovaginal fistulae may be encountered but are less common in the cow than in the mare. Most perineal lacerations occur in conjunction with forced extraction of an oversized fetus or delivery of a fetus through an inadequately lubricated or dilated birth canal. Both first-degree and second-degree lacerations are usually treated with local antiseptic and emollient creams. Systemic antibiotics are indicated in cases of necrotic vaginitis. Indications for surgery include removal of necrotic perivaginal fat and correction of malocclusion of the vulvar labia with episioplasty. Third-degree lacerations are best treated by local application of emollients until swelling and necrosis of the injured

tissue subsides at about 6 weeks after the insult. At that time surgical correction of the defect can be accomplished by the procedure of the operator's choice. Most cows with perineal lacerations are infertile due to chronic irritation of the vagina and cervix until the condition is corrected. The prognosis for fertility after surgical correction is generally fair to good.

Vaginal Prolapse

Prolapse of the vagina most frequently occurs during late gestation and the early postpartum period. The condition may be associated with previous injury of the tissues, intake of large volumes of poor quality forage, and excessive perivaginal fat. Although the condition occurs sporadically in all breeds of cattle, vaginal prolapse is more common in Holsteins than other dairy breeds and a hereditary predisposition has been suggested in Herefords.

In the early stages of vaginal prolapse, the floor of the vagina is everted only when the cow is recumbent and returns to its normal position when the cow rises. Continued irritation by contaminants and dessication lead, in most cases, to constant eversion of the vaginal mucosa. The prolapsed mass may contain the retroverted urinary bladder. Rectal prolapse may accompany neglected cases.

The goals in treating vaginal prolapse are to return the tissue to its normal position, maintain the vagina in its normal position, and allow unimpeded delivery of the fetus. Replacement of the prolapsed tissue usually requires epidural anesthesia. The prolapsed mass is washed as gently as possible, coated with a lubricating ointment and massaged into place. Catheterization and draining of the urinary bladder may be required should that organ be filled with urine and included within the prolapsed mass. Persistence and patience are required in longstanding cases.

Once the vagina has been replaced, the operator is faced with choosing a method of retaining the prolapsed tissue in its normal position. While several dozen different methods have been described for correction of vaginal prolapses, several contemporary authors have expressed a preference for the method in which, under epidural anesthesia, a special needle is used to place a loop of nylon tape in the subcutaneous tissue around the vulva. Close observation of the affected cow for signs of impending parturition is mandatory. In cases where the breeding date is accurately known, the clinician may consider the artificial induction of parturition with corticosteroids or prostaglandin $F_{2\alpha}$ (PGF). The tape is cut or untied to allow delivery and can be replaced after calving to prevent postpartum vaginal prolapse. Although it is frequently recommended that affected cows be culled from the herd because the condition will likely occur during the next gestation and may be hereditary, the tape can be left in place for several months in cows that are to be retained in the herd. Natural service and artificial insemination are not impeded by a properly placed suture. The fibrous tissue deposited in response to the tape is frequently sufficient to prevent further prolapses and may indeed be sufficient to cause obstructive dystocia at the next parturition.

NEOPLASMS OF THE GENITAL TRACT

Ovarian Tumors

A variety of ovarian neoplasms have been described in cows including carcinomas, dysgerminomas, and ovarian teratomas. However, the most commonly described ovarian neoplasm in the cow is the granulosal-thecal cell tumor. Granulosal-thecal cell tumors are generally unilateral and benign. Older animals are more commonly affected but granulosal-thecal cell tumors have been seen in heifer calves less than 1 year of age. The clinical signs depend upon the steroid hormones produced by the tumor and range from nymphomania to anestrus to virilism. Udder development and lactation may occur in heifers with granulosal-thecal cell tumors. The affected ovary may range from slightly larger than normal to several kilograms. The ipsilateral ovary is usually small and inactive; however, cows are reported to become pregnant even when unilateral granulosal-thecal cell tumors are present. The treatment suggested for these tumors is surgical removal of the affected ovary although there is little information on the subsequent fertility of affected animals.

Tumors of the Tubular Genital Organs

Neoplasms of the tubular genital organs of the cow appear to be rare. Leiomyomas arise from the myometrium, are usually solitary, and benign. Endometrial carcinomas may be single or multiple, vary in size, and may metastasize to regional lymph nodes and the lungs. Bovine leukosis may involve the uterus with diffuse or nodular lesions of the uterine horns or body. The clinician should be aware of the possibility of uterine tumors and should not mistake a neoplastic lesion for one of the positive signs of pregnancy (placentome or fetus).

OVULATORY DEFECTS

Delayed Ovulation

Cows are unique among the common farm animals in that they ovulate spontaneously after the signs of estrus have ended. Ovulation occurs an average of 12 h after the end of behavioral estrus (range 2–26 h). Delayed ovulation has been suggested as a cause of infertility in cows but the condition appears to be infrequent. Examination of cows suspected of being infertile because of delayed ovulation at 24 h after the end of estrus and reinsemination of those that have not yet ovulated has been advocated. This procedure may not be of benefit since some normal cows may not have ovulated by 24 h after the end of estrus and the operator may not be able to differentiate accurately between a soft preovulatory follicle and a developing corpus hemorrhagicum. Another mode of therapy that has been suggested for delayed ovulation is administration of GnRH at the time of insemination (see page 111).

Cystic Ovarian Disease

Cystic ovarian disease (COD) is an important cause of abnormal estrous behavior and infertility in dairy cows. Among the synonyms that have been used for the condition are cystic follicular degeneration, cystic graafian follicles, ovarian cysts, luteal ovarian cysts, and 'cystic cows'.

Ovarian cysts are defined as follicle-like ovarian structures that are 2.5 cm in diameter or larger and persist for 10 days or more in the absence of a corpus luteum. Pathologic ovarian cysts may occur as single or multiple structures on one or both ovaries. While a single large cyst is most common, some cows may have smaller multiple and multilocular cysts. Ovarian cysts may be thin-walled (follicular cysts) or have thickened areas in the wall due to partial luteinization of granulosa cells (luteinized cysts).

Cystic corpora lutea are nonpathologic ovarian cysts, defined as corpora lutea that contain a fluid-filled central cavity of varying size. An ovulatory papilla may be palpable on the surface of cystic corpora lutea. Cystic corpora lutea are capable of normal progesterone synthesis and do not alter the length of the estrous cycle.

Prevalence

The reported prevalence of COD in dairy cows ranges from 10 to 30%. The disease may occur in beef breeds of cattle but appears to be rare. An increased prevalence of COD has been associated with stresses such as retained placenta, metritis, and hypocalcemia around the time of parturition. Cows affected with COD tend to produce more milk than their herdmates. Cystic ovarian disease is a significant cause of reproductive inefficiency because the interval from calving to first service is prolonged in affected cows.

Etiology

Cystic ovarian disease appears to be caused by the inadequate release of gonadotropins and/or ovarian dysfunction that results in failure of ovulation, but the exact mechanism by which cysts develop is not known, although a hereditary predisposition has been suggested. The development of COD before the first postpartum ovulation may be explained by the hypothesis that the hypothalmic–hypophyseal axis may not be responsive to estradiol secreted by follicles that may begin to develop as early as 1 week after calving in dairy cows. Alternatively, there may be insufficient luteinizing hormone (LH) stores in the anterior pituitary to provide an ovulatory stimulus. The lack of an ovulation-inducing LH surge in response to estradiol would result in failure of ovulation. This hypothesis does not, however, explain the development of COD in cows that have previously had normal estrous cycles. There is probably no single cause of all cases of COD; indeed, COD may be a clinical sign with multiple causes.

Clinical Signs

The behavior of cows with COD ranges from anestrus (lack of detectable estrous behavior) to nymphomania (frequent and/or intense estrous behavior). Early descriptions of the condition indicate that nymphomania was the more common behavioral change; however, more recent reports indicate that approximately 70–80% of cows with COD are anestrous while the remaining 20–30% display nymphomania.

The physical appearance of cows with COD depends upon the length of time the condition has existed. In cases of short duration, there are no obvious changes, whereas in longstanding cases relaxation of the pelvic ligaments results in a prominent appearance of the tailhead ('sterility hump'), along with the development of masculine characteristics such as a crested neck.

Diagnosis

The diagnosis of COD is based on a history from accurate reproductive records and clinical examina-

tion. A history of constant or frequent estrus, short interestrous intervals, or anestrus is consistent with a diagnosis of COD.

Palpation per rectum of the ovaries reveals the presence of fluid-filled, round, cystic structures raised above the surface of the ovary. Ovarian cysts are larger than preovulatory follicles; cysts up to 5 cm in diameter or larger are not uncommon. The thickness of the wall of the cyst is variable, ranging from the easily ruptured thin wall of follicular cysts to thicker walls in cysts that are partially luteinized. The examiner may not be able to differentiate between a single large cyst or several smaller cysts on the same ovary. Recognition of the presence of partial luteinization of follicular cysts (based on peripheral concentrations of progesterone) by palpation per rectum is inaccurate.

Ovarian cysts appear to be dynamic structures. Those that occur early in the postpartum period often regress without treatment, and a normal estrous cycle may follow or another cystic structure may develop.

Endocrine Profile

Plasma progesterone concentrations are low in cows with simple follicular cysts but are higher in cows with partially luteinized cysts. Ovarian cysts may undergo partial luteinization, and progesterone concentrations may increase over time but remain lower than those of cows with normal corpora lutea. The concentrations of estrogen in the plasma of cows with COD are variable and may be similar to or higher than those of normal cows. Testosterone concentrations in the plasma of cows with follicular and luteal cysts are similar to those found during the normal estrous cycle. Concentrations of LH in cows with COD are generally higher than those of normal cows and are inversely correlated to concentrations of plasma progesterone.

Differential Diagnosis

Several normal ovarian structures may complicate the diagnosis of COD by palpation of the ovaries. A normal preovulatory follicle may approach 2.5 cm in diameter and have palpable characteristics similar to those of a small follicular cyst. The palpable uterine changes during the follicular phase of the estrous cycle may aid the clinician in differentiating a normal follicle from a small cyst. During estrus the uterus is characterized by increased tone and responsiveness to palpation while the uterine tone of a cow with COD is similar to that found during diestrus. Mucometra may develop in cases of COD that are neglected for a long time, and the uterine enlargement caused by the accumulation of mucus must be differentiated from pregnancy.

Corpora lutea in various stages of development and regression may be confused with ovarian cysts. During the first 5–7 days of the estrous cycle, the corpus hemorrhagicum is smooth and soft. As the corpus luteum matures, it becomes more liverlike in consistency and is more easily differentiated from an ovarian cyst. Sequential examinations may be useful in differentiating ovarian cysts from corpora lutea. Normal and cystic corpora lutea are characterized by an ovulation papilla, which is frequently palpable.

Causes of ovarian enlargement that must be differentiated from ovarian cysts include adhesions between the ovary and the surrounding structures, salpingitis, hydrosalpinx, oophoritis, ovarian abscesses, ovarian neoplasia, and cysts of the fimbria. Histories that may erroneously suggest COD include mistaken detection of estrus during the luteal phase of the estrous cycle and shortened interestrous intervals caused by daily administration of oxytocin during metestrus and early diestrus for the purpose of stimulating milk letdown.

Treatment

The goal in treating COD is to induce luteinization of the cyst and reestablish normal ovarian cycles. Treatments suggested for COD include spontaneous recovery, manual rupture, LH, GnRH, and PGF.

Spontaneous Recovery Spontaneous recovery from COD is more likely in cases that occur during the first 30 days after calving. As many as 60% of cows that develop COD prior to the first postpartum ovulation may spontaneously initiate normal ovarian cycles. In contrast, spontaneous recovery may be expected in only 20% of cases that develop after the first postpartum ovulation. The phenomenon of spontaneous recovery may confound the evaluation of therapeutic agents.

Manual Rupture One of the earliest treatments described for COD is manual rupture of the cystic structure(s) by palpation per rectum. Thin-walled follicular cysts may be easily ruptured and unintentional rupture may occur during examination of the ovary. The rates of recovery following manual rupture vary and generally are within the range reported for spontaneous recovery, although some are higher. The procedure may be less effective if the condition is prolonged. Hemorrhage and adhesions may follow manual rupture which could further

contribute to infertility. Although manual rupture has been advocated as a useful treatment for COD, effective pharmacological treatments are available, and many clinicians believe that manual rupture of ovarian cysts is an archaic form of treatment

Luteinizing Hormone Preparations high in LH-like activity have been effectively used to treat COD for several decades. Human chorionic gonadotropin (hCG) and pituitary extracts from sheep and swine are common sources of exogenous LH. Recommended doses of hCG range from 5000 i.u. given either intravenously (i.v.) or intramuscularly (i.m.) to 10 000 i.u. given i.m. Luteal tissue develops either by luteinization of the cyst or other follicles with or without ovulation in cows that respond to treatment with LH. Luteinization and secretion of progesterone in response to LH may be monitored by measurement of progesterone in the milk or plasma of treated cows. Following a single treatment with LH, 65–80% of treated cows develop a normal estrous period within 20–30 days. A second or third treatment may be required in cases that do not respond within 3–4 weeks or where nymphomania persists. Cows that exhibit a normal estrus after treatment should be inseminated. Those cows that do not conceive or those from which service is withheld may develop subsequent ovarian cysts.

Although anaphylaxis appears to be uncommon following treatment with LH, such reactions to protein hormones are possible. Another undesirable response is the development of antibodies that may diminish the effectiveness of subsequent treatments. The use of different LH products at subsequent treatments is suggested if the clinician is concerned about antibody formation.

Gonadotropin Releasing Hormone Synthetic GnRH is the most recently introduced product for treatment of COD. Exogenous GnRH acts on the pituitary gland to stimulate the release of endogenous LH. Response of cows to GnRH appears to vary with the dose administered. In the United States, the standard dose of GnRH is 100 µg/cow. Following treatment with this dose, concentrations of plasma progesterone increase due to luteinization of the cyst. When GnRH is used at doses of 0.5–1.5 mg, some cows respond with luteinization of the cyst, while others respond with ovulation and luteinization of follicles present at the time of treatment. Most cows that respond to treatment with GnRH display estrus 18–23 days after treatment.

Anaphylaxis following treatment with GnRH has not been reported. Antibody formation is unlikely due to the small molecular weight of GnRH, so

GnRH may have some advantage over hCG in treatment of COD. Even though GnRH shortens the interval from treatment to estrus, inadequate breeding practices on some farms may contribute to continued infertility in treated cows.

Prostaglandin $F_{2\alpha}$ Ovarian cysts that luteinize in response to GnRH administration appear to undergo regression at a time similar to that of normal corpora lutea. The luteolytic activity of PGF may be used to reduce the interval from treatment with GnRH to the first estrus from 18 to 23 days to an average of 12 days by administering PGF on day 9 after GnRH treatment. Fertility of cows given PGF 9 days after GnRH is similar to that of cows given only GnRH.

Cows with partially luteinized cysts respond favorably to initial treatment with a luteolytic dose of PGF. Unfortunately, most clinicians are only about 50% accurate in determining the degree of luteinization of the cyst by palpation per rectum. Measurement of the concentration of progesterone in the plasma or milk of affected cows allows the clinician to select accurately GnRH or hCG for treatment of cows with follicular cysts and PGF for treatment of cows with luteinized cysts. If progesterone assays are not available, initial treatment of COD with GnRH (or hCG) should be followed by treatment with PGF 9–14 days later.

Control and Prevention of Cystic Ovarian Disease

The clinician must determine the optimum time for treating COD based on the expected frequency of spontaneous recovery, the number of days since parturition, and the intervals between scheduled examinations. Spontaneous recovery is more common in the early postpartum period (< 30 days) but it may be more expensive to wait for spontaneous recovery than to treat the condition at the time of diagnosis.

Treatment of cows with GnRH 12–14 days after calving reduces the prevalence of COD under some management conditions, and the number of cows culled for infertility. Although reduction in the prevalence of COD would require several generations due to the low heritability of the condition, breeding of dairy cows to bulls whose offspring have been shown to have a low prevalence of COD and culling of affected cows and their daughters should be considered as a method of control. Use of genetic selection to reduce the prevalence of COD in the national dairy herd has been effective in Sweden where artificial insemination centers have selected bulls only from cows with no history of COD.

Multiple Ovulations

Pregnancy rates are lower in cows with multiple ovulations than in cows with single ovulations. This form of infertility in cows may be due to an endocrine imbalance that results in multiple ovulations in a normally monotocous animal or to defects of the ova. Twinning is undesirable in cattle under most conditions, so the infertility associated with multiple ovulations may be a protective mechanism.

FUNCTIONAL INFERTILITY

Infertility in dairy herds results in reduced milk production and income for the producer, increased involuntary culling, and increased costs for replacement animals as well as semen and drugs. Similarly, in beef herds infertility results in reduced income due to fewer and/or lighter weight calves available for sale at weaning.

Anestrus

A common problem in bovine reproduction is failure of the cow to display, or the herder to observe, the normal signs of estrus. When artificial insemination is used, the more common problem is failure to observe estrus, while in herds using natural service infertility may be due to failure of the cow to have a normal estrous cycle. When the history given by the herder suggests anestrus (failure to cycle), the clinician must determine if the problem of anestrus is due to failure to detect estrus in normal cows or suspension of the estrous cycle due to some pathological process. In dairy herds, approximately 90% of the anestrous cases presented for examination are due to unobserved estrus while only about 10% are due to an abnormality that suspends the estrous cycle.

Unobserved Estrus

Failure to detect estrus accurately is an important cause of delayed insemination and prolonged calving intervals. Twice as much time is lost due to failure to detect estrus as is lost due to conception failure. Nearly 90% of dairy cows initiate normal-length estrous cycles by 60 days after calving, but only about 60% are detected correctly in estrus by that time. For efficient detection of estrus the herder must be able to recognize multiple signs of proestrus and estrus, have sufficient time to observe all animals, and observe the herd for signs of estrus at least twice daily. Rates of detection by twice-daily observation vary with the skill of the observer and range from 50 to 70%, with observers able to identify more accurately those cows showing strong signs of estrus.

At the onset of estrus cows become more active and spend less time grazing and ruminating; milk yield usually declines. The single definitive behavioral characteristic of estrus is standing immobile while being mounted by a bull or female herdmate. Secondary signs of estrus include increased switching of the tail, frequent urination, aggressive behavior toward herdmates (butting), investigative behavior (sniffing, rubbing, licking, and chin-resting), and disoriented mounting.

Estrous behavior is more common between 1800 and 0600 h than between 0600 and 1800 h and more mounts per hour occur in the evening than in the morning. The average number of mounts per hour ranges from two to eight and the total number of mounts during estrus ranges from 11 to 56. The number of mounts during estrus increases with increasing numbers of cows simultaneously in estrus. Thus, grouping of cows by production level is beneficial since the highest milk yield usually occurs during the early postpartum period when most cows are not pregnant.

Environmental factors affect the display of estrous behavior. Estrous behavior and mounting activity are reduced by hot and cold ambient temperatures and during milking and feeding times. Slippery surfaces reduce mounting activity; nearly twice as many mounts are observed in cows on a dirt surface as are observed in cows on a concrete surface.

Various aids have been used in attempts to improve detection of estrus. Increased physical activity associated with estrus can be measured by the use of pedometers, and the efficiency and accuracy of detection improved; but pedometers may not be a practical method because of the cost of the apparatus and the need for frequent repairs. Pressure-sensitive mount detectors and tailhead paint and measurement of changes in vaginal pH, vaginal temperature, milk yield, and heart rate may be useful aids to detection of estrus by directing the herder's attention to cows that are expected to be in estrus, but these are not as accurate as simple observation of cows standing to be mounted. Electronic vaginal probes may be a useful adjunct under some management situations, but are too labor-intensive in large herds and may not be a practical aid in timing insemination. Expectancy charts and accurate records of individual reproductive histories are also useful aids in the detection of estrus. Observation of cows for standing estrus, at least twice daily,

for a sufficient length of time to observe all animals, is the most reliable and practical method. Insemination of cows on the basis of standing to be mounted results in a higher pregnancy rate than does insemination on the basis of secondary signs of estrus.

Insemination during the luteal phase of the estrous cycle is not likely to result in conception; however, mistaken identification of cows in estrus may be a problem in some herds. Insemination of pregnant cows erroneously thought to be in estrus may be followed by abortion. Herds in which infertility is due to inaccurate detection of estrus are usually characterized by one or more of the following: prolonged interval between calving and first service; prolonged intervals between services; breeding intervals of 10–15 days and 30–35 days; examinations that confirm that progressive ovarian changes occur but estrus is not observed; and more than 10–15% of the cows are found to be nonpregnant when examined at 35–50 days after breeding.

Treatment of Unobserved Estrus   Prior to the 1970s, a number of drugs and hormones were used to treat unobserved estrus, but critical evaluation showed that none were superior to the prediction of the time of the next estrus following palpation of the temporary ovarian structures by an experienced clinician. More recently, PGF has been widely used in the clinical management of unobserved estrus in dairy cows. Treatment with PGF shortens the intervals from treatment to first breeding and from treatment to conception, but does not affect fertility.

The effectiveness of PGF in the clinical management of unobserved estrus can be limited by inaccurate palpation, failure of the cow to respond to the drug, and failure of the herder to detect estrus in treated cows. Although treating cows with PGF is no more effective than efficient observation for estrus in reducing the time from calving to conception, PGF treatment makes the time required for observation more compact.

The response of cows to PGF appears to vary with the stage of diestrus at the time of treatment. Cows treated in early diestrus (days 5–7) may respond less frequently than cows in middle (days 8–11) or late (days 12–15) diestrus. However, those that do respond to PGF treatment during early diestrus may have a shorter and less variable interval from treatment to estrus than those that respond to treatment in middle or late diestrus. The pregnancy rate in PGF-treated cows with an aged corpus luteum is higher than that in cows with a young corpus luteum. This variation in response can be expected to reduce fertility when cows are inseminated at a predetermined time after treatment without detection of estrus (insemination by appointment), and may reduce the number of cows responding to the second dose of PGF if a two-dose synchronization scheme is used. Single or multiple doses of PGF do not reduce subsequent fertility of cows that do not conceive when estrus is induced. Accurate examination for pregnancy must precede treatment with PGF because misuse of PGF will induce abortion when cows are pregnant at the time of treatment.

Milk Progesterone Assays Enzyme immunoassays (EIA) for measuring concentrations of progesterone in milk and plasma can be used to aid in the diagnosis and clinical management of a variety of reproductive abnormalities. The corpus luteum is a temporary endocrine organ that secretes progesterone during most of the estrous cycle and during pregnancy in the cow. The secretory activity of the corpus luteum can be monitored by measurement of progesterone concentrations in plasma, or in milk which, although higher, parallel those in plasma (Fig. 6.1a). These assays are sensitive and specific, do not require the use of specialized equipment, trained personnel, or radioactive chemicals, and the results are rapidly available and correlated with those of validated radioimmunoassays.

One of the earliest practical applications of milk progesterone assays was early pregnancy diagnosis. Progesterone secreted by the corpus luteum is required to maintain pregnancy throughout most of the gestation period; so cows with elevated concentrations of progesterone in their milk may be pregnant, and those with low concentrations of progesterone in their milk or plasma are not likely to be pregnant. In most schemes for pregnancy diagnosis, a milk sample is taken at the time of the first expected postservice estrus (or some multiple thereof) and the progesterone concentration measured (Fig. 6.1b). Cows with high concentrations of progesterone in their milk are assumed to be pregnant while those with low concentrations are assumed to be nonpregnant. Measurement of the progesterone concentration in a single milk sample taken between 20 and 24 days after service is 70–80% accurate in identifying pregnant cows and nearly 100% accurate in identifying nonpregnant cows. Therefore, measurement of milk progesterone concentrations at the first expected postservice estrus should be considered to be an accurate indicator of nonpregnancy.

Successful service can take place only during a short time during the estrous cycle of the cow. Frequently, cows are identified as nonpregnant by a single milk progesterone assay only after the optimal time for service has passed. The herder then has two

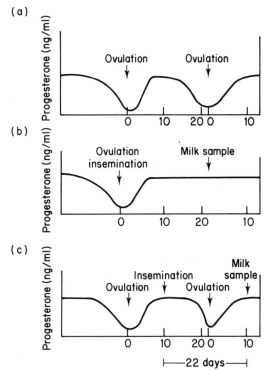

Fig. 6.1 Patterns of progesterone concentrations during a normal estrous cycle, early pregnancy and insemination in the luteal phase of the estrous cycle. (a) Normal pattern of peripheral progesterone concentrations during a nonfertile estrous cycle. (b) Normal pattern of peripheral progesterone concentrations during a fertile estrous cycle and early pregnancy. Measurement of the concentration of progesterone on day 20–24 after insemination accurately predicts pregnancy. (c) Pattern of peripheral progesterone concentrations when insemination during the luteal phase of the estrous cycle results in a 'false positive' diagnosis of pregnancy by milk progesterone assay 22 days after insemination.

choices in dealing with the nonpregnant cow; observe the cow closely for estrus at the time of the second expected postservice estrus (day 42 after the first unsuccessful service), or wait until the corpus luteum becomes responsive to PGF (days 7 or 8 after ovulation), administer PGF, and inseminate at the observed estrus (days 30–35 after the first unsuccessful service).

Cows that have high progesterone concentrations at 20–24 days after insemination may be pregnant (70–80%) or the result of the progesterone assay may be a false positive due to a number of causes, some of which are:

1. Insemination during the luteal phase of the cycle (Fig. 6.1c).
2. Long or short estrous cycles.

3. Prolonged luteal function (uterine disease).
4. Embryonic death (after days 16 or 17).
5. Ovarian cysts.
6. Management errors (mistiming of sample, mistaken identification of cows and/or samples).
7. Laboratory errors.

Because of the inaccuracy in identification of pregnant cows, those that have a high concentration of progesterone in milk at the first expected post-service estrus should be examined for pregnancy by palpation per rectum at the earliest opportunity.

Errors in estrus detection lead to missed opportunities for insemination, the insemination of 10–20% of cows during the luteal phase of the estrous cycle when conception is unlikely, and insemination of pregnant cows. Intervals between calving and first breeding can be reduced and normal pregnancy rates can be achieved without detection of estrus if milk progesterone concentrations are determined daily by EIA and if cows are inseminated once, 2 days after the characteristic decrease in milk progesterone associated with luteolysis.

Assay of progesterone concentrations in milk samples taken on the day of breeding is useful in some herds with a history of poor fertility to confirm that the cows being inseminated are not in the luteal phase of the estrous cycle. If more than an occasional cow presented for insemination has a high concentration of progesterone, the methods used to detect estrus should be reviewed and appropriately modified.

Stress around the time of breeding may stimulate secretion of progesterone (or a progesterone-like compound) by the adrenal glands. Ovariectomized cows given ACTH may have concentrations of progesterone similar to those of intact cows during the luteal phase of the estrous cycle. This phenomenon might lead to elevated progesterone concentrations in cows that are indeed in the follicular phase of the estrous cycle if they are stressed prior to obtaining a sample for assay.

Early embryonic death is often diagnosed as infertility since most embryo loss occurs early in the gestation period and the cow returns to estrus at a normal interval. Embryonic loss prior to the maternal recognition of pregnancy does not prolong luteal function and is not accurately detected by measurement of milk progesterone concentrations. Loss of the embryo or fetus after maternal recognition of pregnancy prolongs the estrous cycle and the degree of embryonic loss from days 16 to 17 onward may be estimated by repeated measurement of progesterone concentrations in milk.

In cases where an abortus is found among a group of cows previously known to be pregnant, progesterone concentrations may be measured in several suspect cows if no other clinical signs are obvious. Low progesterone concentrations in cows previously known to be pregnant are consistent with a diagnosis of abortion.

Milk progesterone assays have been used to diagnose more accurately reproductive abnormalities in dairy cows. Laboratory assistance is useful in identifying nonpalpated luteal tissue and to detect cases in which a structure resembling a corpus luteum is palpated but is not secreting progesterone. Milk progesterone profiles around the time of breeding might be used to determine the cause of unsuccessful inseminations.

Unobserved estrus may be differentiated from acyclicity by measuring milk progesterone concentrations at weekly intervals during the postpartum period. If low concentrations are found in each of four weekly samples, it may be assumed that the cow has not established normal estrous cycles. If the progesterone concentration in one of the samples is low and those in the other three samples are high, the cow is likely to be having normal estrous cycles. Uterine disease (or pregnancy) should be suspected if all four weekly samples contain high concentrations of progesterone.

The response of cows to endocrine therapy can be monitored by progesterone profiles. In the case of COD, luteinization of the cyst in response to GnRH treatment is characterized by increased progesterone concentrations. Cows that have not responded to GnRH therapy after 10–14 days can be identified and retreated without further loss of time. The response of cows to treatment with PGF can be monitored by serial measurement of progesterone concentrations.

Pathological Causes of Anestrus

A number of pathological changes affect ovarian function and suspend the estrous cycle.

Prolonged Luteal Function The corpus luteum normally regresses near the end of an infertile estrous cycle but is maintained by pregnancy or the presence of abnormal material within the uterine lumen. Retained corpora lutea without uterine disease do not occur in cows. Pyometra is characterized by suspension of the estrous cycle, prolonged luteal function, and anestrus. Most cases of pyometra respond promptly to treatment with PGF. Mummification of the fetus in the cow is also characterized by prolonged luteal function and anestrus. When fetal death is not followed by abortion, the retained fetus may mummify if the uterine contents are not invaded by pyogenic microorganisms. A mummified fetus may be retained within the uterus for a period longer than a normal gestation, and cases are usually brought to the attention of the clinician when cows previously known to be pregnant do not deliver at the expected time. Treatment with PGF is usually followed by expulsion of the mummified fetus in 3–5 days. The prognosis for future fertility following delivery of the mummy is generally good but it may not be economical to maintain the cow in the herd for another gestation period.

While pregnancy is not usually considered to be an abnormal condition in cows, conception at an unknown, undesired, or unrecorded service may be misinterpreted as anestrus. Pregnancy must be included in the differential diagnosis of each case of anestrus regardless of the history given by the herder. Examination for pregnancy must precede the administration of PGF.

Ovarian Abnormalities Abnormal conditions of the ovary that cause anestrus include congenital defects, COD and ovarian tumors. Ovarian atrophy may be caused by prolonged exposure to exogenous hormones.

Postpartum Anestrus

Normal ovarian cycles resume later after calving in beef cows than in dairy cows due to the influence of frequent suckling. Most dairy cows resume regular estrous cycles within the first 3–4 weeks after calving, while suckled beef cows have a postpartum anestrous period of 6–8 weeks. These periods of postpartum acyclicity are influenced by the nutritional management of the cow. High-producing dairy cows may experience a delay in resumption of the estrous cycle during their peak lactation because they cannot consume enough energy to meet the needs of both lactation and reproduction. Although treatment with gonadotropins has been suggested, hormonal therapy has not been shown to be of any consistent benefit in these cases and regular estrous cycles resume when milk production decreases later in lactation. Deficiencies in energy prolong postpartum acyclicity in beef cows and may severely affect the reproductive performance of a herd. Cows should be fed so they gain weight through the last trimester of pregnancy, and through the calving and breeding seasons. Cows that are gaining weight are more likely to have regular estrous cycles and are more likely to conceive than are cows that are losing weight. Enough energy must be provided to first-calf heifers to meet their needs for continued growth

and lactation. Pregnancy rates in cows during their second breeding season (while nursing their first calf and continuing their own growth) are frequently low due to inadequate nutritional management. Replacement heifers should be bred so as to calve 3 weeks prior to the cow herd so they can be closely observed for dystocia and be allowed a longer postpartum interval than older cows prior to the start of the breeding season. The nutritional management of beef cows is especially important if estrous synchronization with PGF is anticipated.

Prepubertal Anestrus

Body weight and age are significant factors in determining the onset of puberty. Heifers should be managed so they reach puberty before 15 months of age if they are to calve for the first time at 2 years. There is considerable variation among breeds in the weight and age at the onset of puberty, but heifers should be fed to reach at least 65% of their expected mature weight before the start of their first breeding season.

Undernutrition Puberty is clearly delayed by undernutrition. Deficient energy intake is the most significant nutritional factor in delaying the onset of puberty in both female and male cattle. Puberty occurs earlier in adequately fed heifers than in underfed heifers and the pregnancy rate in adequately nourished animals is higher than that in animals receiving energy-deficient diets. Undernourished heifers that become pregnant are more likely to have calving difficulties and have a reduced chance of conceiving while nursing their first calves. Conversely, overfeeding young animals to the point of obesity results in the deposition of excessive amounts of fat in the mammary gland and pelvic canal and reduces the animal's lifetime production of offspring.

Dietary Deficiencies Protein deficiency is a cause of delayed puberty only when severe underfeeding is practiced and is frequently complicated by vitamin A and phosphorous deficiencies. Rations that provide adequate protein for maintenance and growth are also adequate for reproduction.

Mineral deficiencies and imbalances that retard growth secondarily delay puberty. Deficiencies of phosphorous (P), manganese (Mg), cobalt (Co), copper (Cu) and iron (Fe) have been reported to cause abnormal reproductive performance. Infertility is not a clinical sign of calcium deficiency in cattle.

Deficiencies of vitamin A are associated with the

delivery of dead or weak calves and retained placentas. While vitamin A deficiency may result in cornification of the vaginal mucosa, irregular estrous cycles and delayed breeding, infertility is not a common clinical sign of vitamin A deficiency. Similarly, deficiencies of vitamin E may be associated with retained placenta but have not been shown to result in abnormalities of the estrous cycle or infertility.

If heifers are near puberty, the onset may be hastened in some cases by treatment with an implant of 6 mg norgestomet and an injection of 3 mg norgestomet and 5 mg estradiol valerate (Synchro-Mate B). The implant is removed after 9 days and estrus is expected within 120 h after implant removal. Insemination at the induced estrus results in pregnancy rates of up to 50% which may be acceptable under some circumstances.

CONCEPTION FAILURE/REPEAT BREEDERS

A frequent complaint of dairy producers is that inseminated cows are found to be nonpregnant when examined at 35–60 days after breeding or that cows continue to return to estrus after having been bred. In the case of the nonpregnant cow, it is usually impossible to determine if the cow failed to conceive or if conception was followed by embryonic death. The repeat breeder cow is one of the most frustrating reproductive problems in a dairy herd.

Defining a Repeat Breeder

A repeat breeder cow is defined as one that:

1. Has returned to estrus after a third infertile service.
2. Has had a minimum of one calf to exclude those with congenital defects that prevent conception (although some authors have expanded the definition to include heifers).
3. Is less than 10 years of age (to exclude those with senile changes).
4. Does not have any abnormalities of the reproductive organs detectable by physical examination.
5. Has no abnormal discharges from the genital tract.
6. Has normal interestrous intervals.

Embryonic Death

Most embryonic death develops at 6–7 days after insemination and cannot be clinically differentiated from fertilization failure because the interestrous interval is usually normal. Embryonic death after day 16 prolongs luteal function, resulting in a prolonged interestrous interval. Cows inseminated once usually have high fertilization rates; however, the percentage of cows that maintain pregnancy decreases as the time between breeding and detection of pregnancy increases. Hormonal asynchrony (resulting in an abnormal uterine environment), retarded embryonic development, and abnormal maternal karyotype may be reasons for reproductive failure after fertilization. Another possibility is that many embryonic deaths are due to genetic abnormalities, are unavoidable, and are the normal means by which unfit genotypes are eliminated at a low biological cost. Repeat breeding following service by bulls with histories of high fertility is usually due to embryonic death while repeat breeding following service by bulls with histories of low fertility is due to both fertilization failure and embryonic death. Although lower maternal plasma progesterone concentrations have been associated with abnormal embryos, lack of differences between normal and repeat breeder cows has also been reported.

Embryologic and Maternal Factors

The embryologic and maternal factors that contribute to repeat breeding are not well-defined. In one study, when embryos from healthy donors were transferred to normal or repeat breeder recipients, the pregnancy rate at day 60 was the same in both groups of recipients. Conversely, in other experiments when embryos from healthy or repeat breeder donors were transferred to healthy recipients, the pregnancy rate was higher than when embryos from healthy or repeat breeder donors were transferred to repeat breeder recipients. Cows culled as repeat breeders have a slightly lower fertilization rate than do healthy cows; however, embryo survival can be normal if fertilization occurs, suggesting that errors in detection of estrus contribute substantially to repeat breeding. Cows with a history of repeat breeding during one season may conceive readily during the next breeding season.

The breeding efficiency of the herd affects the percentage of cows requiring three or more services per pregnancy. In herds with low pregnancy rates, the prevalence of repeat breeding is high; while in herds with high pregnancy rates, the prevalence of repeat breeding is lower (Table 6.1).

Bacterial Infections

Nonspecific bacterial infections of the uterus have

Table 6.1 Percentage of cows remaining nonpregnant after one, two, or three services at various herd pregnancy rates

	Cows remaining nonpregnant (%)		
	After one service	After two services	After three services
Herd pregnancy rate (%)			
20	80	64	51.2
30	70	49	34.3
40	60	36	21.6
50	50	25	12.5
60	40	16	6.4
70	30	9	2.7
80	20	4	0.8

not been shown to be a significant cause of repeat breeding. Histologic lesions of endometritis are not correlated with the isolation of nonspecific bacteria from the endometrial cavities of repeat breeder cows nor are bacteria isolated more frequently from opaque estrual mucus than from clear estrual mucus. The infusion of antiseptics and antibiotics into the uterus of cows after insemination has been shown to be of no benefit in improving pregnancy rates and has, in fact, been shown to reduce pregnancy rates in most groups of cows. Postbreeding infusions have been shown to be beneficial only after the fifth service and are least detrimental in cows over 6 years old.

Improving the Pregnancy Rate

The pregnancy rate of repeat breeding dairy cows (but not first service pregnancy rates) can be improved by administering GnRH at the time of insemination. The mechanism by which GnRH administration improves the pregnancy rate has not yet been determined, but synchronization of ovulation and increased luteinization of follicular cells have been suggested. Administration of hCG on days 10, 11, and 12 after insemination delays return to estrus but does not improve pregnancy rates. Repeat breeder cows are also reported to become pregnant after lavage of the uterine cavity with saline solution.

Abnormalities of the Musculoskeletal System

Abnormalities of the musculoskeletal system have an adverse effect on conception. Lameness has been associated with increases in the intervals between calving and first breeding, and between calving and conception and a decrease in the pregnancy rate. This may result from decreased ability or willingness to display estrous behavior. Correct conformation of the feet and legs must be considered when selecting sires.

HERD HEALTH PROGRAMS

Some type of planned productive herd health program is offered by many veterinary practices. In most programs, dairy cows are examined at intervals appropriate for the size and management of the herd. Typical intervals are fortnightly or monthly, but daily or weekly visits may be necessary in some large herds. Cows routinely examined during herd health visits are:

1. Those that have calved from 14 to 45 days previously (postpartum examination).
2. Those that have been inseminated more than 35 days previously and have not returned to estrus (pregnancy examination).
3. Cows that have not been detected in estrus by the time of desired breeding or found to be nonpregnant at the previous examination (anestrus).
4. Cows that have a history of an abnormality of the reproductive organs such as cystic ovarian disease, metritis, retained placenta, pyometra, and dystocia.

Most reproductive failure in cattle herds is due to deficiencies in management. The most significant benefit of a reproductive herd health program is the

Table 6.2 Normal fertility levels in dairy cattle based on a sample of 322 herds in England, 1985

	Whole sample	Top 10%†	Bottom 10%†
Herd size	136	129	111
Days from calving to assumed conception*	99	81	130
Days from calving to first service	71	64	80
Number of services per assumed conception*	1.82	1.65	2.22

* Conception assumed if no repeat service date recorded within 60 days of service.

† Top and bottom 10% selected from the interval from calving to assumed conception.

From: Milk Marketing Board of England and Wales' Checkmate Report 1985 by Tony Poole and James Booth.

stimulation of improvements in the detection of estrus that decrease the interval from calving to conception.

Reproductive herd health programs increase the efficiency of production, and thus net income of participating dairy herds. The yearly cost of veterinary service per cow is higher in herds responding maximally to preventive programs compared to herds using emergency services only, but significant improvements in net income have been demonstrated in favor of herds using preventive programs.

A summary of normal fertility levels in dairy cattle is shown in Table 6.2.

Complementary References

Ayalon, N. (1981) Embryonic mortality in cattle. *Zuchthygiene*, **16**, 97–109.

BonDurant, R. H. (1986) Examination of the reproductive tract of the cow and heifer. In *Current Therapy in Theriogenology II*, ed. Morrow, D. A., pp. 95–101. Philadelphia: W. B. Saunders.

Eyestone, W. H. & Ax, R. L. (1984) A review of ovarian follicular cysts in cows, with comparisons to the condition in women, rats and rabbits. *Theriogenology*, **22**, 109–125.

Grunert, E. (1986) Etiology and pathogenesis of retained bovine placenta. In *Current Therapy in Theriogenology II*, ed. Morrow, D. A., pp. 237–242. Philadelphia: W. B. Saunders.

Hemeida, N. A., Gustaffson, B. K. & Whitmore, H. L. (1986) Therapy of uterine infections: alternatives to antibiotics. In *Current Therapy in Theriogenology II*, ed.

Morrow, D. A., pp. 45–47. Philadelphia: W. B. Saunders.

Hopkins, S. M. (1986) Bovine anestrus. In *Current Therapy in Theriogenology II*, ed. Morrow, D. A., pp. 247–250. Philadelphia: W. B. Saunders.

Hudson, R. S. (1986) Genital surgery of the cow. In *Current Therapy in Theriogenology II*, ed. Morrow, D. A., pp. 314–352. Philadelphia: W. B. Saunders.

Jubb, K. V. F., Kennedy, P. C. & Palmer, N. (1985) The female genital system. In *Pathology of Domestic Animals*, 3rd ed., vol. 3, pp. 305–407. Orlando: Academic Press.

Kesler, D. J. & Garverick, H. A. (1982) Ovarian cysts in dairy cattle: a review. *J. Anim. Sci.*, **55**, 1147–1159.

Olson, J. D., Bretzlaff, K. N., Mortimer, R. G. & Ball, L. (1986) The metritis–pyometra complex. In *Current Therapy in Theriogenology II*, ed. Morrow, D. A., pp. 227–236. Philadelphia: W. B. Saunders.

Paisley, L. G., Mickelsen, W. D. & Anderson P. B. (1986) Mechanisms and therapy for retained fetal membranes and uterine infections of cows: a review. *Theriogenology*, **25**, 353–381.

Woicke, J., Schoon H.-A., Heuwisser, W., Schulz, L.-Cl. & Grunert, E. (1986) Morphologische und funktionelle Aspekte plazentarer Reifungsmechanismen beim Rind. 1. Lichtmikroskopische Befunde. *J. Vet. Med. A.*, **33**, 660–667.

Youngquist, R. S. & Bierschwal, C. J. (1985) Clinical management of reproductive problems in dairy cows. *J. Dairy Sci.*, **68**, 2817–2826.

Youngquist, R. S. & Braun, W. F. (1986) Management of infertility in the cow. *J. Amer. Vet. Med. Assoc.*, **109**, 411–414.

Zemjanis, R., Fahning, M. L. & Schultz, R. H. (1969) Anestrus—the practitioner's dilemma. *Vet. Scope*, **XIV**, 14–21.

7

Management of Noninfectious Problems in Reproduction of the Ewe and Female Goat

RANDALL S. OTT

Goats and sheep were the first animals to be domesticated by man. The symbiotic relationship between man and small ruminants that developed has remained intact for thousands of years and, throughout the world, is the basis for our most important animal industry. Breeds of each species are utilized for production of meat, wool or hair, and milk. Reproduction could be considered the most important aspect of sheep and goat production. Without regular and successful reproduction, there is no product to use or sell.

FLOCK MANAGEMENT

Successful flock management consists of:

1. Selection of the breeds and family lines within these breeds that are genetically best able to perform under available environmental, nutritional, and managemental resources.
2. Provision of the optimal *and* most economically feasible nutrition, management, and prophylactic immunity.
3. Selection of replacement animals from among those that perform best.
4. Slaughter of those that either do not perform well or that require therapy or special management practices that are not cost-effective.

Procedures which increase costs such as special mating, feeding, or vaccination practices must result in a benefit greater than the cost incurred. Therefore, new products or methods may not always be cost-effective.

BREEDING

Exploitation of the genetic variation of different breeds and strains within breeds of goats and sheep provides the opportunity to increase output from existing resources. Utilization of estrus synchronization regimens, artificial insemination, and embryo transfer has the potential of greatly accelerating genetic change. While it is very important for stockmen to identify animals with superior reproductive and productive characteristics, it is equally important to recognize animals with heritable defects. For many such conditions, carriers are difficult to identify because they may be normal as judged by outward appearance. Thus, it is very difficult to control recessive defects. An accurate diagnosis as to whether a congenital defect was genetically or environmentally induced enables the stockman to adjust the selection of breeding animals *or* modify nutrition or management. Since this is seldom possible, it is advisable to consider all congenital defects as heritable, until proven otherwise. Propagation of a genetic defect causes, sooner or later, a decrease in production and a reduction in profit.

A recent and very interesting development of animal breeding has been the attention given to improvement of fertility of females by selection of males with large testicular size. Work with mice, sheep, and cattle shows promise that males with larger testicular size early in life, sire female offspring that reach puberty and conceive at an earlier age and have a higher ovulation rate.

On an annual basis, individual rams and bucks should be assessed for fitness for breeding before they are joined with females. Highly fertile rams and male goats impregnate more females during a shorter breeding period. Breeding soundness examinations can be valuable procedures to help diagnose breeding problems in the flock. Finding that the males are satisfactory breeders may 'rule out' this parameter and cause one to consider infertility of the ewes, or infectious, management or nutritional problems. Many times breeding soundness examinations confirm a suspected case of male infertility and may allow the owner to receive compensation or a replacement animal from the seller if the ram or male goat is under warranty. Two of the most important traits of breeding males are scrotal circumference (an indirect measurement of testicular size which is positively related to sperm production) and serving capacity (the male's ability to inseminate females).

GOATS

Optimum Mating Time

The length of the estrous cycle in dairy goats is usually 20–21 days. Abnormally short (5–8 day) estrous cycles may occur in female goats early in the breeding season. In one study of Nubian goats, 55% of short cycles averaging 6.8 ± 0.5 days observed at the beginning of the breeding season were anovulatory.

Selective or hand mating is a common practice in dairy goat herds. The duration of estrus in females is approximately 32–40 h. Female goats are usually mated with males at the onset of estrus and at 12 h intervals until estrus subsides. In artificial insemination programs, the female is usually inseminated at the onset of estrus, and again 12 h later.

Proper detection of estrus is a very important aspect of goat breeding when either hand mating or artificial insemination is practiced. Females in estrus actively seek the presence of the male. Males are sometimes de-scented at the time of de-horning by burning and destroying the odor glands located posteriorly and medially to the horn buds. This is a bad practice because females, when given a choice, will usually prefer a scented male to a deodorized one.

Detection of estrus in females is best accomplished with the aid of a male. An intact male should be confined in an area where females in estrus can be observed congregating near the pen. Males with breeding aprons, vasectomized males, or testosterone-treated females, wethers, or intersex goats can be used to aid estrus detection. Signs of estrus in females include tail-wagging, bleating, and urination near the male. There may be swelling of the vulva and mucous discharge. The reaction of the male to the female being teased is an indication of estrus in the female. Some females show few signs of estrus other than limited tail-wagging and standing for mounting by the male and these signs may be observed only after teasing. Females will occasionally stand for mounting by other females; however, the level of homosexual activity in goats is low in reproductively normal females, so observation of this activity is not useful for estrus detection. Females that frequently engage in homosexual activity may suffer from the intersex condition.

Male Effect on Initiation of Breeding

The mere presence of a male goat has been shown to initiate and even synchronize the cyclic activity of females early in the breeding season. A profound influence of the male was demonstrated in a study in which males were introduced to a group of 17 females that were in late seasonal anestrus. Estrus was detected within a mean of 5.5 days in 16 of the 17 females within 21 days after exposure to males (Fig. 7.1); 13 of these 16 females had progesterone profiles characteristic of normal estrous cycles during the 35 day observation period as compared with only one of 17 control females (Fig. 7.2). None of the females in the control group exhibited signs of behavioral estrus during the 35 days of the experiment. However, 15 of 17 exhibited estrus by a mean (± SE) of 7 ± 1.5 days after introduction of males to this group. Four of the females initially exposed to males had short interestrous intervals of 6 days (Fig. 7.3). Other studies have confirmed that these short cycles are usually anovulatory. The strong odor of the male goat may play a role in the induction of estrous behavior; however, other exteroceptive factors may also be involved.

Intersexes

An important cause of infertility in dairy goats is the

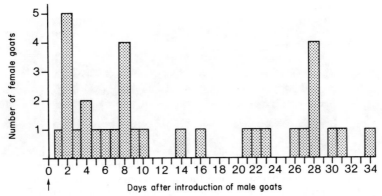

Fig. 7.1 Number of female goats showing behavioral estrus after introduction of male goats on day 0 (↑ = males introduced). Of 17 female goats, 16 exhibited estrus within 21 days of exposure to males (mean 5.5 days). (From Ott, Nelson and Hixon (1979), reprinted with permission.)

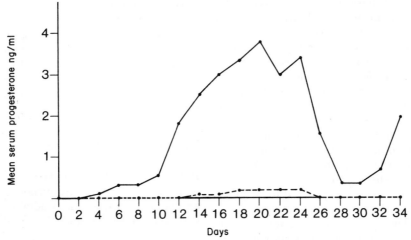

Fig. 7.2 Mean serum progesterone concentrations of 17 female goats exposed to males (solid line) and 17 control females (broken line). (From Ott, Nelson and Hixon (1979), reprinted with permission.)

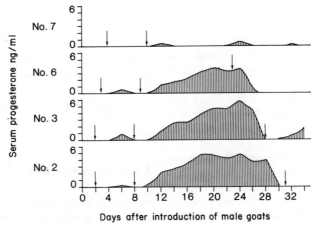

Fig. 7.3 Serum progesterone concentrations of four female goats experiencing short interestrous intervals after exposure to males. Onset of estrus(↓). (From Ott, Nelson and Hixon (1979), reprinted with permission.)

(a)   **(b)**   **(c)**   **(d)**

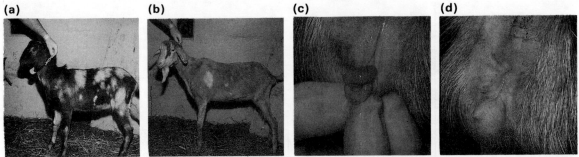

Fig. 7.4   (a) A polled intersex goat with a slightly enlarged clitoris and a short atretic vagina; this goat was found to be a 60,XY with testes located in the abdominal cavity near the inguinal rings. (b) A polled intersex goat with (c) a penile clitoris (d) obscured by the ventral labia. This goat had a hypoplastic uterus and was 60,XX. The gonads were testes. (From Ott (1982), reprinted with permission.)

intersex condition. Intersex goats often have a normal-sized vulva but an enlarged clitoris and a short or atretic vagina. A penile clitoris or even ovotestes can occur in females that otherwise appear phenotypically female. Affected animals are usually genetic females with a normal female chromosome (60,XX) complement. Intersex goats and congenital hypoplasia of the reproductive tract are most often associated with naturally hornless (polled) goats and are more likely to occur when both parents are polled. The use of a horned male is advised, since intersexes are rare when at least one parent is horned. XX,XY chimerism rarely occurs in goats.

A polled intersex goat that appeared to be a normal female had a slightly enlarged clitoris and a short vagina (Fig. 7.4a). Chromosome analysis revealed this animal to be 60,XY; examination of the reproductive tract post mortem showed a highly masculinized tract with testes located near the inguinal rings. A second goat was phenotypically female with a penile clitoris obscured by the vulva (Fig. 7.4b,c,d). The uterus appeared hypoplastic with the left uterine horn ending blindly; gonads were testes. The karyotype of this animal was 60,XX. A third goat was a highly masculinized female with strong male odor, masculine behavior, and a penile clitoris. The reproductive tract was rudimentarily female; testicular tissue only was found in the gonads. The karyotype of this goat was 60,XX.

Gonads of intersex goats are almost always testes. Some polled intersex goats have a near normal male phenotype with the exception of small or hypoplastic testes. These goats are aspermic but may exhibit normal male libido. More intersex goats are reported to occur in the Saanen, Toggenburg, and Alpine breeds.

Cystic Ovaries

Cystic ovaries are thought to occur in dairy goats with a clinical history of nymphomania; however, inability to palpate the ovaries by rectal examination makes diagnosis difficult. Suggested treatment has been gonadotropins injected at one-quarter of the bovine dose.

Retained Fetal Membranes

Retained fetal membranes and metritis occasionally occur in dairy goats. Intravenous broad spectrum antibiotic therapy is usually administered to females with acute infection and elevated body temperature.

Pseudopregnancy and Hydrometra

Pseudopregnancy occurs in the female in which a large volume of clear fluid is passed at 'parturition'. Subsequent fertility is usually normal. A more common condition that occurs in females is hydrometra, in which as much as several liters of a clear fluid may be present in the female's enlarged and thin-walled uterus. The animal exhibits abdominal distention and ultrasonography fails to discern a fetus.

Abortion and Stress

In Angora goats 'abortion storms' 1 or 2 days after stress such as changes in weather or transport have been reported to involve as many as 16% of the flock.

EWES

Sheep breeds vary in prolificacy. Selection of a productive breed that is adaptable to a particular environmental and managemental situation is an important initial consideration. Under most environmental conditions, increased litter size contributes to the profitability of sheep production. Crossbred dams have been shown to have production advantages over purebreds; therefore, programs for maximum lamb production will most likely utilize a crossbreeding system.

Mating Systems

The length of the estrous cycle in ewes is 16–17 days. The duration of estrus in the ewe ranges from 10 to 40 h with an average of 24 h. The duration of estrus is shorter in ewe lambs than in mature ewes. Ewes in estrus actively seek the ram. Ewes appear to vary in attractiveness to rams and may compete among themselves for proximity to the ram. The need for learning how to find and successfully compete for the ram is thought to account for the poor performance of maiden ewes in pasture mating. In one trial where rams were tethered in order to investigate the ram-seeking ability of ewes in estrus, only 43% of two-tooth ewes were mated compared to 73% of the older ewes. Rams with high libido and serving capacity may be even more important for flocks comprised of young ewes.

Most ewes are bred by natural service although selective or hand mating and artificial insemination are used in certain situations. A suggested mating system for maximum ewe fertility is the use of three rams in each breeding unit. It has been shown that significantly more ewes are detected in estrus when three rams are working together rather than individually. An average of two to six matings per estrous period of the ewe has been reported, and when more than one ram is present multiple sire matings occur. Males with good libido can mate 20 to 30 times a day. Breeding pastures should be large enough so that dominant rams do not prevent or 'block' subordinate rams from mating. While dominant rams mate more often than subordinate rams, the differences between dominant and subordinate rams decrease when more ewes are present or when ewes are more dispersed. A limit of 50 ewes per ram is given as a general recommendation; however, the optimal mating ratio depends on a number of factors including age of ewes, serving capacity of the rams, size and terrain of the mating pasture, etc.

One hundred or more ewes have been successfully mated per ram. Satisfactory performance of mature rams with high libido and good semen quality utilized in ram : ewe ratios of 1 : 350 and even 1 : 400 have been reported under optimal conditions. Ewes are less likely to be serviced by more than one ram when the ewe : ram ratio is high. In rams, high libido appears to be heritable and positively correlated with prolificacy. Serving capacity is a useful predictor of the sexual performance of a ram in the flock. Higher pregnancy rates result from an increased number of services per estrus ewe. Apparently sight is important to the ram, since, in one study, depriving rams of smell and hearing had no effect on sexual behavior, while blindfolded rams were limited in mounting ability. Poor nutrition of the ram may result in a decline in libido. Rams are frequently harnessed with tupping crayons so that ewes that have been served by the ram can be identified. The crayon color can be changed every 14–15 days.

Male Effect on Initiation of Breeding

The observation that introduction of the ram to the breeding flock at the beginning of the breeding season resulted in partial synchrony of ovulation in the ewes several days later, led to investigation of what has since been termed 'ram shock' or the 'ram effect'. It has been well-established that the introduction of rams will induce ovulation in seasonally and lactationally anovular ewes and will induce puberty in ewe lambs. The breeding season can be extended when introduction of rams is used to stimulate earlier cyclic activity of ewes in the late anestrous period. The ewes must have been isolated from the rams for a period of time prior to reintroduction. Isolation of the ewes from the sight and odor of the rams for at least 1 month has been recommended. The induced ovulation is not usually accompanied by estrus. Ewes may experience a short cycle of 5–6 days after introduction of the rams. Neither the induced ovulation nor the second ovulation following the short cycle may be accompanied by signs of estrus in the ewe. Therefore, the first estrus of the ewe may not be seen until 24 days after introduction of the rams. At the beginning of the breeding season, sheep tend to ovulate without showing overt signs of estrus, whereas goats tend to exhibit signs of estrus without ovulation. Some investigators have reported that intact rams were more effective at inducing ovulation than vasectomized rams; however, testosterone-treated wethers or ewes have been utilized successfully. One investigation of this 'pheromone' effect revealed that exposure of ewes to the wool and wax, but not urine, of rams resulted in the same effect as exposure to intact rams.

Nutritional Factors

A common practice in sheep breeding is to flush the ewes just before and during the breeding season. Flushing ewes is thought to stimulate more ovulations during the early and late breeding season, but is probably of little benefit during the middle of the season. Failure to meet energy requirements during gestation may result in pregnancy toxemia (ketosis) in late gestation in ewes (or female goats) with more than one fetus. Pregnancy toxemia is seldom effectively treated, particularly in those ewes in which anorexia is already present. A proper assessment of the general state of health and the nutritional status of the entire flock is indicated. It may be more important to improve the nutrition of the other sheep, some of which may not be showing symptoms of pregnancy toxemia but may be in the early stages of the disease.

Puberty

Early-born ewe lambs can become cyclic and conceive in their first breeding season. Lambs born later may not reach puberty until their second year. Bringing ewe lambs into production as early as possible reduces maintenance costs before the start of production. Range ewe lambs which are cyclic in their first year have better lifetime reproductive performance than those not experiencing estrus in their first year. In order to accomplish early breeding, lambs must be large enough (65% of mature weight is suggested) and in good condition. Ewe lambs reared on a high plane of nutrition reach puberty earlier than those reared on a low plane of nutrition. Rams with larger scrotal circumferences at an early age sire ewe lambs that reach puberty earlier. Age at puberty varies greatly among breeds.

Prevention of Infectious Disease

Care should be taken that animals added to the flock come from herds that practice disease control. A program of reproductive disease prevention would include strict sanitation, early diagnosis of disease, and proper vaccination programs.

Use of Pregnancy Diagnosis

Determination of pregnancy in ewe lambs can be a cost-effective procedure because it enables the non-pregnant ones to be culled and marketed while they can still command slaughter lamb prices.

MANAGEMENT OF REPRODUCTION IN FEMALE GOATS AND EWES

Effects of Photoperiod

Goats and ewes are considered 'short-day breeders' because they initiate reproductive activity in response to a decreasing length of daylight. Female goats and ewes are classified as seasonally polyestrous. They usually stop exhibiting estrus either because they become pregnant or the breeding season ends. Although temperature and the presence of the male influence the seasonality of the estrous cycle, effects of the photoperiod are felt to be the most important. Control of the photoperiod with artificial lighting has received a great amount of attention in research studies involving sheep but not much application in either species. Some goat dairies have utilized the practice of exposing breeding animals to total darkness for 17 h/day after the beginning of June to induce early onset of cycling. In the Northern hemisphere the breeding season for sheep and goats generally extends from August to February; however, breed differences and geographical area account for a wide variation. In both species there is interest in developing breeds and strains that under proper management might reproduce without seasonal restrictions, allowing accelerated lambing in ewes and year-round milk production in goats.

Induction of Estrus

Administration of exogenous progestagens and prostaglandins has been successfully used to control reproductive events of goats and ewes. Progestagens can induce early mating of female lambs that have attained adequate weight and body development. Early mating of lambs can enhance subsequent fertility and increase lifetime productivity. Puberty occurs in lambs around 9 months of age. Estrus can be induced several months earlier by progestagen treatment for 10–14 days with 400–600 i.u. of pregnant mare serum gonadotropin (PMSG) injected at the time of progestagen removal.

Synchronization of Estrus

Control of the time of breeding allows control of the time of lambing and kidding, and milk production. Progestagens have been the most widely used agents for ovulation control. Fluorogestrone acetate has been administered by the intravaginal route in both ewes and female goats using a hormone-impregnated polyurethane sponge. In the past, vaginal pessaries were left in place for 14 days in sheep, 21 days in goats, and followed by an injection of PMSG when the pessaries were removed. A successful program of artificial insemination using frozen semen from genetically superior goats has recently been practiced in France. All insemination is performed after estrus synchronization beginning in June using vaginal pessaries that are left in place for 11 days. On day 9 an injection of PMSG (400–600 i.u.) and cloprostenol (100–200 μg) is administered. Insemination is performed on days 12 and 13. The protocol is varied slightly depending upon the breed of female treated (Alpine or Saanen). A 60% kidding rate was achieved in 1985 following insemination of 17 000 female goats. Replacement goats are largely selected from the group of artificial insemination-sired kids, thereby enhancing genetic progress.

Prostaglandin $F_{2\alpha}$ or one of its analogs will induce luteolysis in the cycling ewe or female goat during the breeding season. A two-injection scheme of prostaglandin administered 11 days apart has been used for estrous synchronization of cyclic female goats in research trials with excellent fertility results. A dose of 2.5 mg $PGF_{2\alpha}$ has been shown to be adequate for estrus induction in the female goat. For ewes, the injections should be 9 days apart. Dosages ranging from 6 to 15 mg have been used for estrus induction of ewes. However, fertility of ewes at the induced estrus has been reported to be reduced by some workers. Prostaglandins are limited in their use for estrus synchronization of goats and ewes because an active corpus luteum must exist at the time of treatment and, in most instances, estrus control of goats and ewes is utilized when most of the females are anestrous.

Induction of Parturition

Control of the time of parturition in goats and ewes enables closer supervision of kidding and lambing during planned time periods when labor could be used more efficiently. In one study, dexamethasone (16 mg) administered to ewes on day 143 of gestation resulted in lambs born on days 144–146 with the largest litters being delivered earliest. The use of exogenous prostaglandin has been demonstrated to be the drug of choice to induce parturition in the goat. In a recent study, female goats receiving either 2.5 mg or 5.0 mg $PGF_{2\alpha}$ on day 144 kidded within 28–57 h. Retained fetal membranes have not been reported to be associated with induced parturition

Table 7.1 Normal fertility levels in sheep

Type	Hill	Upland	Lowland
Average flocksize	767	607	438
Ewe lambs in flock (%)	0	10	
Ewes (per 100 ewes put to the ram)			
Empty	5	6	Not known
Dead	4	5	Not known
Lambed	93	92	93
Lambs (per 100 ewes put to the ram)			
Born dead	9	8	Not known
Born alive	110	138	159
Died after birth	5	7	Not known
Reared	105	131	153

From: Sheep Year Book 1986. Meat and Livestock Commission, Milton Keynes, England.

Under normal conditions, where rams are at free range with ewes, 75–80% of ewes conceive at first mating and more than 90% after the second and third services.

Using liquid semen less than 10 h old for single insemination in the normal breeding season, average conception rates of 70% have been obtained. (R. M. Curnock, personal communication.)

of ewes or female goats. The latter should not be induced to kid earlier than 144 days of gestation because the kids born as triplets or quadruplets might be too small for survival. Induction on days 145–149 should work satisfactorily.

Most female goats induced to abort using prostaglandin experience consecutive interestrous intervals of 2–15 days. Progesterone concentrations in these female goats have indicated that ovulation usually did not occur. Female goats would not be expected to conceive if mated during an estrous period preceding a short cycle.

Normal levels of fertility in sheep are summarized in Table 7.1.

References

Gonyou, H. W. (1984) The role of behavior in sheep production: a review of research. *Appl. Anim. Ethol.*, **11**, 324–358.

Ott, R. S. (1982) Dairy goat reproduction. *Compendium on Continuing Education for the Practicing Veterinarian*, **4**, S164–S172.

Ott, R. S. & Memon, M. A. (1980) *Sheep and Goat Manual*. Hastings, Nebraska: Society for Theriogenology.

Ott, R. S., Nelson, D. R. & Hixon, J. E. (1979) Effect of presence of the male on initiation of estrous cycle activity of goats. *Theriogenology*, **13**, 183–190.

8

Noninfectious Causes of Reproductive Failure in the Female Pig

G. D. DIAL and G. W. BEVIER

Most successful operating businesses have established a corporate mission with strategic plans, goals, market plans, and sales targets. These functional areas are frequently reviewed and revised by management staff. For example the corporate mission of a pig farm might be 'to produce quality, lean meat efficiently'. Each department within the farm has specific strategic plans. For example, the breeding and gestation department manager targets a specific herd inventory, replacement rate, number of matings and farrowing rate. The farrowing house manager targets lactation lengths, amount of sow feed, number of pigs weaned, stillbirths, and mortality. Each strategic plan among all departments may have a profound influence on overall herd profitability. In addition, an awareness of these factors is often instrumental in the elucidation of perceived problems. The following example of the influence of replacement rate upon sow herd parity will illustrate how management strategy can create problems. It is often tempting for producers and veterinarians to implicate other etiologic agents in these problems.

HERD PARITY STRUCTURE: AN EXAMPLE

This case involves a newly populated pig farm. For the first 6 months of operation the manager reports many of the following problems to varying degrees: reduced litter size, delayed puberty, delayed return to estrus, increased stillbirths, reduced farrowing rate, reduced lactational ability, and reduced appetite (all compared to previously established targets). As time elapses, replacement gilts are delivered into the herd at the rate of 33% per annum. The farrowing distribution as depicted in Fig. 8.1 begins to develop over a 4-year period.

Next, a change in the economy such as declining market prices of slaughter pigs and rising corn prices combined with increasing interest rates may change the financial position of the business. As this occurs, the strategic plan changes and the senior management staff decides to reduce the replacement gilt rate to zero for 2 years. This will conserve capital investment in the operation. After two years, the parity distribution curve might appear as Fig. 8.1.

Curve (b) depicts young and old animals with very few in the optimum productive stages of second to sixth parity. Similar problems as itemized above (when the herd was young) will also be prevalent with this particular parity distribution. This example illustrates how the management decision to alter the replacement rate will have an adverse effect on herd performance and may create prob-

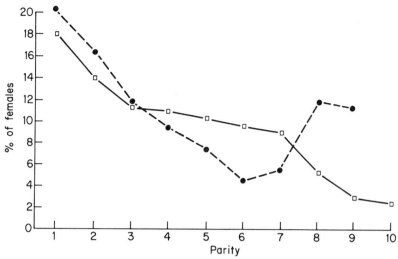

Fig. 8.1 Parity distribution of a herd having a replacement rate of 33% per annum (□——□) and that of a herd in which the replacement rate was transiently reduced before normal replacement schedules were reestablished (●– –●).

lems erroneously confused with infectious disease. It will take time to resolve this problem and recommendations for an effective replacement schedule should be initiated.

Establishing parameters for performance evaluation and decision-making models can serve as useful guidelines for the veterinary consultant. It is important to use targets in order to monitor performance effectively. There are numerous ways in which the productivity of a sow herd can be assessed, including:

1. Number of pigs born alive/sow/year.
2. Number of pigs weaned/sow/year.
3. Number of feeder pigs produced/sow/year.
4. Piglets produced/farrowing crate/year.
5. Kilograms of pork produced/sow/year.
6. Number of sow days/pig produced.
7. Number of pigs weaned/sow life.
8. Net margin ($) over feed cost/sow.

For the purposes of this chapter, the number of pigs born alive/sow/year has been selected as a parameter which is easily understood and in frequent use to compare reproductive performance between pig farms. The number of pigs born alive/sow/year is the product of two readily available components: litters/sow/year and number of pigs born alive/litter. The total number of pigs born/litter sets the upper limit for the number of pigs born alive/litter. The difference between these two figures represents the number of stillbirths per litter. Numerous management and environmental factors and many infectious diseases may contribute to peripartum and postnatal mortality. Many of these cannot be attributed to sow reproductive failure but they do influence herd productivity adversely. The following section deals with the principal factors which influence sow fertility, namely the number of litters/sow/year and the number of pigs born alive/litter. Causes and factors influencing postnatal mortality will not be discussed.

COMMON CLINICAL PROBLEMS

The introduction has set the stage for a more detailed consideration of some clinical cases which are often management-related. When investigating reproductive failure in the pig it is important to look at both the pigs and the records and to remember that one misses more by not looking than for not knowing.

Number of Litters/Sow/Year

When the annual productivity of a sow herd is suboptimal, litter size averages are often the first parameter examined. Table 8.1 depicts the relationship between litters/sow/year and the number of pigs produced/sow/year. At the level of nine pigs weaned/litter there are 0.9 additional pigs produced annually by each sow for every 0.1 increase in the number of litters/sow/year. The number of litters/sow/year is highly and positively correlated ($r = 0.83$) with the number of pigs weaned/sow/year. Similarly, litter size at weaning is highly

Table 8.1   Influence of litters/sow/year and pigs weaned/sow/litter on pigs weaned/sow/year

| | Litters/sow/year | | | | | | | | | |
Pigs/litter	1.6	1.7	1.8	1.9	2.0	2.1	2.2	2.3	2.4	2.5
7.5	12.0	12.8	13.5	14.3	15.0	15.8	16.5	17.3	18.0	18.8
8.0	12.8	13.6	14.4	15.2	16.0	16.8	17.6	18.4	19.2	20.0
8.5	13.6	14.5	15.3	16.2	17.0	17.9	18.7	19.6	20.4	21.3
9.0	14.4	15.3	16.2	17.1	18.0	18.9	19.8	20.7	21.6	22.5
9.5	15.2	16.2	17.1	18.1	19.0	20.0	20.9	21.9	22.8	23.8
10.0	16.0	17.0	18.0	19.0	20.0	21.0	22.0	23.0	24.0	25.0
10.5	16.8	17.9	18.9	20.0	21.0	22.1	23.1	24.2	25.2	26.3
11.0	17.6	18.7	19.8	20.9	22.0	23.1	24.2	25.3	26.4	27.5

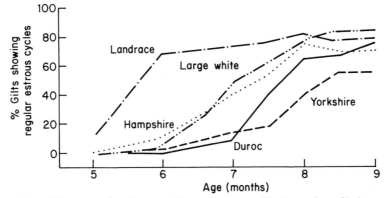

Fig. 8.2   Estrous activity relative to age for gilts reared in confinement. (Redrawn from Christenson and Ford, 1979.)

related ($r = 0.82$) to the number of pigs produced/ sow/year. Because the correlations are the same, it can be concluded that both contribute equally to sow productivity and that neither should be ignored when investigating problems related to herd productivity.

The number of litters a sow has during each year is dependent upon the following factors: age at puberty, lactation length and the weaning-to-estrus interval. While some of these factors cannot be altered in every herd to improve farrowing interval, they must not be overlooked when problems related to sow herd productivity are evaluated. The relative contributions of each factor to a herd's overall litters/sow/year average are not known and are certain to vary among herds.

Age at Puberty

A delay in the onset of puberty is often diagnosed when a gilt of the 'correct weight' has been in the herd for several months and has failed to breed or show pregnancy. The primary causative factors to be considered include stocking density, age at first

mating, estrus detection procedures, and genetics. With a high stocking density or large number of gilts per pen (> 30), submissive females may exhibit delayed puberty. Age is more important than weight as a determinant for onset of puberty. By 7 months of age, $> 90\%$ of gilts should show estrual activity. As genetic selection for performance traits improves daily weight gains, it may be common for a 100 kg gilt to be 150 days of age. It is probably best to wait until 170 days of age prior to first mating. This procedure will increase ovulation rates and ensure adequate acclimatization to the breeding herd flora. Additionally, delayed puberty is more common in Duroc and Yorkshire gilts than in Landrace, Hampshire, or Large White breeds. Figure 8.2 illustrates the breed differences among age at puberty. Other factors to consider with this dysfunction include time and duration of boar exposure and environment. Gilts are also more likely to experience delayed puberty in the summer months. A case pertaining to delayed puberty in a group of 12 gilts presented the following history. Twelve gilts ranging in age from 9 to 13 months of age were described as 'never cycling'. Ultrasonic pregnancy detection was performed prior to slaughter and one gilt was

Table 8.2   Ovarian structures found at slaughter in apparent anestrous gilts

| Gilt | Ovarian activity | | Approximate day of cycle | Tract |
	left	*right*		
300	9 CL	2 CL	6	N
301	10 CL;CA	3 CL;CA	9	N
302	8 F;CA	8 F;CA	18	N
303	4 CL;CA	5 CL;CA	2	N
304	10 CL	4 CL	2	N
305	6 F;CA	9 F;CA	18	N
306	4 CL;CA	9 CL;CA	2	N
307	6 CL;CA	6 CL;CA	2	N
308	7 CL;CA	7 CL;CA	2	N
309	4 F;CA	8 F;CA	18	N
310	12 CL	2 CL	9	N

Key: CL = corpora lutea; CA = corpora albicantia; F = follicles; approximate day of estrous cycle = an estimate of the phase of the cycle (day 0 = day of ovulation) based upon the size of the follicles and the appearance of the CL; tract = N (normal gross appearance).

found to be pregnant. The 11 gilts listed in Table 8.2 were slaughtered on a Friday. A gross examination of their reproductive tracts supplied the following information.

These gilts appear to have 'normal' tracts and were experiencing cyclic ovarian activity. Three were in the follicular phase of the cycle and 8 were in the luteal phase. There was evidence of previous cyclicity on 8 of the gilts based on the presence of CAs. Also, notice that the average ovulation rate was 13 based on the number of follicles or corpora lutea present. These were normal cycling gilts and better estrus detection procedures should be initiated. This may have been apparent early in the case history when an alleged anestrous gilt was found to be pregnant. There is still more information available from these reproductive tracts. Notice that there were three groups of gilts in relation to the day of the estrous cycle; those around day 2, those around day 9, and those around day 18—each at approximately weekly intervals. Since the gilts were slaughtered on a Friday, those at day 2 of the estrous cycle ovulated on Tuesday or Wednesday and were in behavioral estrus on a Sunday or Monday. The other groups also experienced estrus at a similar day of the week, indicative of a weekend management problem. Appropriate prophylaxis for delayed puberty includes boar exposure, culling gilts not showing behavioral estrus within 45–60 days following exposure to the boar, improved genetics, and better environment.

Farrowing Rate

Conception rate and farrowing rate are terms commonly but incorrectly used interchangeably. Conception rate refers to the proportion of bred sows having fertilized ova and can be estimated as the proportion that fail to return to estrus at the anticipated time (approximately 18–24 days postbreeding). In the absence of accurate follow-up estrus detection, conception rate can be estimated as the proportion of bred sows that are found to be pregnant by ultrasound, usually 30–40 days postmating. In contrast, farrowing rate refers to the proportion of bred sows that farrow and includes sows that conceive and maintain their pregnancy until term. Since pregnancies are often interrupted after conception, conception rate is reflected in farrowing rate but remains a distinct measure of reproductive performance. Factors which may contribute to reductions in conception rates are different from those that affect the capacity of the sow to maintain pregnancy. Consequently, the veterinary consultant should separate these two parameters when evaluating fertility problems on commercial swine enterprises.

A decline in conception rate, as reflected by an increased number of sows having regular returns to estrus, may occur with the following circumstances: the entire 'crop' of ova fails to be fertilized, all the ova die within hours of fertilization, or insufficient numbers of blastocysts survive until days 12–15 postcoitus.

Whole herd targeted levels for farrowing rate should be 85–90%, however the results of several large surveys in the US pig industry indicate that farrowing rates average 72% on an annual basis. This is an area of great importance and offers an opportunity for significant increases on most farms.

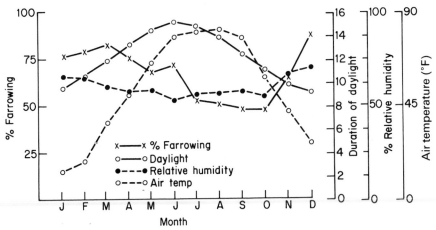

Fig. 8.3 Monthly farrowing rates and corresponding changes in ambient parameters for a 500 sow, total confinement facility in the midwest United States.

Figure 8.3 presents the farrowing rate during a 2 year period on a 532 sow totally confined gestation crate facility in the midwest United States. Note the variation with no apparent trends.

In order to elucidate cause(s) for a reduced farrowing rate, it is necessary to determine specifically when the female returns to estrus postcoitus. For example, the sow may return to estrus 'on cycle' at 21 ± 3 days (or at 21 day intervals such as 42, 63 etc.), or she may return at irregular intervals postweaning. Figure 8.4 depicts these two patterns of postweaning returns to estrus.

To identify more completely the noninfectious causative variable(s) which may reduce farrowing rate it is important to consider the management, nutrition, environment, and genetic components.

Management

Timing of Mating In order to optimize conception rate it is important that mating is timed relative to ovulation. In the pig, optimal conception rates are achieved when mating occurs 12 h prior to ovulation. This is usually 28 h after the onset of estrus. In order to approximate the onset of estrus, accurate and frequent estrus detection procedures should be initiated. Since estrus detection protocol on most US pig farms is generally once per day, it is important to practice double mating in order to have sperm present at the correct time for optimum conception rates.

Asynchronous breeding may occur: if estrus detection is delayed following weaning, or if it is practiced infrequently; if a mature boar is not used to evaluate behavioral signs of estrus; when there is overreliance on the boar's ability to detect an

estrous sow; if group sizes are too large to accurately identify sows in estrus (> 30 per pen), or when submissive sows are housed with dominant sows. Such factors reduce farrowing rates and ultimately litters/sow/year.

Matings per Estrus Multiple matings per sow per estrus are often initiated in order to increase the likelihood that one or more of the matings will occur near the time of optimal fertility. Many studies have demonstrated that females mated once per estrus have reduced farrowing rates relative to those mated multiple times per estrus. Several studies have shown no increase or only a marginal but nonsignificant increase in conception rates when sows were naturally or artificially inseminated three times per estrus rather than twice.

Type of Service When more than one mating occurs per estrus, the producer may have the choice of using the same boar (homospermic insemination) or a different boar(s) (heterospermic insemination). Homospermic matings are used in purebred operations and on some commercial farms where producers are attempting to identify and remove subfertile boars. Homospermic matings could potentially be used to estimate the relative fertility among boars. There is a perception that homospermic matings result in reduced conception rates when compared to heterospermic matings. Some studies show improved conception rates when semen is mixed from several boars via a process referred to as competitive fertilization. Other studies have shown no differences when different boars are mated to the same sow during one estrus. Though mixing semen from several boars is distinctly differ-

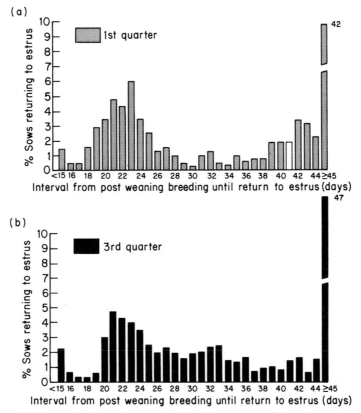

Fig. 8.4 (a) Regular and (b) irregular intervals to estrus following unsuccessful mating.

ent from naturally mating several boars to the same female, additional research in this area is needed before recommendations can be made.

Quality of Mating For natural mating to be effective it is important to have a fertile and receptive female. In addition, it is important to have a sexually aggressive boar, able to mount successfully, copulate, and ejaculate sufficient number of fertile spermatozoa in an adequate seminal volume. Matings of poor quality may result from a failure in any one of these areas.

Pen mating frequently results in lower conception rates than hand mating. This may be associated with factors such as excessive frequency of ejaculation by sexually aggressive boars, less than optimal matings/estrus, inadequate estrus detection resulting in asynchrony between ovulation and insemination or incomplete ejaculation.

Hand mating systems also may have reduced conception rates if the producer fails to assure that intromission has been successful and that ejaculation is completed before the boar withdraws from the sow. A breeding area having slippery floors, elevated ambient temperature, distractions, poor hygiene, or improper boar handling by the herdsman may cause incomplete ejaculation.

Artificial Insemination It is generally accepted that artificial insemination with fresh semen results in lower conception rates when compared to natural service. Farrowing rates following insemination with frozen semen are usually lower than that obtained with a fresh ejaculate. The observation that 40% of herds ($n = 172$) using artificial insemination had $> 80\%$ conception rates suggests that fertility may be similar to that obtained with natural service for some herds. On some farms there may be inadequate boar inventory to allow multiple natural matings/estrus/sow. In these cases, a common practice is to follow the first natural service in 18–30 h by artificial insemination. This second service is with fresh, extended semen. Farrowing rates comparable to those obtained when sows receive several natural matings have been achieved.

Parity The introduction to this chapter described a case concerning herd parity structure. It has been clearly demonstrated that lower parity sows, especially gilts and primiparous sows, have reduced farrowing rates when compared to higher parity females. In addition, the percentage of sows returning to estrus by 30 days after breeding is greater for low parity sows. Differences in these parameters among parities are more pronounced during summer months than during the other seasons. It appears that parity influences both the ability of female pigs to conceive as well as to maintain pregnancy.

Failure to Farrow Pseudopregnancy and the not-in-pig syndrome may result in reduced farrowing rates. This category of sows is very costly in the number of open days between farrowings. They are often 'lost in the herd'. A variety of factors must be ruled out when comprising a differential diagnosis list. The history should include such questions as when the females were mated, method for follow-up estrus detection, ultrasonic detections or any clinical signs (discharges). If the history indicates a failure to farrow there are several alternatives to consider: testing for estrone sulfate to determine the presence of a viable fetoplacental unit, termination of pregnancy with prostaglandin, or recovery of reproductive tracts at slaughter for gross and microscopic examination. The pathogenesis of the problem could include inaccurate estrus detection protocol, incomplete fetal absorption following a transient infectious etiology, or estrogenic mycotoxins which are luteotropic in the pig.

Nutrition

Feed Nutrition during lactation may have a great influence on litter size and return to estrus following weaning. Of notable interest are the effects of feed and caloric intake during the lactation period. Although it has been suggested that thin sows and those having the greatest lactational weight losses have reduced fertility, the influence of lactational feed intake remains unclear. The starvation of gilts during pregnancy for periods exceeding 1 month does not influence pregnancy rates or embryonic development. This might indicate that feed consumption during gestation has no obvious detrimental effects on the ability of the sow to maintain pregnancy. High level feeding of gilts and increased feed intake by primiparous sows, but not multiparous sows, during this interval from weaning to breeding improves farrowing rates. Thus the practice of flushing may be useful in improving the conception rates of low parity females but is unlikely to be beneficial in older sows.

Complete feed and/or water deprivation is a common practice often used by swine producers during the rebreeding period to shorten the interval between weaning and rebreeding. However, feed and/or water deprivation has been found to have no influence on conception rate, farrowing rate, or the rebreeding interval. In fact, feed deprivation may increase rather than shorten the weaning-to-rebreeding interval in primiparous sows.

Although remaining controversial, the addition of supplemental choline and biotin to lactation and gestation rations has been suggested to improve conception rates as well as decrease the weaning-to-rebreeding interval and to increase the number of pigs born alive.

Mycotoxicosis Contamination of feed grains with the mycotoxin zearalenone may result in reproductive failure. Among the multiple manifestations are dramatically reduced farrowing rates in accompaniment with irregular returns to estrus following breeding. It appears that while zearalenone interferes with conception and disrupts normal ovarian cyclicity, it promotes the artificial maintenance of corpora lutea for highly variable lengths of time. Zearalenone may also influence farrowing rate through its detrimental effects on sperm production and semen quality. Other manifestations of zearalenone toxicosis include reduced litter sizes and delayed puberty.

Environment

Temperature The exposure of females to increased ambient temperatures (> 90 °F) after mating is associated with decreased conception and farrowing rates and increased embryonic mortality. There is some debate regarding the time at which elevated temperature causes the greatest reduction in embryonic survival. One study implicated the time around mating, while a second study indicated that temperature elevation has its most pronounced detrimental effect prior to day 15 postmating, and the greatest embryonic mortality between days 8 and 16 postmating in a third study. Since nidation commences between 12 and 15 days after breeding in the pig it might be concluded that the highest rate of embryonic mortality occurs when sows are heat-stressed around the implantation interval. As a result, temperature stress in the sow may be manifested as lowered conception rates with regular returns to estrus if all the litter is killed. Cycles may be extended to irregular periods such as day 26, or small litters may occur if embryonic mortality is limited.

Elevated ambient temperatures have similar

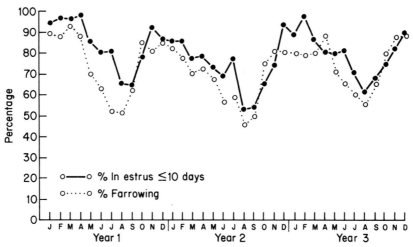

Fig. 8.5 Farrowing rate and percentage of weaned, mixed-parity sows returning to estrus ≤ 10 days post farrowing during each quarter of the year over a 3 year period on a 1500 sow, curtain-sided confinement herd in the southeastern United States.

detrimental effects on the boar. Sperm motility, quantity and morphology may be adversely affected by as few as 3 days of elevated temperature. If long-term exposure of the boar to elevated ambient temperature occurs, reductions in fertility may be seen for as long as 8 weeks. This roughly corresponds to the normal interval for spermatogenesis. Thus, when breeding boars are exposed to elevated temperatures, a decline in conception rates of mated females will occur. The decline may often occur 6–8 weeks following the initial temperature elevation. Lowered ambient temperature can have a negative influence on male fertility. Scrotal frostbite may occur in boars housed in extensive facilities during inclement weather in the midwest United States. It is rare to find this situation in confined housing units.

Season There have been numerous retrospective investigations in several countries throughout the world which document decreases in farrowing rates of sows that are mated during the summer months. Summer decreases in farrowing rates are greater in lower parity females when compared to older parity sows (Fig. 8.5). The summer decline in farrowing rate is in accompaniment with increases in the percentage of sows returning to estrus at irregular intervals following breeding. The irregular return may be due to spontaneous abortion after the luteotropic signal for pregnancy has been given. The summer decrease in farrowing rates is often attributed to elevated ambient temperatures characteristic of this season. Since elevated ambient temperature reduces both conception rates and litter size it is interesting

to note that litter size reductions are not usually seen with seasonal infertility.

During the summer to early fall period there is an increase in the incidence of spontaneous abortion and sows failing to farrow (not-in-pig). Abortions in the pig are often associated with infectious agents, however, the 'autumn abortion syndrome' has been documented without an apparent infectious etiology. Figure 8.6 is a summary of data from five farms (2500 sows) in the United Kingdom experiencing this apparently noninfectious phenomenon.

The abortion rate on many US swine farms averages between 1 and 2%. Figure 8.7 shows data collected from a client 'worried about an abortion problem' on his farm. Is there a problem?

Housing There is a debate regarding the influence of sow housing during the postweaning period and/or during gestation on farrowing rate. Some research has shown no significant influence of housing on fertility while other research indicates that sows housed in groups following breeding had higher farrowing rates relative to sows housed in stalls. Other studies suggest that sows placed in individual stalls following breeding have both higher fertility and shorter rebreeding intervals. It has been suggested that the stress response of social stimulation versus individual stall housing may mediate differences in fertility. Much variation exists among farms on management, environment, and facilities. There are cases where farrowing rates on group-housed sows exceed those of individual stall-housed sows. It is important to remember this farm by farm effect. Sow housing seems to influence the sow's re-

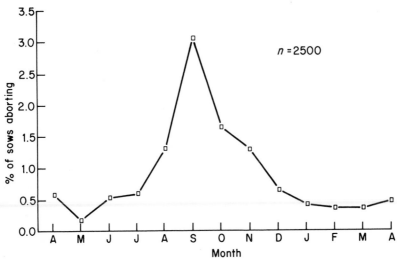

Fig. 8.6 Mean monthly abortion rate for five farms (2500 sows) in the United Kingdom. (Redrawn with permission of Pig Improvement Company, R&D Report no. 12, Franklin, Kentucky.)

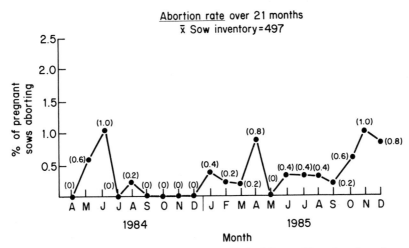

Fig. 8.7 Monthly abortion rates for a farm in the midwestern United States. Note that there is no obvious pattern to the occurrence of abortions and that abortion rates remained below suggested interference levels (1–2%).

productive response to changes in season. Sows housed in totally enclosed facilities have less seasonal fluctuations in fertility than those housed in open-front facilities.

Genetic

Breed Differences Some purebreds have higher conception rates than others and conception rates vary among different crossbred sow lines. Estimates of the heterosis of conception rate vary considerably with breeds used in the cross. For example, Yorkshires are associated with a conception rate heterosis of approximately 9.7% whereas Hampshires are

about 1.7%. The average individual heterosis for conception rates across all breeds, which excludes heterosis in the parents, is about 3.5%. This indicates that the crossbreeding heterosis may be used to improve the trait by an average of approximately 2.8 percentage units. Conception rates tend to be higher when crossbred boars are used rather than purebreds.

Boar Differences It has been of great interest to identify the fertility of boars. If it were possible to identify boars that were responsible for either reduced conception rates or litter sizes, a potential for increased productivity would be realized. In

Table 8.3 Herd mean conception rate (percentage of sows)

Conception rate (%)	90%	80%
97.5–100	4	0
92.5–97.5	24	1
87.5–92.5	44	8
82.5–87.5	24	24
77.5–82.5	4	34
72.5–77.5	0	24
67.5–72.5		8
<72.5		1

Table 8.4

Age at weaning (days)	Year					
	1979	1980	1981	1982	1983	1984
			Percentage of herds			
Under 19	4	5	10	11	8	7
19–25	38	41	44	45	54	57
26–32	13	13	18	18	19	22
33–39	37	32	22	20	15	10
Over 39	8	8	6	6	4	3
Number of herds	594	653	720	766	739	725

contrast to other species, regular semen evaluations on large numbers of boars in commercial swine operations are not done routinely and are usually not sufficiently accurate in determining differences in fertility among boars. It is generally accepted that differences in fertility exist between individual boars and that there can be significant differences in both farrowing rates and litter sizes. A breeding soundness examination/fertility evaluation is an important procedure for new boars coming into a commercial unit. It is not clear how much variation exists between groups of boars on commercial farms. One study indicates that 4% of the boars had < 60% farrowing rates whereas 87.5% had rates > 80%. When there are large variations in the fertility of groups of boars it is important to look at the records. Table 8.3 illustrates the variation expected by chance alone in mean conception rate of groups of randomly mated sows. The number of matings per boar equals 50. The data represent the expected distribution of conception rates among sows for two different herd mean conception rates (80% and 90%).

For some boars that mate only one to three times/week, it may take 6 months or longer to evaluate their fertility. Since fertility may change with the season, ambient temperature, or management factors, there is a risk of culling boars that have a transient infertility or boars who have not yet reached peak fertility.

Lactation Length

With the advent of better weaning rations and the desire to increase throughput on facilities there has been a trend towards earlier weaning. Table 8.4 is taken from the *MLC Pig Yearbook* (1985) showing these trends in the United Kingdom.

Notice the increase in the percentage of herds weaning between 19–25 days postfarrowing. Table 8.5 illustrates the influence of lactation length on

Table 8.5 Effect of weaning age on pigs/sow/year

Age at weaning (days)	14	21	28	35
Weaning to service (days)	8	8	8	8
Gestation (days)	116	116	116	116
Total days	138	145	152	159
Litters/sow/year	2.64	2.52	2.40	2.29
Pigs weaned/litter	9.0	9.0	9.0	9.0
Pigs/sow/year	23.8	22.7	21.6	20.6

some important parameters including pigs/sow/year.

Lactation lengths are usually established via the desired animal flow rate, number of farrowing crates, and management protocol. On farms weaning once per week, Thursdays are a common day to wean because sows will be in estrus Monday, Tuesday, or Wednesday of the following week. Figure 8.8 illustrates a 'typical' distribution of lactation lengths. Figure 8.9 depicts a herd having two separate populations in regards to lactation length. This variation may lead to other problems such as increased preweaning mortality in earlier weaned piglets and perhaps delayed returns to estrus from sows not having extended lactational intervals.

There is an inverse relationship between the length of time that a sow is allowed to lactate and the interval between weaning and return to estrus. The relationship is curvilinear with increases in lactation length up to at least 6 weeks resulting in shorter intervals from weaning to rebreeding (Fig. 8.10) It has been estimated that for each 10 day reduction in lactation length, there is an increase of

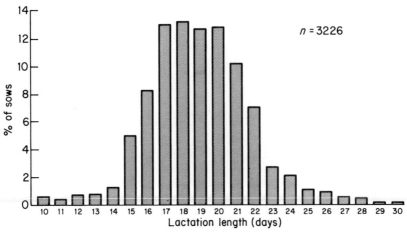

Fig. 8.8 Typical distribution of lactation lengths of sows on a herd in which pigs are weaned at '3 weeks' following farrowing. (Reproduced with permission of Pig Improvement Company, R&D Report no. 50, Franklin, Kentucky.)

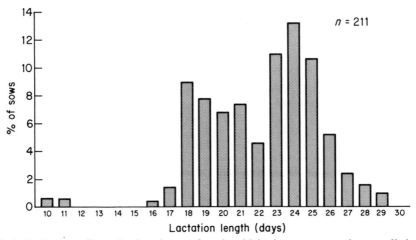

Fig. 8.9 Atypical distribution of lactation lengths on a farm in which pigs were weaned at two distinct ages.

about one day in the weaning-to-conception interval.

Techniques which have been used to optimize lactation length include split weaning of a group of sows in order to keep the sows more evenly spaced, split weaning of the litter (weaning the heaviest pigs several days early), and prostaglandin-induced farrowing.

Weaning-to-Estrus Interval

Prior to weaning there is modest follicular growth, however, once piglets are removed from the sow at weaning, an abrupt acceleration in follicular growth occurs. This appears to be in response to removal of inhibitory feedback influences present during the lactational period. The gradually increasing circu-

lating levels of estradiol following weaning eventually precipitate the onset of estrus and trigger the preovulatory discharge of luteinizing hormone which initiates the ovulatory process.

The sow will typically return to estrus 4–8 days following weaning. Figure 8.11 is from data collected on six farms in the United Kingdom. Notice the large percentage of females returning to estrus by day 10. In addition, there seems to be a second grouping of females in estrus between days 20 and 28. This second group of females may have been in physiologic estrus yet behaviorally anestrous at the correct time (days 4–8) and were undetected by the herdsman. One might speculate an additional group between days 40–46 using a similar rationale.

Several factors can affect the ability of the sow to return to estrus at the correct time following weaning. Their importance will vary among farms.

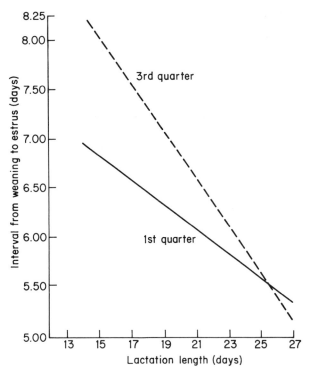

Fig. 8.10 Influence of lactation length on interval from weaning to rebreeding during two seasons of the year (first quarter = January to March and third quarter = July to September).

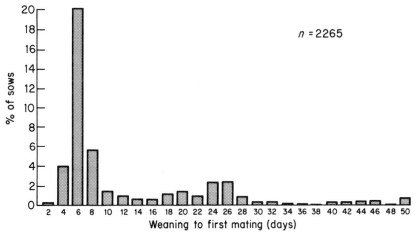

Fig. 8.11 Pattern of return to estrus following weaning in crossbred sows on six farms in the United Kingdom. (Reproduced with permission from the Pig Improvement Company, R&D Report no. 50, Franklin, Kentucky.)

Parity Primiparous sows have a longer mean interval from weaning to estrus and a lower proportion of sows returning to estrus within 7 days following weaning than higher parity sows. The introductory section of this chapter presented a case of a newly populated herd with delayed returns to estrus as a common event. In addition, herds that have high

mortality and/or high culling rates ($> 35\%$) will tend to have a younger average parity, thus creating an opportunity for prolonged interval to the first postweaning estrus.

Environment During the summer months there is a decline in the percentage of sows returning to estrus

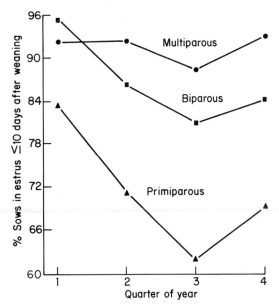

Fig. 8.12 Influence of season on return to estrus following weaning on three herds in the southeastern United States.

within 7 days following weaning and an increase in the incidence of sows remaining anestrous. Primiparous sows are affected to a greater degree when compared to older parity sows (Fig. 8.12) As with fertility, the seasonal delays in return to estrus appear to be more pronounced in sows housed in completely enclosed buildings versus those housed in open-front buildings. It is not uncommon for feed consumption to be reduced during the warm summer months. The evaporative cooling of sows will help increase feed intake thus minimizing weight loss during lactation.

Genetics There is variation in the interval from weaning to estrus among different purebreds and among different crossbred lines. A recently completed study suggests that the interval from weaning to estrus is influenced by breed, parity, and an interaction between them. Table 8.6 is a summary of this information. Furthermore, some breeds have a higher proportion of sows that remain persistently anestrous following weaning than others.

Nutrition Feed and/or caloric intake during lactation is related to the interval from weaning to estrus. It appears that intakes of at least 12 Mcal/sow/day will minimize the incidence of sows having delayed returns to estrus postweaning. During lactation, sows having reduced caloric intakes lose more weight and backfat than sows fed higher

levels. But it is not clear if body condition measurements are useful to identify those sows who will have delayed returns to estrus postweaning. The addition of dietary fat to the lactation ration will increase the caloric density and palatability of the ration which minimizes lactational weight loss. This is of particular interest in the warm summer months when sow appetite declines. While data in the literature provide conflicting evidence on the benefits of high nutrient intake during lactation and the postweaning period on subsequent fertility, it is recommended that sows be fed at a high level during this critical period. This is especially important for the primiparous sow which is still experiencing some general growth.

Boar Exposure It is very important to begin boar exposure commencing at weaning. The sight, sound, and smell of the boar are important stimuli which mediate the onset of estrus postweaning. Also, such procedures will minimize the number of anestrous females postweaning. It is important to cull females failing to return to estrus postweaning within 30–45 days to reduce the number of open sow days on the farm.

Farrowing Schedule Continuous farrowing schedules require appropriate facilities and a significant demand on labor and husbandry skills. Though a continuous farrowing schedule may appear as the most biologically efficient, it may not be the most cost-effective. The past trends in the United States have been towards more intensive rearing of swine which has influenced producers to invest capital in fixed assets. Currently, there is a greater awareness regarding employed capital with a move among some producers towards more extensive and traditional pig-keeping methods. With this change, sows are often grouped to farrow at regular 2, 3 or 4 week intervals. Some may even farrow sows at irregularly spaced intervals. In many cases, with minor modifications in the farrowing schedule combined with facility changes to handle the added throughput, the farrowing intervals can be reduced with commensurate increases in litters/sow/year.

Number of Pigs Born Alive/Litter

A parameter which sets the upper limit for the number of pigs weaned/litter is number of pigs born alive/litter. With currently available technology, targeted levels for number of pigs born alive should range between 10.5 and 11.5/litter. It usually follows that procedures which maximize farrowing rate will also maximize litter size and vice versa. It is

Table 8.6 Interval to postweaning estrus for first, second, and third parity Large White, Landrace, Yorkshire, and Chester White sows

Parity	Large White	Landrace	Yorkshire	Chester White	All breeds
1	7.8 (0.6)	6.6 (0.6)	9.3 (0.8)	14.0 (1.0)	9.4 (0.4)
2	6.0 (0.6)	4.9 (0.6)	6.0 (0.8)	7.0 (1.0)	6.9 (0.4)
3	6.4 (0.7)	5.2 (0.7)	6.8 (0.9)	4.6 (1.2)	5.8 (0.4)
Total	6.7 (0.4)	5.6 (0.4)	7.4 (0.5)	8.6 (0.6)	
Overall					7.1 (0.2)

Key: Numbers are days expressed as mean (±SE); total number of animals in the study = 598; lactation length = 28 days.

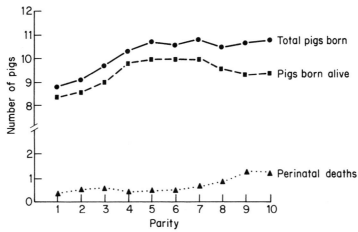

Fig. 8.13 Changes in total number of pigs born, number of pigs born alive, and number of stillborn pigs with parity in a 500 sow purebred Large White herd in the southeastern United States.

not uncommon, however, to have reductions in litter size without having reductions in other parameters of fertility. It is important to investigate the records completely to identify the distinct differences which may be elucidated.

There are several events during the reproductive process which may affect the number of pigs born alive/litter: ovulation rate, fertilization rate, embryonic mortality, and peripartum mortality (stillbirths). In order to investigate the area of dysfunction more specifically, it is important to clarify the management, nutritional, environmental, and genetic parameters which may influence the number of piglets born alive.

Management

Parity As discussed previously, parity can have a profound influence on fecundity. The results of numerous studies have indicated that litter size is smallest at the first parity, rises to a maximum

between the third and sixth parity, and then remains constant or declines slightly with additional parity increases. Figure 8.13 is taken from a large compiled sample of information and demonstrates the proportion of sows having maximum litter size at each parity.

On page 125 and in Fig. 8.1 an example is provided of a skewed parity distribution with comments on litter size reductions. It is important to remember that there is not an ideal parity distribution for all farms. That is, a parity distribution which optimizes litter size on one farm with specific facilities and husbandry skills may vary from that of another farm. Figure 8.14 illustrates three possible patterns of born alive/sow versus sow parity. Figure 8.14a shows a typical pattern of litter scatter with a decline in later parities; Fig. 8.14b shows the pattern of a large increase in number born alive from the first to second farrowing, and Fig. 8.14c shows a 'second litter dip' seen in some herds.

This decline in litter size seen on some herds is not

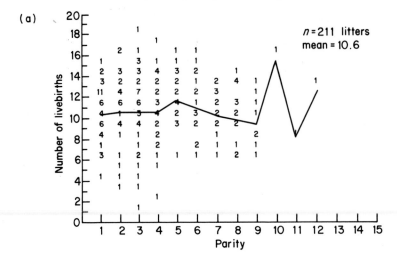

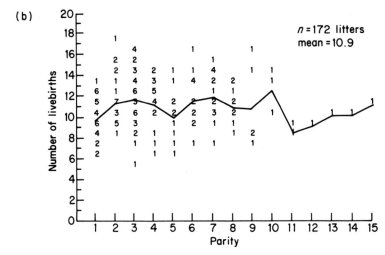

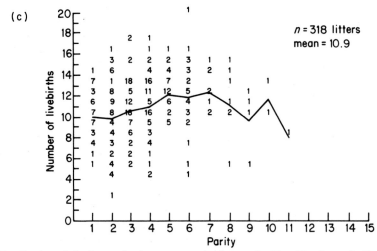

Fig. 8.14 (a) Distribution of pigs born alive/sow over parity in a typical herd having a decline in liveborn litter size at higher parities; (b) a herd having an increasing litter size from the first to second farrowings; (c) a herd having a decrease in litter size from the first to second farrowings.

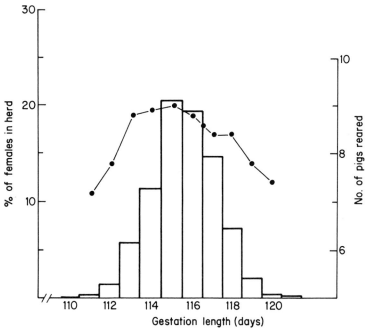

Fig. 8.15 Relationship between gestation lengths and number of pigs reared per litter. Bars indicate percentage of females farrowing at day indicated; line indicates number of piglets reared. (Redrawn with permission from Pig Improvement Company R&D Report no. 15.)

obligatory. That is, there are a number of herds which do not experience this problem. Tentative evidence on retrospective analysis of data may lead the veterinary consultant to recommend not mating first parity females when they return to their first estrus postweaning. Instead, the suggestion has been made to wait until the second estrus postweaning to improve subsequent litter size. There does not seem to be enough evidence to make this recommendation for all herds at the present time.

Gestation Length There is a relationship between the gestation length and the number of pigs reared per litter. Sows gestating > 116 days tend to have lower number of total pigs born, born alive, and reared than those < 116 days. Figure 8.15 depicts this relationship between gestation length and number of pigs reared per litter. One possible solution is to induce farrowing with prostaglandin treatment on day 114.

Lactation Length While there is a negative relationship between lactation length and rebreeding interval postweaning, lactation length is related positively to size of subsequent litter. Reductions in weaning age from approximately 6 weeks are accompanied by a concomitant reduction in litter size. The reduction in litter size becomes more pro-

nounced with lactation lengths of less than 4 weeks. It has been estimated that there is a reduction of 0.1 pig/day for each 1 day decrease in lactation below 28 days. This relationship is graphically presented in Fig. 8.16.

The reduction in litter size with shortened lactation lengths is generally thought to be attributed to increased embryonic mortality around the time of implantation. Exogenous steroid hormone therapy has been used experimentally around the time of nidation to reduce the extent of these losses. This procedure has not been adequately tested in commercial situations to make a specific recommendation at this time.

Time of Breeding Optimum fertilization rates occur when gilts are inseminated 12 h prior to ovulation which usually corresponds to 28 h after the onset of standing estrus. Because of inadequate estrus detection procedures and variation among individual sows it is important to practice multiple matings per estrus to optimize the chance that fertile sperm are deposited at the correct time. Similar to conception rate, litter size increases when sows are double mated when compared to single mating. There appears to be differences among farms on the influence that the number of matings per estrus has on litter size. On some farms, there is no difference in

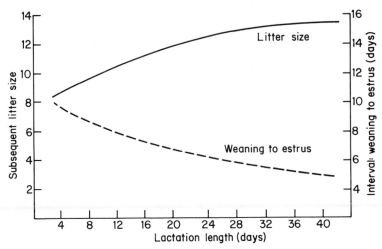

Fig. 8.16 Influence of lactation length on interval from weaning to rebreeding and on litter size at the subsequent farrowing. (Redrawn from Cole, Varley and Hughes, 1975.)

the litter sizes of sows mated once, twice or three times during estrus. On others, there is an advantage of multiple over single matings. It is difficult to triple mate sows on some farms if boar numbers are insufficient, or if sows do not stand long enough for the last service. As with conception rate, there is a controversial influence regarding homospermic and heterospermic inseminations on litter size. That is, some studies indicate an increase with heterospermic inseminations on litter size and others have shown no effect. Unless breeding records are being effectively monitored on commercial farms it is advisable to utilize heterospermic inseminations to optimize litter size.

Peripartum Mortality   Peripartum mortality is a significant component which reduces the number of pigs born alive/litter. In the United States about 7% of all piglets are presented dead at birth. These piglets were alive prior to the onset of parturition and can be distinguished from those piglets presented alive and expiring soon after birth by a lung flotation test. This information is confirmed by hysterotomy observations from hundreds of sows which indicates that literally all the piglets are alive. In utero death can be attributed to many causes such as female constipation, overweight females, piglets located near the distal ends of the uterine horn, piglets born in the last third of the litter, carbon monoxide levels in the farrowing house, female parity plus many others. Observed farrowings will minimize the incidence of this problem. In addition the advent of prostaglandin usage to predict more accurately the time of parturition induction can be a useful management tool to assist with this prob-

lem. Care must be exercised, however, since use of this drug too soon prior to expected farrowing can also reduce survival of piglets. In general it should not be given prior to 111 days of gestation.

Nutrition

Even though caloric and feed intake during lactation influence the rebreeding interval of sows, there appears to be no effect on ovulation rate, embryonic mortality or litter size at the subsequent farrowing. Primiparous sows fed at a high rate (> 3.5 kg/day) during the weaning to rebreeding interval have higher ovulation rates and greater litter sizes that those fed lower amounts of feed (< 2.0 kg/day). There appears to be no influence of rebreeding interval feed level on the litter sizes of multiparous sows. The practice of *ad libidum* feeding (flushing) gilts for 3 weeks prior to breeding has been shown to increase ovulation rates and litter sizes. Following flushing, feed level and caloric intake should be reduced to minimize the chance of increased embryonic mortality.

Environment

In contrast to other manifestations of season, there is considerable controversy over the influence of season on litter size. Seasonal variations in total pigs born and pigs born alive per litter have been shown in some studies but not in others. When variations in litter size are reported it does not seem to be restricted to the summer months. As with other variations mentioned previously, there are many differences between farms. Elevations in ambient

Table 8.7 Variation expected in mean litter size

Rank	Mean litter size/boar
1	11.61
2	11.40
3	11.26
4	11.15
5	11.05
6	10.95
7	10.85
8	10.74
9	10.60
10	10.39

Table 8.8 Reported changes in pigs weaned/litter

Years	Pigs weaned/litter
1949–51	6.4
1959–61	7.3
1969–71	7.2
1974	7.2
1984	7.4

Source: Illinois FBFM Recording System.

temperature can adversely affect both estrous cyclicity and conception rates. In addition, some studies have shown an adverse effect on litter size while others reveal no effect. Again, there may be a sensitive time around the period of nidation.

Genetics

Boars Numerous studies have demonstrated that boars influence the total number of pigs born, the number of pigs born alive, and/or the number of pigs weaned. It has been suggested that sire differences in litter size are associated with differences in semen quality. Although not yet demonstrated, it cannot be ruled out that qualitative differences in sperm production and morphology may also contribute to differences in litter size.

Boar usage appears to influence litter size similarly to its effect on conception rate. Litter size does not appear to be adversely affected if boars are used fewer than six times per week. It has been suggested that litter size is less sensitive to overuse of boars than farrowing rate. When records are investigated regarding litter size problems and possible 'boar effects' it is important to consider the variation expected by chance alone. Table 8.7 lists the variation expected in mean litter size for each boar in a group of ten boars. The average litter size for the herd was 11 piglets per litter and the number of matings per boar was 50. The ranking is from best to worst (1–10) for the ten different boars.

Notice that there is an expected variation of about 1.2 piglets between the best and the worst boar. When differences of this order are described the veterinary consultant must be careful to put things in perspective and appreciate the normal variation in a group. The veterinary consultant can provide very useful input by using such information to cull boars and raise the mean litter size in the herd.

Breed Differences There are considerable variations in the prolificacy among purebred and crossbred lines. As with other reproductive traits, crossbreeding has been used to increase the fecundity of commercial swine in many parts of the world. The United States has been particularly slow to adapt to the genetic improvement programs which are currently available to make this change. Table 8.8 is from data in Illinois, and illustrates the slow increase in pigs weaned per litter in a major swine producing state during a 35 year period.

The heterosis resulting from crossbreeding varies with the crossbreeding program used (for example, three-breed rotation, four-way terminal) and with the breeds used in making the cross. The average individual heterosis for litter size at birth is approximately 2.4%, which relates to an improvement of about 0.23 pigs/litter. There does not appear to be an improvement in litter size by using crossbred over purebred boars.

ECONOMIC IMPLICATIONS

The purpose of this section is to give some examples to provide an economic perspective for the previous sections. Among the variety of ways in which the economic implications can be viewed, is to look at the large increases in output which result from small yet significant changes in fertility. Pigs weaned/sow/year will be used in the following example as a base measure for output monitoring.

Assume 100 sows are producing 18 pigs/sow/year yielding an annual production of 1800 pigs. If the feed cost and medication cost to rear a 20 kg pig is US $8.00 and if the feeder pig market is $35.00, then each extra pig is worth an additional $27.00 assuming no extra sow feed, labor, or facility costs. If pigs/sow/year could be improved by one piglet to 19, total output would be 1900 pigs. The extra 100 pigs would generate an additional $2700.00.

Another concept which integrates productivity, efficiency, and cost control into one value is margin

Table 8.9   Influence of pigs/sow/year on margin over feed costs (MOFC)

Farm identification	A	B	C
Herd size (number of sows)	300	300	300
Farrowing/sow/year	1.75	1.85	2.30
Pigs weaned/litter	7.6	7.7	10.0
Pigs weaned/sow/year	13.3	14.3	23.0
Pigs slaughtered/year	3990	4361	6900
Weight (kg) at slaughter	100	100	100
Total kg of pork ($\times 10^5$)	3.99	4.36	6.90
Market price ($/kg)	1.00	1.00	1.00
Revenue ($)	399 000.00	436 000.00	690 000.00
Feed costs			
Total kg of pork ($\times 10^5$)	3.99	4.36	6.90
Feed conversion ratio	3.9	3.9	3.9
Total kg feed ($\times 10^4$)	155.61	170.04	269.1
Feed price/kg	0.16	0.16	0.16
Total feed cost ($)	248 976.00	272 064.00	430 560.00
MOFC/sow ($)	500.08	546.45	864.80
MOFC/herd ($)	150 024.00	163 936.00	259 440.00
Economic advantage		+13 912.00	+109 416.00

over feed cost (MOFC). Great differences in MOFC by changes in farrowings/sow/year and pig weaned/litter are shown in Table 8.9. The total increase in MOFC between herd A and herd C is $364.72/sow or $109 416.00 over all 300 sows per annum.

SUMMARY

The recognition and evaluation of noninfectious reproductive problems on commercial swine farms is difficult and often tedious work. Since the majority of US swine producers do not effectively utilize individual sow records and farm information systems, the veterinary consultant is challenged to make suggestions without having a basis for understanding. When a herd experiences reproductive failures, it is important to define clearly the parameters measured and to collect all pertinent data in order to avoid any confusion between the veterinary consultant and the herdsman. Next, the approach should consider normal variation and management factors as major influences on the data set collected. Once the problem has been clarified, it may be categorized as either of probable infectious etiology and pathogenesis or of a noninfectious nature. Infectious problems are generally easier to identify, diagnose, and treat medically than noninfectious problems. However, infectious problems represent a small component of the overall reproductive biologic inefficiencies which a pig herd may experience. Though significant improvements in output can often be achieved with incrementally smaller levels

of input costs, the veterinary consultant should try to achieve a balanced approach to problem-solving.

For example, the major components influencing decision-making in most businesses include the following: level of output, input costs, throughput rate, and overall financial position. If the veterinary consultant approaches reproductive failure solely from the perspective of increased output, the effect on input costs might be exorbitant. Similarly, overall financial position influences many of these key decisions. In most instances, the reproductive potential is limited by management, genetics, environment, and nutrition. As our awareness and understanding of these key areas is increased, it will be possible to consider achieving optimum sow herd productivity.

References

Anderson, L. L. (1975) Embryonic and placental development during prolonged inanition in the pig. *Amer. J. Physiol.*, **229**, 1689.

BeVier, G. W. & Backstrom, L. (1980) Seasonal infertility pattern during 1978 in 22 swine herds in Iowa and Nebraska, USA. *Proc. 6th Int. Congr. Pig Vet. Soc., Copenhagen, Denmark*, p. 321.

Bichard, M. (1983) Litter size and sow productivity. In: *New Developments in Scientific Breeding No. 3, Pig Improvement Supplement*, pp. 2–6, April.

Brooks, P. H. & Cole, D. J. A. (1972) Studies in sow reproduction 1. The effect of nutrition between weaning and remating on the reproductive performance of primiparous sows. *Anim. Prod.*, **15**, 259–264.

Brooks, P. H., Smith, D. A. & Irwin, V. C. R. (1977) Biotin-supplementation of diets; the incidence of foot lesions, and the reproductive performance of sows. *Vet Rec.*, **101**, 46–50.

Chang, K., Kurtz, H. G. & Mirocha, C. J. (1979) Effects of mycotoxin zearalenone on swine reproduction. *Amer. J. Vet. Res.*, **40**, 1260–1267.

Christenson, R. K. & Ford, J. J. (1979) Puberty and estrus in confinement reared gilts. *J. Anim. Sci.*, **49**, 743–751.

Cole, D. J. A., Varley, M. A. & Hughes, P. E. (1975) Studies in sow reproduction 2. The effect of lactation length on the subsequent reproductive performance of the sow. *Anim. Prod.*, **20**, 401–406.

Dziuk, P. J. (1970) Estimation of the optimum time for insemination of gilts and ewes by double-mating at certain times relative to ovulation. *J. Reprod. Fertil.*, **22**, 277–282.

Esbenshade, K. L., Britt, J. H., Armstrong, J. D. *et al.* (1986) Body condition of sows across parities and relationship to reproductive performance. *J. Anim. Sci.*, **62**, 1187–1193.

Ford, J. J. (1978) Effect of floor space restriction on age at puberty in gilts and on performance of barrows and gilts. *J. Anim. Sci.*, **47**, 828–832.

Foxcroft, G. R. and Van de Wiel, D. F. M. (1982) Endocrine control of the oestrous cycle. In: *Control of Pig Reproduction*, eds Cole, D. J. A. and Foxcroft, G. R., pp. 161–178. London: Butterworths Scientific.

Hemsworth, P. H., Salden, N. T. C. J. & Hoogerbrugge, A. (1982) The influence of the postweaning social environment on the weaning to mating interval of the sow. *Anim. Prod.*, **35**, 41–48.

Hilley, H. D., Dial, G. D., Hagan, J. *et al.* (1986) Influence of the number of services and season on the litter size and farrowing rate of primiparous sows. *Proc. Int. Pig Vet. Soc. Congr. Barcelona*, p. 23.

Hilley, H. D., Dial, G. D., Hagan, J. *et al.* (1986) The influence of parity, season of the year, number of matings, and previous lactation length on the number of pigs born alive to multiparous sows. *Proc. Int. Pig Vet. Soc. Congr., Barcelona*, p. 24.

Hunter, R. H. F. (1977) Physiological factors influencing ovulation, fertilization, early embryonic development and establishment of pregnancy in pigs. *Brit. Vet. J.*, **133**, 461–468.

Hurtgen, J. P. (1982) Reproductive diseases. *Symposium on Diagnosis and Treatment of Swine Diseases, Vet. Clin. N. Amer., Large Anim. Pract.*, **4**(2), 277–229.

Hurtgen, J. P., Leman, A. D. (1980) Seasonal influence on the fertility of sows and gilts. *J. Amer. Vet. Med. Assoc.*, **177**, 631–635.

Irgang, R. & Robinson, Q. W. (1984) Heritability estimates for ages at farrowing, rebreeding interval and litter traits in swine. *J. Anim. Sci.*, **59**, 67–73.

Johnson, R. K. (1981) Crossbreeding in swine: experimental results. *J. Anim. Sci.*, **52**, 906–923.

King, R. H. & Williams, I. H. (1984) The effect of nutrition on the reproductive performance of first-litter sows 1. Feeding level during lactation, and between weaning and remating. *Anim. Prod.*, **36**, 241–247.

Love, R. J. (1981) Seasonal infertility in pigs. *Vet. Rec.*, **109**, 407–409.

MacLean, C. W. (1965) Observations on noninfectious infertility in swine. *Vet Rec.*, **85**, 675–682.

Maurer, R. R., Ford, J. J. & Christianson, R. K. (1985) Interval to first postweaning estrus and causes for leaving the breeding herd in Large White, Landrace, Yorkshire and Chester White females after three parities. *J. Anim. Sci.*, **61**, 1327–1334.

Meat and Livestock Commission (1985) *Pig Yearbook.* April. Bletchley, UK: Meat and Livestock Commission, Economics Livestock and Marketing Services.

Omtvedt, I. T., Nelson, R. E., Edwards, R. L. *et al.* (1986) Influence of heat stress during early, mid and late pregnancy of gilts. *J. Anim. Sci.*, **32**, 312–317.

Rasbech, N. O. (1969) A review of the causes of reproductive failure in swine. *Brit. Vet. J.*, **125**, 599–614.

Reese, D. E., Moser, B. D., Peo, E. R., *et al.* (1982) Influence of energy intake during lactation on the interval from weaning to first estrus in sows. *J. Anim. Sci.*, **55**, 590–589.

de Sa, W. F., Pleumsamran, P., Marcom, C. B., *et al.* (1981) Exogenous steroid effects on litter size and early embryonic survival in swine. *Theriogenology*, **15**, 245–255.

Signoret, J. P., (1971) The mating behavior of the sow. In: *Pig Production*, ed. Cole, D. J. A., pp. 295–313. University Park: Pennsylvania State University Press.

Singleton, W. L. & Shelby, D. R. (1972) Variation among boars in semen characteristics and fertility. *J. Anim. Sci.*, **34**, 762–766.

Svajgr, A. J., Hays, V. W., Cromwell, G. L. & Dutt, R. H. (1974) Effect of lactation duration on reproductive performance of sows. *J. Anim. Sci.*, **38**, 100–105.

Teague, H. S., Roller, W. L. & Grifo, A. P., Jr. (1968) Influence of high temperature and humidity on the reproductive performance of swine. *J. Anim. Sci.*, **27**, 408–411.

Tilton, J. E. & Cole, D. J. A. (1982) Effect of triple versus double mating on sow productivity. *Anim. Prod.*, **334**, 279–282.

Varley, M. A. & Cole, D. J. A. (1978) Studies in sow reproduction 6. The effect of lactation length on preimplantation losses. *Anim. Prod.*, **27**, 209–214.

Warnick, A. C., Wallace, H. D., Palmer, A. Z., *et al.* (1965) Effect of temperature on early embryo survival in gilts. *J. Anim. Sci.*, **24**, 89–92.

Wetteman, R. P., Wells, M. E. & Johnson, R. K. (1979) Reproductive characteristics of boars during and after exposure to increased ambient temperature. *J. Anim. Sci.*, **49**, 1501–1505.

9

Breeding Programs in the Mare

R. M. LOFSTEDT

with a section on Endometritis with T. W. A. LITTLE

NORMAL LEVELS OF FERTILITY IN MARES

In most cases, conformation and athletic ability are more important to owners than fertility. Therefore, mares are not usually selected for fertility. In addition, they are often bred very early in the breeding season when conception rates are low. During early springtime, in the temperate zones, single estrus conception rates are approximately 30%, but this increases to 50–55% in the summertime. By contrast, mares that are selected for fertility and bred in summertime have first estrus conception rates as high as 65–70%.

By the end of a 6-month breeding season, at least 85% of thoroughbred or standardbred mares should have conceived. In fact, the conception level for the whole season is usually over 95% on well-managed farms. The number of services per ovulation is approximately 1.6, and the number of ovulations per conception 1.7 or less. Young mares are usually less fertile than older mares. This has been demonstrated by the poor success of embryo collection in 2-year-old mares and studies in wild horses which showed that 2-year-olds seldom had foals and the foaling percentage increased until the broodmares were 6 years or older. In addition, computations from well-managed breeding farms have shown that conception levels in 2-year-olds were significantly lower than in older mares. Fertility increased until the mares were 8–10 years old then decreased after

15 years of age. A loss of 10–15% of embryos can be expected before 50 days of gestation, the majority of losses occurring before 35 days. The cause of embryonal death is unknown in most cases, but if the mare is similar to the human and the pig some embryos probably die because of chromosomal abnormalities. In the second and third trimester of pregnancy, the abortion rate should not exceed 5% of all pregnancies.

THE INFLUENCE OF MANAGEMENT ON FERTILITY

Early Season Breeding

Mares have estrous cycles throughout the year in the tropics, but experience a limited breeding season at temperate latitudes because they stop cycling or experience irregular cyclicity in periods of short daylength. The administration of the racing industry dictates that the official birthdate of thoroughbred and standardbred mares should fall in the middle of the short daylength period, that is January 1 in the northern hemisphere or August 1 in the southern hemisphere. Therefore, breeders of racehorses require newborn foals as soon as possible after the official birthdate so that these offspring have a maximum physical advantage over their cohorts at yearling sales and on the race track. This dictates that mares also have to be bred during the short daylength period because the modal length of their gestation is just over 11 months which creates a biological imposition for the breeding industry. A minority of mares cycle normally at the beginning of the breeding season (February 15, northern hemisphere, or September 15, southern hemisphere), while the majority experience prolonged or occasional split estrous periods and a high incidence of failure of ovulation. As a result, the general level of fertility is low. In addition, stallions may become overworked because of increased use during the prolonged estrous periods experienced by the mare. In those cases, the libido of the stallion may be even more severely depressed than it normally is at this time of year, especially in young animals.

Light Treatment

On many breeding farms these problems have been controlled by treating mares with an artificial long daylength photoperiod which begins approximately 8–10 weeks before the intended onset of breeding. The photoperiod may be a combination of natural as well as artificial light and it need not necessarily increase gradually up until the time of breeding. For example, a 40 watt fluorescent tube or 200 watt incandescent bulb can be suspended in the mare's stall so that the floor of the stall is brightly illuminated and a timing device can be used to regulate the photoperiod to 15 or 16 h of light and 8 or 9 h of darkness per 24 h. A very wide range of illumination levels are effective in inducing cyclicity, and consequently the light level in the stall is not very critical. However, the timing of the light *is* critical. Furthermore, continuous lighting will retard the onset of cyclicity and is not recommended.

Light treatment will induce cyclicity significantly earlier in treated than in untreated mares, but estrous cycles are still irregular and ovulation unpredictable when cyclicity begins; therefore it is recommended that the cycle be modulated by daily injection of progesterone (25 mg/kg i.m.) or feeding of altrenogest (0.44 mg/kg/day) for 15 days prior to the onset of breeding. These treatments will decrease the incidence of prolonged or split estrus and failure of ovulation, resulting in a higher level of conception per unit time than in untreated mares. Due to the fact that these treatments do not induce cyclicity but merely modulate it, it is important to ensure that mares are having normal estrous cycles or are on the verge of cyclicity before progestagenic treatments are initiated. To ensure that this is the case, candidates for the treatment should have demonstrated estrous behavior with a teaser stallion or have one or more follicles greater than 20 mm in size.

Breeding at Foal Heat

The uterus of the mare usually involutes to its nongravid size by 2 weeks postpartum, but conception at foal heat which occurs within 20 days of foaling may be marginally lower than at subsequent estrous periods. Conception rates can be 5–10% lower during foal heat as compared to later estrous periods, but in some cases there may be no difference at all. Therefore, the conception rate at foal heat probably depends on when it occurs after parturition and the degree of uterine involution at that time.

Some investigators have tried to delay foal heat for a few days to allow for additional uterine involution to occur. This has been done by using altrenogest or a combination of progesterone and estradiol but the benefits when compared to untreated mares were questionable. 'Short cycling' the mare by administering prostaglandins in the luteal phase following foal heat to advance the time of the subsequent estrus was also of questionable value. Therefore, if foaling has been uneventful and the mare and foal are in good health, the mare should be rebred during foal heat. Foal heat occurs predictably regardless of the time of the year, and ovulation rate is normal even during late winter (although it may be marginally delayed when compared with foal heat during summertime). This provides an excellent management opportunity for early season breeding.

Detecting Estrus

Due to the fact that mares show no overt signs of estrus unless they are exposed to a male animal, it is essential to practice an effective teasing method for good breeding results. Owners are frequently convinced that their mares are in estrus because they may be urinating frequently, may squat or appear to be excited. Sometimes these mares are bred artificially or they may even be hobbled and forced to mate naturally, but due to the absence of physiological estrus, they fail to conceive. Such contamination of the uterus during the luteal phase may cause endometritis and compromise future fertility. This practice can also lead to breeding accidents and human injury.

Breeding of mares at inappropriate times is not a common problem on large breeding farms but may be encountered when horse owners are relatively inexperienced, when a stallion is unavailable for teasing or when only a few mares are bred each year. When a stallion is not available for teasing, or if there is any question as to whether or not a mare is in physiological estrus, a serum sample should be analyzed for its progesterone level. Rapid ELISA tests for progesterone determination are now available allowing one to determine whether an animal has a functional corpus luteum. During the spring-time transitional period, a single low serum progesterone value may be misleading because the mare may not have started to cycle. Therefore, a second sample taken 7–8 days later should also be examined. If the mare is in estrus, breeding should occur every 48 h until a prebreeding serum sample indicates that progesterone is increasing.

Even if one is adept at rectal palpation and makes use of transrectal ultrasonography to examine ovarian structures, the physiological status of the mare may still be difficult to determine, especially if she is a maiden mare and does not exhibit cervical changes that are typical of estrus, such as erythema, moistening and relaxation. Further confusion may arise due to the fact that ovarian follicles frequently grow to preovulatory size during the luteal phase as well as during estrus. A special effort must be made to detect luteal tissue in the ovary by ultrasonography in those cases, but even if it is detected, its functional status may be difficult or impossible to determine. For example, ovarian stroma can easily be confused with small corpora lutea, and corpora lutea and corpora albicantia can also have a similar appearance on ultrasonography. These diagnostic problems illustrate the need for a reliable teasing stallion and a conscientious teasing program. With the help of such a program, the estrous cycle of most mares can be well-defined. Mares should be teased on a daily basis.

Most mares respond to almost any stallion by winking, squatting or not kicking when they are in heat: the three cardinal signs of estrus. Some mares do not squat during estrus, but winking and absence of kicking are invariable components of estrous behavior. Some mares, especially if timid or inexperienced, may kick in the presence of very aggressive stallions even when they are in heat but this is unusual and seldom poses a problem in diagnosing estrus. However, a few mares show definite stallion preference despite the fact that they are in estrus. They will kick or strike out at one male, but exhibit classical signs of estrus when teased with another. One study indicated that stallion preference can be expected in less than 5% of broodmares; therefore it is not a significant problem but it may occasionally lead to some confusion if it is not recognized in a teasing program.

The method of teasing is of great importance if maximum fertility is to be achieved. For example, mares are frequently teased by leading a stallion past their paddocks or stable doors, but this method is only satisfactory if mares show obvious signs of estrus and is of little value when they are apparently disinterested onlookers. Objective study has shown that almost 50% of mares in estrus may not be detected when these methods are employed. Even when mares are tested by 'nose-to-nose' exposure over a stable door they may not display signs of estrus. Therefore, it is essential to 'force tease' uncommitted mares to determine their reproductive status. During force teasing, the mare is restrained in teasing stocks and the stallion is allowed to examine her completely. He may nudge the mare or even nip her over the neck and rump regions, usually eliciting an obvious response. During the anestrous and transitional phases, however, some mares receive the stallion's advances passively and ultrasonography or progesterone analysis is required to ascertain their physiological status.

The author is unaware of any data that compares the efficacy of geldings and stallions when they are used as teasers. In fact, there is also little objective information on the efficacy of geldings that are used for this purpose. The maintenance of masculine behavior varies from one gelding to another and while some geldings appear to be effective teasers others do not exhibit sufficient libido. Testosterone treatment (for example, 2.5 mg/kg of testosterone propionate i.m. for 7–10 days followed by injections of testosterone enanthate at 5 mg/kg i.m. at 10–14-day intervals, as necessary) may improve the performance of a gelding as a teaser. However, the performance of a teaser is so important to a breeding program that if the libido of a gelding is questionable, it may be advisable to acquire a pony stallion solely for the purpose of teasing.

Estrus Detection Records

When a mare has been teased, her behavior should be plotted on a breeding chart so that the normalcy of her cycle is recorded for prospective and retrospective analysis. For example, prolonged estrous periods are often associated with failure of ovulation and a record of such an estrous period may explain why a particular mare did not conceive. In some cases, mares will also experience embryonal death and this can be reflected by prolonged diestrous periods on their teasing charts. The teasing chart also serves as a cue for more intensive teasing at the time of expected return to estrus, or for pregnancy determination by ultrasonography at 12–15 days postovulation. The records can also be used prospectively to determine the time of foaling.

Hormonal Manipulations that Facilitate Estrus Detection

Mares that are timid and do not show well-expressed estrous behavior, may not receive adequate attention on large breeding farms and can conceive late in the breeding season or be bypassed altogether. In these cases, or when artificial insemination is to be performed under 'backyard' conditions in the absence of a teaser male, controlling the time of estrus and ovulation can facilitate estrus detection and breeding. When breeding farm personnel expect an animal to be in heat they are far more likely to detect estrus, no matter how poor or bizarre its expression. An additional benefit of controlling estrus is that the mare can be delivered to a breeding farm shortly before she is due to ovulate thereby avoiding the substantial expense which is normally incurred for longterm boarding.

For crude control over the time of estrus and ovulation, altrenogest can be administered for 15 days at 0.44 mg/kg per os and estrus will usually begin 3–5 days after cessation of treatment. Ovulation occurs at the usual time during estrus, or about 8–10 days after the cessation of treatment. However, the time of ovalation can vary between day 1 and 15 after treatment; therefore diligent monitoring of the mare by ultrasonography and per vagina examination must follow altrenogest treatment when it has been used for this purpose.

For similarly crude control over the time of estrus and ovulation, prostaglandins (prostaglandin $F_{2\alpha}$, fluprostenol, alfaprostenol, prostalene, etc.) can be administered to a mare 15 days apart but she must be delivered to the breeding farm at the time of the second prostaglandin injection and teased and examined immediately, because some of these mares will be in estrus at the time of the second injection and can ovulate 1 or 2 days later. Alternatively, serum progesterone can be measured by rapid ELISA, and if it is elevated prostaglandins can be administered and the mare delivered to the breeding farm a day or two later. When prostaglandins are given during the luteal phase, estrus usually begins within 3–5 days and ovulation occurs 5 or 6 days later.

Timing and Frequency of Breeding

Due to the fact that follicles measuring 35–40 mm in diameter, periovulatory in size, can be present at the onset of estrus, and because the expression of estrus is variable, breeding should begin on the first or second day of estrus even if estrus detection charts or hormonal manipulations predict a later date for ovulation. Occasionally, these large follicles persist for 4 or 5 days and ovulate shortly before the end of estrus suggesting that the inseminations earlier in estrus are wasted. However, estrus can be abbreviated and these follicles can ovulate much sooner than expected. After the first insemination (natural or artificial), it is advisable to reinseminate a mare every 48 h until she is no longer receptive or until ovulation has been confirmed by rectal palpation. When transrectal palpation or ultrasonography are used to monitor the progress of estrus, breeding can be delayed until the largest follicle on the ovaries reaches a diameter of 35 mm or more.

The author is unaware of any objective data that substantiates the fertility of postovulation inseminations. However, conceptions that followed single postovulation inseminations during estrus have been recorded by some veterinarians. Presumably the equine oocyte remains viable for at least 24 h after ovulation, but the prudence of inseminating only after ovulation has occurred is questionable because the need for capacitation of stallion spermatozoa is still unknown. There has also been considerable interest in whether or not conception rates can be increased by insemination every 24 h rather than every 48 h. Experimental results have been mixed but suggest that insemination every 24 h may provide a slight increase in conception rates. This is understandable in terms of the early embryonal death which has been associated with aged gametes. However, such frequent breeding does not appear to be justified in terms of personnel and expense and the increased usage of the stallion.

A current consensus of opinion indicates that although frequent breeding of the mare involves a substantial bacterial challenge to the uterus it does not have significant potential for inducing endometritis because normal equine uteri are immunologically equipped to cope with such challenges. This immunological protection is especially well-developed in the high estrogen and low progesterone milieu of behavioral estrus. Furthermore, it has been shown that mares may be bred very frequently by stallions under paddock conditions, with no adverse effects on conception rates.

CONGENITAL DEFECTS THAT DECREASE FERTILITY

Poor Vulvar Conformation

When the vulvar opening is tilted cranially, the vulvar seal is usually compromised and the mare becomes predisposed to genital infection. Tilting of the vulvar labia is accentuated in older mares because the perineal region is more flaccid and stretches with age and each successive foaling. The uterus is also heavier in pluriparous mares causing the perineal body to be pulled cranially, thereby repositioning the vulva into a more horizontal plane over the ischial arch. This causes the vulvar labia to sag apart, breaking the vulvar seal. This abnormality is most pronounced in mares with congenitally poor vulvar conformation, but injury, undernourishment and neoplasia can also disrupt the vulvar seal.

This leads to air entering the vagina, initially only at estrus, but eventually there may be a permanent pneumovaginitis and air is sometimes heard passing out of the vagina when the animal is trotting or during urination or defecation. Once the vulvar seal has been broken, contaminated aerosols from the perineal area enter the uterus when negative abdominal pressure develops during respiration. During the initial stages of this syndrome, which is called 'windsucking', contamination of the uterus is controlled by the mare but eventually she succumbs to this challenge and acute or chronic endometritis ensues. This is initially characterized by luminal epithelial pleomorphism and leukocyte infiltration in the lamina propria, but as the condition becomes more chronic, lymphocytes and plasma cells begin to infiltrate into this region. Periglandular fibrosis can be mild, or very severe in advanced cases, constricting the glands and reducing the flow of embryotroph into the uterus. Lymphatic lacunae are also characteristic of advanced endometritis.

Endometritis can preclude conception if the process is still active because of bacterial toxicity to the gametes or embryo; but in chronic, inactive cases, conception, early embryonal and fetal development usually proceeds normally until the yolk sac stores have been depleted at 60–70 days of gestation. After this time, the fetoplacental unit relies entirely upon the endometrium for its sustenance, but sufficient fetotrophic support is not available because of periglandular fibrosis and other compromises in the endometrium. Therefore, the fetus dies causing abortion. The stage of pregnancy at which the fetus dies is dependent on the severity of the chronic changes in the endometrium, but these abortions usually occur towards the end of the first trimester.

Due to the heritability of conformation, it may be possible to decrease the incidence of windsucking by eliminating affected mares from breeding programs. However, the athletic potential of most of these animals precludes this consideration. Instead, the problem of windsucking is controlled by suturing or stapling together the dorsal two-thirds of the vulvar labia, called a Caslick's operation. The labia can be joined after debridement of the mucocutaneous junction or can be apposed in a temporary fashion, using metal staples. If the vulvar seal is severely compromised, the vulvar labia should be sutured in the conventional manner instead of using staples; but once the mare is pregnant and the cervical seal is well formed, the seal created by the Caslick's operation can actually be removed, usually not until late in pregnancy or shortly before foaling.

Karyotypic Anomalies

Freemartinism is rare in horses, but spontaneous aneuploidy such as XXX, XO or XXY is a relatively common cause of infertility in mares. Sometimes it is obvious that an individual is abnormal because there may be clitoral enlargement and varying degrees of vulvar and vestibulovaginal dystrophy. The vagina may end blindly and there may be no cervix and uterus. Various combinations of ovaries and testes may also be found. In other cases, the clinical findings may be more subtle. For example, the tubulogenital tract of a mare may be normal but her ovaries may be small and inactive. This is typical of the XO or Turner's syndrome in mares. However, many genital phenotypes are associated with aberrant genotypes, and a particular phenotype does not necessarily indicate that a mare has a certain genotype. The behavior of these animals is also variable. Some show male behavior or do not cycle at all, while others are persistently receptive to the stallion despite the absence of palpable follicles on their ovaries.

In the event that an abnormal karyotype is suspected, the clinician should submit a noncooled, heparinized blood sample to a laboratory that specializes in karyotyping. However, requirements for sampling procedures may differ from one laboratory to another, so the laboratory should be contacted prior to sending the blood sample.

Persistent Hymen

Persistent hymen is not as common in mares as it is in heifers, and unlike the situation in cattle there is usually little or no fluid accumulation cranial to the hymen. The hymen can be taut, or in some cases, greatly stretched so that it resembles a membranous sock lying within the vagina. The blind end of this sock-like structure may even lie outside the vulva like a polyp hanging from the vulva lips. When a speculum is inserted into the vagina, the hymen can cover the blades of the speculum and although the instrument can be inserted to its full depth, the cervix may be invisible. It is always advisable to examine a mare for persistent hymen prior to breeding because natural breeding can result in severe trauma to the vagina if the hymen is not transected prior to copulation.

Segmental Aplasia

Unlike the situation in ruminants and pigs, segmental aplasia of the tubulogenital tract is very rare in horses, and is therefore seldom a consideration in infertility.

The Role of Parovarian Cysts in Infertility

From an examination of postmortem specimens, it can be concluded that cystic structures up to 10 mm in diameter occur on the ovary and mesovarian ligaments in the majority of normal mares and are therefore unlikely to affect ovarian function. These cysts are the remnants of various embryonic structures but their specific origin is obscure in most cases. If such a cystic structure was to occur in the ovulation fossa or infundibulum, it could theoretically interfere with oocyte transport. However, this appears to be rare and generally unimportant.

ACQUIRED INFERTILITY

Vestibulovaginal Tears

Foaling injuries involving the vestibulum and vulvar lips are fairly common, especially in maiden mares where the tissues are less distensible than in older animals. The injuries sustained by these mares usually occur when the front hooves of the foal penetrate the dorsal vaginal wall during the second stage of labor. The forelimbs of the foal may then drop back from the rectum and be born normally through the vulvovaginal tract, but an injury is created that results in formation of a fistula between the rectum and the vagina. More commonly, however, there is complete destruction of the perineal body and a single 'cloaca' is formed where the anus and vulva once existed. On rare occasions, the foal can even be born through the anus.

The destruction which occurs in vaginal–rectal tears is usually retroperitoneal, is seldom associated with severe hemorrhage and, despite its dramatic appearance, is almost never life-threatening. Routine antitetanus treatment should be used but the use of antibiotics is of questionable value. Never-

theless, it may be prudent to administer broad-spectrum antibiotics by a parenteral route for 7–10 days after the accident. The wound usually heals uneventfully by second intention but the mare is then highly susceptible to airborne contamination of the uterus because the vulva and vestibulovaginal seals are destroyed and fecal material may even be deposited into the vagina. Despite this challenge to the uterus, the immunological system of normal mares can prevent significant damage to the endometrium for months or even years. Therefore, the perineum should not be reconstructed immediately after the accident because surgery is seldom successful at that time.

Many surgical techniques have been described for the repair of perineal lacerations and details of these techniques can be found in surgery texts. None of these methods are very successful if they are employed immediately after foaling. Instead, the wound should be allowed to heal by second intention so that viable wound margins can be located for surgery. The foal should also be weaned before surgery, because the dietary restrictions which are recommended to alter the consistency and volume of feces during the postoperative period usually cause a significant drop in milk production and the foal can suffer accordingly. Although this means that fecal material will be present in the vagina for up to 6 months, these mares usually reconceive quite readily, bearing testimony to the remarkable defense mechanism in the normal equine uterus. Nevertheless, prudence dictates that mares with vaginal–rectal tears should be given a guarded prognosis for future fertility, and that they should also be examined by uterine biopsy and culture before they are rebred. Perineal damage seldom recurs in subsequent foalings.

Vaginal Varicosities

Varicose veins in the vagina are seldom mentioned in the literature and their importance in infertility is questionable. Nevertheless, they are occasionally a source of hemorrhage from the vulva and may be of great concern to the owner or inexperienced veterinarian. These veins can be up to 4 or 5 mm in diameter and are usually most obvious in the dorsal vaginal wall, just cranial to the urethral opening. They are most common in older mares and appear to distend during estrus and the last half of pregnancy, presumably because of increased blood flow to the genitalia under the influence of estrogens. Occasionally these vessels will rupture, resulting in the appearance of blood at the ventral vulvar commissure. During pregnancy, this hemorrhage may give the impression that the mare is about to abort, but if hemorrhage occurs during estrus it may have more significance because blood has been shown to decrease the fertility of semen. Therefore, rather than natural service, artificial insemination is recommended so that the semen is not contaminated with blood.

Varicosed vessels can be ligated if the hemorrhage is severe or persistent, but usually no treatment is required because the condition resolves spontaneously when pregnancy ends or the mare enters a luteal phase.

Vaginal and Cervical Adhesions

Unlike the vagina of the cow, the vagina of the mare is acutely sensitive to physical irritation and after prolonged obstetrical procedures, a plasma transudate will cover the vaginal surface. Within 24 h, fibrinous adhesions will form and by 10–14 days these adhesions will have organized into fibrous tissue that causes permanent transluminal adhesions. If the adhesions are extensive enough, complete vaginal and cervical occlusion may occur. Sometimes these adhesions can be broken down manually but occasionally the cervix and vagina may be blocked. To prevent this from happening, it is essential that the vagina should be examined 1 or 2 days after an obstetrical procedure. At this time, any adhesions can be broken down and the vagina can be treated with an oily antibiotic preparation (such as a cow mastitis formula) which lubricates the vagina and may help in preventing further adhesions. This procedure should be repeated every 2 or 3 days or until fibrinous adhesions are no longer encountered. More frequent vaginal examination may irritate the vagina and could be counterproductive.

Cervical Tears

Cervical tears are an infrequent complication of foaling. If the tear is severe, complete cervical closure may be impossible when healing is complete and fertility is likely to be compromised. However, it is often impossible to predict how fertility will be affected unless a cervical tear is very severe, because pregnancy can be maintained in mares that have obvious cervical tears. Nevertheless, if an endometrial biopsy indicates the presence of endometritis or if there is evidence of early embryonal death, cervical reconstruction should be attempted. This procedure has been described but is difficult and requires special instrumentation.

Some caution must be exercised in diagnosing cervical tears, especially when mares are in estrus because cervical relaxation can disguise even large tears, even if both gloved hand and speculum examinations are performed. Therefore mares should preferably be examined during the luteal phase for the most accurate identification of cervical tears. At that stage of the cycle, the cervix is well organized and tears can be seen and felt easily.

Urine Pooling

In old mares and those in poor condition, splanchnoptosis or ventral displacement of the vagina may cause urine to accumulate in the anterior vagina and flow through the cervix, resulting in chemical endometritis and infertility. Apparently a significant proportion of mares can be cured of this condition by improving their body condition but if this does not help, a surgical cure should be attempted. The surgical cures that have been described involve either the creation of a low transverse wall created from the vaginal mucosa just cranial to the external urethral orifice, or in more severe cases extension of the urethra using longitudinal vestibular folds. However, before a surgical cure is attempted, it may be prudent to examine the endometrium by biopsy, cytology and culture to establish the need for such an operation.

Non-specific Endometritis

Endometritis in the mare is a disease of great economic importance and one of the most important causes of infertility.

Non-specific endometritis may be due to windsucking or to iatrogenic contamination during diagnostic procedures. The uterus may become contaminated with bacteria at coitus, but this infection is normally rapidly eliminated and usually does not interfere with either fertilization or implantation. In some cases however, the infection will persist leading to endometritis and infertility. In other cases, outbreaks of endometritis appear to have occurred where the stallion has been a carrier of either klebsiella or pseudomonas.

Other cases of metritis are caused by difficult parturition or retention of the placenta. In most mares the uterus becomes infected at this time even if they have foaled normally, but as long as involution of the uterus takes place normally the infection is eliminated rapidly. Sometimes metritis may be a sequel to vaginitis.

It can also be related to the chemical irritation which accompanies urine pooling. However, recent evidence suggests that bacterial endometritis only becomes established in the uteruses of mares that have impaired uterine defense mechanisms. The cellular and humoral defense mechanisms of the uterus can cope with massive bacterial challenge, to the point where it is actually difficult to induce endometritis in healthy experimental mares. Apparently the immunological defense mechanisms in the endometrium depend on mechanical barriers to the uterus, that is, the vulva, vestibulovaginal seal and the cervix, to keep infection challenges from the perineal environment at tolerable levels. When there is a breakdown of one or more of these mechanical barriers, and the bacterial challenge is chronic or particularly pathogenic, the defense mechanism fails and endometritis becomes established. Sometimes the predisposing cause of endometritis may be obvious—for example, a mare may have poor vulvar conformation or a torn cervix—but often there is no obvious predisposing cause. It has recently been shown that migration, elasticity and killing ability of polymorphonuclear leukocytes are compromised in mares that are susceptible to endometritis, but deficiencies of humoral immunity in susceptible mares are still unclear.

A wide range of bacteria commonly found as normal inhabitants of the genital tract have been implicated in the etiology of endometritis and their importance has been the subject of much controversy. Since 1977 a new condition has appeared, contagious equine metritis (CEM), which has a specific cause, the contagious equine metritis organism (CEMO). For convenience CEM will be discussed later.

The bacteria most frequently implicated in equine endometritis are β-hemolytic streptococci, *Escherichia coli*, *Staphylococcus aureus*, *Pseudomonas aeruginosa*, and both *Klebsiella pneumoniae* and *K. aerogenes*.

The streptococci are normal inhabitants of the skin of perineum, vulva and vagina of the mare and the prepuce of the stallion. The most frequent isolate from cases of endometritis is *Streptococcus zooepidemicus* but *S. equisimilis* also occurs. Both belong to Lancefield group C and produce relatively wide zones of hemolysis. *Staph. aureus* is also a common skin commensal and both *E. coli* and klebsiella are found in equine feces.

Diagnosis

The diagnosis of endometritis is based upon the history and clinical examination aided by the bacteriological and cytological examination of uterine discharge, the use of endometrial biopsy for histological examination, hormone assays to determine underlying endocrinological factors and possibly ultrasound technique.

Uterine secretion for bacteriological examination must be collected with care using any type of sheathed swab or catheter which prevents contamination from the vagina. The swab or uterine secretion should be examined soon after collection or be sent to the laboratory in transport medium.

The majority of organisms can be cultured successfully on blood agar plates but special media are needed for CEMO (see below, page 149). The identity and antibiotic sensitivity of the organisms isolated are important for whilst the β-hemolytic streptococci are very sensitive to penicillins, pseudomonas are sensitive only to other antibiotics as are some strains of *E. coli* and klebsiella. A single sterile sample does not necessarily indicate the absence of endometritis. Smears of secretion should be examined for the number of types of leukocyte present as well as for the presence of bacteria.

Endometrial biospy is also a valuable diagnostic technique, and a number of special instruments have been developed for the purpose. Samples should be collected during diestrus rather than estrus because the chance of iatrogenic infection is lessened.

While the use of ultrasound technique (see page 68) has proved a useful aid to the early detection of pregnancy, it can also, with experience, be used to examine the ovaries for the presence of active follicles or corpora lutea and the uterus for the presence of fluid in the lumen, endometrial cysts, pyometra and some types of endometritis.

Uterine bacterial cultures alone should not be used to diagnose endometritis because many of the bacteria that cause endometritis are also common commensals on the perineum and in the vagina, and contamination of uterine cultures is common despite the use of guarded culture swabs. Bacteria isolated from a single uterine culture should only be considered significant if there are accompanying signs of endometrial fibrosis of uterine biopsy, or inflammatory cells are present on cytologic evaluation of the endometrium. If bacterial culture alone is to be utilized to confirm a diagnosis of endometritis, the same organism should be isolated on at least two or three sequential cultures several days or an estrous cycle apart. It is not clear when culture results are the most reliable in relationship to the time at which they are taken during the estrous cycle. Some uterine defense mechanisms appear to lapse during the luteal phase; therefore, logic suggests that pathogenic bacteria may be easier to isolate at that time. However, uterine defense mechanisms may control general contaminants during estrus and allow only the isolation of bacteria that are specifically involved in endometritis. Furthermore, the uterus is better equipped to cope with iatrogenic contamination during estrus; therefore, it is preferable to perform diagnostic procedures during estrus rather than diestrus. It is also not advisable to culture the flora of the uterus within 48 h after breeding because of misleading results that may arise from airborne contamination of the uterine lumen and natural contamination by the ejaculate.

Endometrial biopsy enables one to determine the significance of endometrial bacterial cultures and give prognosis on the reproductive potential of mares. Its value has been proven in several studies. Prognostication is based primarily on the degree of fibrosis present within the endometrial sample, a factor that is also used to place mares into one of three categories according to their reproductive potential—that is, good, intermediate or poor for categories I, II and III, respectively. These categories have some statistical value when used in pre-purchase examinations or when owners have limited financial resources and must choose whether or not to breed a particular mare. However, when an owner is intent on breeding a specific animal, a poor endometrial categorization should not prevent breeding because many mares classified in category II or even III can conceive and maintain pregnancy normally.

If endometrial fibrosis is severe, lymphatic lacunae may be present and there may even be transluminal adhesions and pockets of fluid accumulated within the uterus. Such advanced changes can usually be appreciated by transrectal ultrasonography or endoscopy and if these changes are extreme, they may even be palpable per rectum.

Treatment

Mares with a tendency towards pneumovagina should be treated surgically by Caslick's operation to stop aspiration of the air (see above, page 144). After vulvar suturing, the vaginitis and endometritis may resolve spontaneously if the mare has normal ovarian cycles, but such mares are usually treated with intrauterine antibiotics. In these, as in other mares with endometritis given antibiotics, the choice of antibiotic is dependent upon the type of organism present and its antibiotic sensitivity pattern. While β-hemolytic streptococci, sensitive to penicillin and other drugs, are the most frequently isolated organisms, other organisms resistant to several antibiotics commonly occur.

When the mare is cycling normally, the normal phagocytic and self-clearing activity of the uterus will lead to resolution of endometritis in some cases without the use of antibiotics. Therefore, use of prostaglandin or estrogens has been advocated when there is reduced follicular activity, and particularly if pyometra is diagnosed, or during the winter months when the mare is not cycling.

In practice, veterinarians often attempt to augment uterine defense mechanisms in susceptible mares by supplying opsonins in the form of immunoglobulins and complement derived from serum or colostrum. Data generated in this way have been from uncontrolled trials but they do suggest that these practices may have some value. At this time it is not clear how such augmentation of the immune system should relate to antibiotic therapy, because many antibiotics are known to inhibit cellular immunity and may even be contraindicated when immunotherapy is used. Acute endometritis should be treated with antibiotics on the basis of bacterial sensitivity, but if that treatment fails, augmentation of the immune system should be attempted.

Antibiotics can be administered to mares by local or systemic routes, but if the local route is used sufficient saline or sterile water must be infused as part of the treatment to ensure adequate distribution of the antibiotic within the uterus. However, before antibiotic or immunologic treatment is initiated, any fluid or debris present within the uterus should be flushed out with hot (50°C) saline until the saline flush becomes clear. The flushing procedure should be repeated daily until the first flush of the day is clear. Immunological or antibiotic treatment can then begin. Hot saline flushes serve as mild irritants to the endometrium, stimulating uterine blood flow and neutrophil migration into the lumen; therefore, they may be beneficial even if there is no debris within the uterus. Guidelines for antibiotic therapy are supplied in Table 9.1. If augmentation of the immune system is to be employed, 100–200 ml of autogenous, heparinized or citrated plasma is infused into the uterus for several days after the saline flushes and the mare is bred during the subsequent estrous period. Plasma or serum can be infused again on the first and second day after ovulation. It is important not to heat-sterilize the plasma or colostrum used for these treatments because complement and antibodies will be denatured at high temperatures.

Instead of using autogenous plasma, some clinicians have used plasma from other mares or even equine colostrum and have reported good results. However, all these data were generated from uncontrolled trials and must be interpreted cautiously.

Contagious Equine Metritis (CEM)

In 1977 a highly contagious venereal disease of horses was described for the first time in mares at stud farms in the Newmarket area of England. The disease, a specific form of metritis in mares, referred to as contagious equine metritis (CEM) had serious repercussions for the racing industry and it has subsequently been described in Ireland, France, the United States, Australia, Japan and in many other countries worldwide. The disease has also been diagnosed in nonthoroughbred horses and it has been shown that it can be transmitted experimentally to donkeys.

The causal organisms for CEM were initially found to be somewhat difficult to isolate and both *Bacterioides* and *Proteus* species were implicated before the disease was clearly ascribed to an unusual gram-negative coccobacillus found in smears of cervical and vaginal exudate which grew on heated blood agar in an atmosphere containing 5–10% carbon dioxide in hydrogen. These findings were confirmed by transmission experiments in ponies.

The classification of the organism has been the subject of debate between bacterial taxonomists. Initially it was found that hematin stimulated the growth of the organism and on this basis it was named *Haemophilus equigenitalis*. However, it is now recognized that it does not belong to the *Haemophilus* genus but to a new genus— *Taylorella*, and the name *Taylorella equigenitalis* has been proposed for the CEMO. *Taylorella equigenitalis* is transmitted venereally to mares from asymptomatic carrier stallions. It causes suppurative endometritis and early embryonic death resulting in a repeat breeding syndrome until the mare becomes immune to the organism. The disease can be devastating to the horse industry because of its effect on conception and pregnancy early in the breeding season. Therefore international quarantine measures have been enforced to curtail the spread of the disease, but because CEM was only discovered in 1977, control measures are still in a state of change and local animal health authorities should be consulted for the most recent regulations pertaining to its control.

The Causal Organism

The organism of contagious equine metritis was defined as a microaerophilic, gram-negative, nonmotile coccobacillus which is positive to both catalase and oxidase tests but otherwise quite unreactive.

The recommended growth medium for primary cultures consists of either a blood agar base or columbia agar with added sodium sulfite and L-cysteine or a commercial CEMO base. To this is usually added 10% chocolated (heated) sheep or horse blood, streptomycin (200 μg/ml) and either pimufucin (0.2 mg/ml) or nystatin (100 units). Some plates without streptomycin should always be included as streptomycin-sensitive strains have been described. A recent improved selective medium has been described containing trimethoprim, clindamycin and amphotericin B.

Cultures are incubated either in an atmosphere of 5–10% carbon dioxide in air or under hydrogen at 37 °C initially for 48 h and then for up to 6 days if no colonies appear. The colonies are small pinpoint to pinhead in size, shiny, smooth and dome-shaped. They are initially offwhite in color turning to a dirty cream on further incubation.

Because the organisms are so unreactive in a wide range of biochemical tests, isolates should be confirmed using slide agglutination test with specific antiserum.

The controversy over the classification arose because initially it was shown that growth was stimulated by hematin (X factor), a classic characteristic of some *Haemophilus* species. However, using a more specific test in which D-aminolevulinic acid (D-ALA) is employed, it was shown later that CEMO was not X-dependent and could not reduce nitrate to nitrite. Also the guanine/cytosine (GC) ratio of CEMO is much lower than for other hemotic-dependent haemophili. For these reasons it could not be classified as a *Haemophilus* species, but included in the *Taylorella*.

Epidemiology

CEM is a highly infectious venereal disease which may also be spread by indirect contact.

The CEMO is found in the urethral fossa and prepuce of the stallion and has been isolated from the preejaculatory fluid. It produces no symptoms in stallions which may remain as apparently healthy carriers for a considerable time. However, 75% of mares covered by such stallions become infected. After the acute phase, they may remain as symptomless carriers with infection persisting in the clitoral fossa; those becoming pregnant may remain as latent carriers. Abortion is not a normal sequel but foals may be exposed to infection at birth and retain the infection until breeding age.

Infection can also be transmitted by attendants or instruments used to treat infected horses.

Symptoms

After mares have been covered by infected stallions

Table 9.1 Common genital infections in mares

Pathogen	Diagnosis	Location	Clinical signs	Drug	Dose	Route	Duration	Comments
Taylorella equigenitalis formerly *Haemophilus equigenitalis*	Contagious equine metritis (CEM)	Uterus, vagina, clitoris	Grayish vulvar discharge, short cycles, repeat breeding	Penicillin procaine	25 000 i.u./kg b.i.d.	i.m.	7–10 days	Mare never considered 'clean' once infected
Escherichia coli	Endometritis	Uterus	Repeat breeding placentitis, abortion, occasionally pyometra	Chloramphenicol	10 mg/kg q 4 h	i.u.	7–10 days	Expensive, very rapid excretion
				Ampicillin sodium	20 mg/kg t.i.d.	i.u.	7–10 days	
				Gentamicin	4 mg/kg s.i.d.	i.u.	7–10 days	Organism often resistant to kanamycin
				Amikacin	4 mg/kg s.i.d.	i.u.	7–10 days	Organism often resistant to kanamycin
Klebsiella pneumoniae (serotypes I and V)	Endometritis	Uterus	Repeat breeding, placentitis, abortion, occasionally pyometra	Chloramphenicol	20 mg/kg q 4–6 h	i.u.	7–10 days	Very rapid excretion; all chloramphenicol is excreted from the mare within 3–4 h; 60–100% of isolates are usually susceptible to chloramphenicol
				Kanamycin	5 mg/kg s.i.d.	i.u.	7–10 days	Aminoglycoside absorption from the uterus is poor but high endometrial levels are attained; most *Klebsiella* spp. isolates are very sensitive to amikacin and least sensitive to kanamycin
				Gentamicin	4 mg/kg s.i.d.	i.u.	7–10 days	
				Amikacin	4 mg/kg s.i.d.	i.u.	7–10 days	
Pseudomonas pyocyanea	Endometritis	Uterus	Repeat breeding, placentitis, abortion, occasionally pyometra	Amikacin	4 mg/kg s.i.d.	i.u.	7–10 days	Kanamycin is frequently ineffective against *Pseudomonas* spp. isolates
				Gentamicin	8 mg/kg t.i.d.	i.m.	7–10 days	
				Carbenicillin	4 mg/kg s.i.d.	i.u.	7–10 days	The absorption of the newer generation penicillins is poor from the uterine lumen; however those products reach high concentrations in the endometrium; the adnexa of the reproductive tract and deeper layers of the uterus may be more adequately treated by high systemic doses of these antibiotics
					8 mg/kg t.i.d.	i.m.	7–10 days	
					60–100 mg/kg s.i.d.	i.u.	7–10 days	
				Ticarcillin	80 mg/kg q.i.d.	i.m./i.v.	7–10 days	
					60–100 mg/kg s.i.d.	i.u.	7–10 days	
				Piperacillin	80 mg/kg q.i.d.	i.m./i.v.	7–10 days	
					60–100 mg/kg s.i.d.	i.u.	7–10 days	

Organism	Condition	Site	Indication	Drug	Dose	Route	Duration	Comments
Staphylococcus aureus	Endometritis	Uterus	Repeat breeding, placentitis, abortion, occasionally pyometra	Chloramphenicol	20 mg/kg q 4–6 h	i.u.	7–10 days	All isolates sensitive to chloramphenicol (see note on rapid excretion of chloramphenicol under *Klebsiella* endometritis)
				Gentamicin	4 mg/kg s.i.d.	i.u.	7–10 days	
				Kanamycin	4 mg/kg s.i.d.	i.u.	7–10 days	
				Lincomycin				*Note*: Lincomycin is effective against most *Staph.* spp. isolates *in vitro*, however it is toxic to the horse and should *not* be used in this species
Streptococcus zooepidemicus β-hemolytic organism	Endometritis	Uterus	Repeat breeding, placentitis, abortion, occasionally pyometra	Penicillin procaine	50 000 i.u./kg b.i.d.	i.m.	7–10 days	Ubiquitous organisms; common on external genitalia. Repeat cultures are required to establish a diagnosis of *Streptococcus* endometritis
				Penicillin sodium/K$^+$	50 000 i.u./kg q.i.d.	i.v.	7–10 days	
				or Ampicillin sodium	15 mg/kg t.i.d.	i.m.	7–10 days	Moderate levels in the uterus with parenteral administration
				or trimethoprim/ sulfamethoxazole	10 mg/kg s.i.d.	i.u.	7–10 days	Unpublished data; dose based on trimethoprim content of drug
					3 mg/kg b.i.d.	p.o.	10 days	
Monilia spp.	Fungal endometritis	Uterus	Repeat breeding, mucopyometra	Clotrimazole	600 mg s.i.d.	i.u.	7 days	Difficult to dissolve; use in propylene glycol base or three to four suppositories
Aspergillus spp.	Fungal endometritis	Uterus	Repeat breeding, mucopyometra	*or* amphotericin B	250 mg s.i.d.	i.u.	7 days	
Mucor spp.	Fungal endometritis	Uterus	Repeat breeding, mucopyometra	*or* nystatin	0.5 mill/ i.u. s.i.d.	i.u.	7 days	
Dermatophytes	Fungal endometritis	Uterus	Repeat breeding, mucopyometra	*or* iodine	0.5%* s.i.d.	i.u.	7 days	*0.5% of 10% stock solution; a diagnosis of fungal endometritis must be substantiated by repeated culture of fungus from the uterus or demonstration of fungal elements within the endometrium

Notes:
1. Although tetracyclines are often used in treating endometritis in mares, they are probably not optimal for that use because many isolates of common uterine pathogens are resistant to them. Caution should be exercised with parenteral administration of tetracyclines to mares because of the possibility of activation of latent salmonellosis. Also, tetracyclines are somewhat irritating to the endometrium. Propylene glycol vehicles serve as an extra irritant.
2. All i.u.-treatments are given in 100–200 ml of sterile water or saline (saline may affect the absorption of aminoglycosides from the uterine lumen).

they may develop a profuse uterine discharge 2–6 days after service. The discharge may be frank pus or a bright, mucopurulent fluid. However, in some mares the discharge is very slight and may not be noticed. There are varying degrees of inflammation of the vaginal mucosa. The result of the infection is a high prevalence of infertility due to interference with fertilization and implantation or to early fetal death. Abortion is not a feature of this disease. As the endometritis subsides most mares become fertile again after several estrous cycles.

Diagnosis

The diagnosis is confirmed by isolation and identification of the causal organism. Guarded or sheathed swabs are taken from either uterine discharge in acute cases or the clitoral fossa and the endometrium in early estrus in suspected carrier mares. In the stallion, swabs should be taken from the sheath, the urethra, the urethral fossa and from pre-ejaculatory fluid. The swabs should be sent to the laboratory in a suitable transport medium such as Amies or Stuart's medium.

Smears should be prepared from uterine discharge and stained by Gram's method. Large numbers of polymorphonuclear leukocytes are indicative of an active endometritis and small gram-negative coccobacillary bacteria may be CEMO.

In some cases endometrial biopsy may be required, but it does not detect latent carriers. In other cases, where contamination by other bacteria or fungi has made cultural examination of stallions difficult, test mating or the collection of smegma and its direct inoculation into a susceptible mare have been used in attempts to demonstrate infection.

A variety of serological tests have been investigated for use in the diagnosis of CEM. If the serum agglutination test (SAT) is used, titers of 1/80 are reached about 3 weeks after infection and may decline to insignificant levels after 6 weeks. With the complement fixation test (CFT), although titers also peaked at about 3 weeks, they declined much more slowly. Thus the SAT may be of value in the diagnosis of acute cases, while the CFT could be used to detect chronically infected animals. Passive hemagglutination and ELISA tests are also useful diagnostic procedures.

Treatment and Control

At the present time, if there is an outbreak of CEM on a breeding farm in the United States, a moratorium is imposed on breeding and all the stallions on the farm treated systemically with penicillin for 10 days. In addition, their genitalia are washed with chlorhexidine scrub and the prepuce packed with furazolidone ointment. Nonpregnant mares are treated with crystalline penicillin via the intrauterine route for 7–10 days, but once infected they are always regarded as potential carriers of CEM and should not be rebred naturally. Treated stallions can only be used again once they have had 6 negative penile and fossa glandis cultures taken at weekly intervals. It is also recommended that two to three maiden mares be bred naturally by a stallion that has undergone treatment, and that the uteruses and clitoral sinuses of those mares should be cultured on three occasions within 14 days postbreeding.

Horses that have never been used for breeding can be imported into the United States from countries where CEM is endemic with only the usual quarantine restrictions. However, mares that have been used for breeding require clitoral sinusectomy, a course of intensive antibiotic treatment and at least 3 negative serological tests for CEM at the port of origin. For that purpose, either a passive hemagglutination test or an ELISA test for CEM should be used as those tests have been shown to be more accurate than tube agglutination or complement fixation tests. Imported mares are retested upon their arrival in the United States. Sexually experienced stallions should have negative serological tests in the country of origin and must also be retested, cultured and test-bred to at least three mares in the United States. Female foals from mares which have been exposed to CEM should be tested for it when they reach puberty by serologic testing and culturing of their uteruses and clitoral sinuses. New regulations pertaining to the control of CEM include possibly withdrawing the need for clitoral sinusectomy because the CEM organism can be harbored for long periods of time almost anywhere in the genital tract.

For routine culturing of the CEM organism, swabs should be placed in Amies transport medium and then placed onto chocolate agar and incubated under 5% CO_2. The organism is fastidious and slow-growing; therefore cultures are not regarded as being negative prior to 10 days of incubation. Most strains of the CEM organism are not sensitive to streptomycin and this antibiotic is used in some bacterial growth media to prevent overgrowth by contaminants (see page 149).

The serious nature of CEM and the threat it posed to the racing industry led to the introduction of a common code of practice in the United Kingdom, the Republic of Ireland and France. (The disease is officially notifiable in the United Kingdom.) The recommendation originally required a series of three negative swabs taken in stallions from preejaculatory fluid, prepuce, urethra and urethral fossa and in mares from the clitoral fossa and sinuses and an endometrial swab taken during estrus. Because of the fall in the prevalence of CEM the number of swabs required from low risk mares has been reduced. Where CEMO is isolated, the horse must be treated adequately, rested for a suitable time and resampled.

Treatment of stallions usually consists of thorough and repeated cleansing of the extended penis and sheath with chlorhexidine followed by the application of furazolidone ointment. In mares, although the condition often resolves spontaneously, latent infection remains and treatment is recommended.

Uterine irrigation with chlorhexidine, nitrofurazone, ampicillin or penicillin for 3–5 days has been used in addition to parenteral administration of penicillin or ampicillin. In symptomless carriers the local cleansing of the clitoral fossa and sinuses with chlorhexidine and application of furazolidone ointment has been used. The overenthusiastic use of chlorhexidine is not to be recommended for treatment of either stallions or mares, or as a prophylactic measure at the time of covering. This can lead to the destruction of the normal flora and the establishment of pseudomonas infection which may be then transmitted venerally leading to further trouble.

Although not widely used in thoroughbred horses, artificial insemination has considerable potential for controlling venereally transmitted infection in horses. Attempts to develop a vaccine against CEMO have been unsuccessful.

Fungal Metritis

If fungi are isolated from uterine fluid or identified in the sediment of such fluid, fungal endometritis should be suspected. This is contrary to the philosophy of some clinicians who only diagnose fungal endometritis on the basis of fungal elements present in endometrial biopsies. Nevertheless, cases will be encountered where there is substantial fluid accumulation in the uterus, and fungi can be seen in this fluid but not in endometrial biopsies from these mares. Fungal elements stain well by the periodic acid Schiff (PAS) reaction but are more easily identified with Gomori's methanamine silver or Grocott's stain. The most common fungi isolated from these cases are *Candida* spp. and *Aspergillus fumigatus*. Many cases of fungal metritis appear to resolve spontaneously, but if the infection appears to be persistent and needs treatment the guidelines and drugs listed in Table 9.1 can be used for that purpose.

Herpes Coital Exanthema ('Spots')

This is a vesicular, then ulcerative venereal disease that causes genital discomfort and reluctance to breed in both sexes. Secondary infection may complicate the condition occasionally but it usually heals spontaneously within 7–10 days. Coital exanthema is caused by equine herpes virus III (EHVIII).

Pyometra

Compared with cattle, pyometra is relatively uncommon, probably because of the rarity of retained placenta in this species, the remarkable rate of postpartum uterine involution in the mare and the distensibility of the equine cervix. Mares with pyometra are seldom debilitated and do not have high circulating leukocyte counts. Therefore, pyometra is often discovered during a routine examination for infertility. Unless there is closure of the cervix by adhesions, mares with pyometra also tend to show a purulent discharge from the vulva, a strong indication of the disease. If the uterus is distended with fluid but no fetus is visible by transrectal ultrasonography, the mare is also likely to have pyometra because mucometra is so rare in horses. The absence of a fetus by ballottement, and low serum estrone sulfate values at 90 days or more after breeding, are further aids in helping to distinguish between normal pregnancy and pyometra, an occasional problem if there has been a history of breeding.

Some mares with pyometra experience long periods of diestrus, but pyometra is also found in mares which are cycling normally. Therefore mares with pyometra do not always have a corpus luteum, and as a result treatment with prostaglandins is not as spectacularly curative as it is in cows. However, long-acting prostaglandin analogs such as fluprostenol, cloprostenol or fenprostalene can cause prolonged contraction of the equine uterus in cycling mares and may also be valuable in the treatment of pyometra. In most cases, uterine lavage with large volumes of fluid is an effective treatment when the purulent material has first been siphoned from the uterus. The lavage should be supplemented by high doses of antibiotics administered by parenteral and intrauterine routes. The most frequent causative organism in equine pyometra is *Streptococcus zooepidemicus*; therefore, penicillin is the antibiotic of choice unless a culture and sensitivity test dictates otherwise.

Fetal Mummification and Maceration

The etiology of fetal mummification and maceration is unknown, and due to the fact that these conditions are rare in mares no research has been conducted in this area. Mummification is usually detected when pregnancy is chronologically advanced but there are no signs of impending foaling. It is also diagnosed when a mare has an unknown breeding history and has failed to conceive to recent breedings. When the fetus dies, the fetal fluids are resorbed and the myometrium contracts down firmly around the conceptus. This mummified conceptus can be a co-twin to a normal fetus or it can occur by itself despite the fact that no placental progesterone is available to maintain the pregnancy. If the cervical seal is disrupted in the latter case, the mummified fetoplacental unit becomes infected and it begins to macerate, producing a purulent vulvar discharge. The diagnosis of such cases rests upon the presence of this discharge together with the history of the case, the characteristic feeling of these fetuses on rectal palpation, and the presence of fetal bones that are visible by transrectal ultrasonography.

The mummified or macerated fetus can be removed by gradual dilatation of the cervix and direct extraction of the uterine contents. The uterus should then be flushed with saline and antibiotics administered according to uterine culture and sensitivity results.

Salpingitis and Periovaritis

These conditions are less common in mares than in cows, possibly due to the valve-like structure of the uterotubule junction that limits the flow of infectious material from the uterus towards the ovaries. The low incidence of salpingitis and periovaritis has been confirmed by postmortem observations.

Neoplasia

The most common forms of genital neoplasia in the mare are squamous cell carcinomas of the vulva and granulosa cell tumors of the ovary. The former are not usually metastatic, but occasionally they cause deformity of the vulva with secondary windsucking and consequent endometritis. Due to the fact that squamous cell carcinomas are locally invasive they should be removed by radical excision if possible.

Melanomas are also encountered in the perineal region but are usually benign and seldom cause genital complications.

Leiomyomas, leiomyosarcomas and lymphosarcomas can be found in the myometrium. Lymphosarcomas are usually multicentric and life-threatening, but smooth muscle tumors of the myometrium are mostly benign. Leiomyomas may impose on the uterine lumen causing infertility and, on rare occasions, leiomyosarcomas may slough neoplastic tissue into the uterus, also causing infertility. Smooth muscle tumors can be excised from the myometrium and normal reproductive function restored.

Granulosa cell tumors, dysgerminomas, arrhenoblastomas, lymphosarcomas, teratomas, cystadenomas and even Sertoli cell tumors have been described in equine ovaries. However the granulosa cell tumor is by far the most common of these tumors. Occasionally the diagnosis of these tumors is subjective and may vary from one pathologist to another. Some pathologists even doubt the existence of arrhenoblastomas in mares.

Granulosa cell tumors occur in young and old mares and usually disrupt ovarian cyclicity. Although they are benign, they produce a variety of sex steroids that exert a negative feedback effect on the hypothalamic–pituitary axis. This results in quiescence of the unaffected ovary and long periods of infertility. Sexual behavior at this time may be masculine, feminine or simply passive. Granulosa cell tumors are usually easy to diagnose on a presumptive basis because an enlarged ovary can be palpated per rectum on one side and a small quiescent ovary on the other side. This is almost unique to this type of tumor because most other ovarian tumors in the mare do not produce sex steroids. Granulosa cell tumors can be small or very large indeed (occasionally up to 30 cm in diameter) and have a typical multicystic appearance when viewed by transrectal real time ultrasonography. The measurement of serum testosterone may be of further diagnostic value in these cases because serum testosterone is often elevated significantly in mares with granulosa cell tumors.

If there is a possibility that a tumor is being confused with an ovarian hematoma, the mare can be reexamined to confirm the diagnosis at a later date because of the benign nature of granulosa cell tumors. When the tumor is removed, the owner should be warned that the mare may take several months to initiate normal ovarian cycles again because of the chronic nature of the negative feedback suppression on the unaffected ovary. On rare occasions these mares never return to cyclicity.

Aberrations in the Estrous Cycle that Lead to Infertility

When the mare experiences prolonged estrous periods early and late in the breeding season, the clinician should always recognize the potential for failure of ovulation and infertility. There are also other physiological and pathological reasons for abnormal cyclicity. Some have been mentioned already—for example, stallion preference, pyometra, granulosa cell tumors and chromosomal anomalies—but others that are common and also worthy of mention include adrenal malfunction, retained corpus luteum or pseudopregnancy, embryonal death after recognition of pregnancy or the formation of endometrial cups, and miscellaneous causes of abnormal estrous cycles.

Adrenal Malfunction

Adrenal malfunction is sometimes quoted as a cause of masculine behavior or irregular cyclicity, but no case reports or objective data are available to substantiate this theory. Acute hyperadrenal states can interfere with ovulation in other species but their significance in the mare is unknown.

Spontaneous Retention of the Corpus Luteum

Pseudopregnancy or spontaneous retention of the corpus luteum is assumed to arise when an ovulation in late diestrus (a common event in mares) results in the formation of a corpus luteum that is too immature to respond to the endogenous prostaglandin surges that occur on days 11 to 15 of the estrous cycle. If luteolysis of this corpus luteum does not occur, the mare will not return to estrus and can remain in a prolonged state of diestrus for up to 4 or 5 months. It is not known why endogenous prostaglandin surges fail to occur for this entire period, because other cyclic events such as follicle development and even ovulation can occur while the corpus luteum is still retained. This is not due to luteal insensitivity to prostaglandins because the offending corpus luteum is responsive to normal luteolytic doses of prostaglandin $F_{2\alpha}$ and its analogs. When prostaglandins are used to treat this condition, rapid luteolysis ensues and the mare returns to normal reproductive function.

A retained corpus luteum is diagnosed by a history of continuous diestrus for longer than 15 days together with findings of a corpus luteum on the ovary by transrectal ultrasonography and a serum progesterone level of greater than 3 ng/ml. There is also uterine tone that is reminiscent of early pregnancy.

Embryonal Death after the Recognition of Pregnancy

Once the mare's uterus has recognized pregnancy, there is no endogenous surge of prostaglandin and the corpus luteum is maintained to support the conceptus. Recognition of pregnancy was thought to occur at the end of the luteal phase, in time to block prostaglandin release and luteolysis but it is now clear from embryo flushing studies that the corpus luteum is protected by the embryo even when it enters the uterus on day 6 after ovulation. If an embryo dies after this protective signal has been received by the corpus luteum, luteolysis may not occur and the mare can enter a period of prolonged diestrus or false pregnancy. The signal for luteal protection in pregnancy appears to become stronger as pregnancy advances, because if embryos die or are removed on day 11 to 12 after conception approximately 25–30% of mares will experience prolonged diestrous periods; however, if embryos die after 20 days of life, luteal protection is complete and nearly all mares will experience significantly prolonged diestrous phases.

From a breeder's viewpoint, it may be impossible to distinguish between this condition and that described for a spontaneously retained corpus luteum, especially if there has been a history of breeding but no early pregnancy detection by ultrasonography. Nevertheless, the clinician may recognize that this is a sequel to early embryonal death because normal luteolytic doses of prostaglandins often fail to cause luteolysis, presumably because of some form of luteal protection. As a result, two or three doses of prostaglandin must be given at 12 h intervals to cause luteolysis.

Embryonal Death after the Formation of Endometrial Cups

The endometrial cups are formed at 28–35 days of gestation and produce equine chorionic gonadotropin (eCG), a glycoprotein hormone formerly known as pregnant mare serum gonadotropin (PMSG). Usually eCG is produced by the endometrial cups until 120 days of gestation but even if an embryo should die off after the endometrial cups have been formed, the production of eCG can continue for its normal duration. During this time, eCG appears to block cyclicity or to cause the mare to cycle abnormally. Even if the secondary corpora lutea are destroyed with prostaglandins, the mare may not begin to cycle normally. In a few cases, there may be early rejection of endometrial cups and the mare may cycle normally and reconceive soon after abortion. If a mare is anestrous or experiencing bizarre estrous cycles but her breeding history is uncertain, a test for the presence of eCG will clarify the mare's condition. Several such tests are commercially available for pregnancy testing in mares. Unfortunately, there is no safe and effective method to terminate endometrial cup function.

Miscellaneous Causes of Abnormal Estrous Cycles

Miscellaneous causes of irregular cyclicity also include ovariectomy and inappropriate use of steroid hormones. Occasionally mares are bought from sale barns with no history at all and some of these mares have been ovariectomized for experimental reasons or to act as recipient mares in artificial insemination programs. Ovariectomized mares can show passive behavior or may exhibit classic signs of estrus without any steriod treatment. Transrectal palpation of the genital tract will provide a diagnosis. Mares are also treated with various anabolic hormones during their racing careers, and although the detrimental effects of these hormones on stallions has been known for some time it has been shown only recently that these hormones can cause reproductive failure in mares as well. These mares can experience irregular cyclicity, ovulation failure and pregnancy failure for up to 3 months after the cessation of treatment. It is likely that all of the anabolic steroids are harmful in this regard, but boldenone undecylenate and laurabolin should be used with extra caution. Estradiol cypionate (ECP) should also be used with caution because this is a conjugated hormone and is slowly metabolized. Therefore it can persist for long periods of time and has been known to cause chronic suppression of ovarian function especially if given by several sequential injections.

ABORTION AND OTHER ACCIDENTS OF PREGNANCY

Common causes of abortion include placentitis, twinning and equine herpes virus infection (EHVI). Placentitis is most frequently caused by bacteria, but fungal and yeast placentitis also have been described in the mare. Other causes of abortion include umbilical abnormalities, tall fescue poisoning, idiopathic thickening of the allantochorion, idiopathic microvillous atrophy, placental infarction and occasional cases of multicentric lymphosarcoma.

Placentitis

Bacterial placentitis may be diffuse because of hematogenous entry into the uterus, or local and ascending due to infection via the cervix. In either case, the fetus dies because of placental compromise and septicemia and often has pneumonia as well from inhaling contaminated amniotic fluid. *Streptococcus* spp., *Staphylococcus* spp., *Pseudomonas aeruginosa*, *Klebsiella pneumoniae* and other bacterial species have been cultured from these abortions. In cases of fungal placentitis, the placenta may be characteristically thickened and severely inflamed. On the histologic sections of the placenta, the fungal organisms can be demonstrated by Gomori's silver stain, Grocott's stain or by the periodic acid Schiff (PAS) reaction. Fungi such as *Aspergillus* and *Mucor* spp., etc. are usually isolated from these cases, but recently a *Histoplasma* sp. was also shown to cause abortion in mares.

Twinning

Twinning is a major cause of early embryonal death, fetal death, late abortion, dystocia and poor neonatal development. Through embryo collection studies and real time ultrasonography, it is now clear that mares have a mechanism for reducing embryo numbers so that they rarely produce twins. This is illustrated by the fact that the mean frequency of twin ovulations can be as high as 15–20% on some thoroughbred farms in midsummer, but the birth rate of twins born is usually less than 1%. Therefore, the birth of twins can be interpreted as a failure of the embryo reduction mechanism. The mechanism for reducing the number of embryos is evident soon after the embryos arrive in the uterus because the success rate in collecting twin embryos is significantly higher at 7 days than at 11 days postovulation. Embryo reduction continues as pregnancy progresses. In fact, it has been reported that the majority of twin pregnancies diagnosed by rectal palpation at 35–40 days were aborted by 70 days of gestation. If twin fetuses survive into the third trimester of pregnancy, the limited availability of endometrial surface starts to retard fetal growth and one or both conceptuses can die from intrauterine starvation. Occasionally normal foals are born accompanied by their dead co-twins that can vary in size from those that are barely detectable to those that are large and well-developed.

Twin conceptions are more common in thoroughbred mares than in other breeds and also more frequent within certain lines of thoroughbreds. So there is undoubtedly a genetic predisposition towards twin ovulations. However, the problem of twin ovulation can be controlled by restricting the breeding of those mares that are predisposed to twinning to the springtime rather than the summer when twin ovulations are more frequent. Embryo transfer can also be used when breed regulations allow it. In addition, great care should be exercised when previously barren mares are examined for pregnancy because these animals are more likely to have twin ovulations than those that are lactating, and early detection of twins is of cardinal importance in the success rate of the treatment of these cases. Attempts to avoid twinning have been made by limiting the energy intake of the mare or by breeding only when a single large preovulatory follicle was present on the ovaries. However, neither of these techniques were successful. On the contrary, it has been shown that when mares were intentionally bred with two preovulatory follicles present, the proportion of twin conceptions was not increased; in fact, fertility was improved. However, the findings in that study disagree with other data and no conclusive recommendations can be made in this regard.

Once a twin pregnancy has been confirmed by transrectal ultrasonography, either one of the twins can be destroyed by crushing. Other methods of embryonic destruction have been described but they are either less practical or less successful than the crushing technique. When crushing is used, the survival rate of the remaining co-twin can be as high as 80% especially if crushing is performed prior to 30 days of gestation, but as pregnancy progresses, the success of the procedure diminishes. The crushed conceptus should be examined by ultrasonography after 3–4 days to insure that it has been destroyed, because embryo survival has been recorded despite vigorous crushing attempts. As described earlier, it is possible for a co-twin to die off spontaneously as pregnancy progresses and this approach is occasionally adopted by those who quote the low success rates that are frequently associated with the crushing procedure. However, most veterinarians prefer embryo crushing because the fate of the pregnancy is known within 7–10 days.

Although it has been shown that administration of flunixin meglumine can prevent prostaglandin release if it is administered shortly before a conceptus is crushed, this compound and other prostaglandin synthetase inhibitors have not been shown to improve the rate of success of the embryo crushing technique. Progesterone administration before and after embryo destruction was not valuable either. Irrespective of the method used for selective abortion of one conceptus, it is essential that the procedure should be performed prior to 35 days of gestation because the endometrial cups start to form at this time and if both conceptuses abort when eCG is being produced, the mare will not cycle normally and the entire breeding season can be lost.

Abortion due to Equine Viral Arteritis (EVA)

It has recently been shown that stallions can shed the EVA virus for prolonged periods of time and can transmit it venereally to mares. Mares that contract EVA in this manner will experience an acute febrile episode 7–10 days later and can become chronic carriers, shedding the virus in their urine. These mares are positive for EVA by a serum neutralization test. Mares that are affected early in pregnancy probably abort occasionally, but abortion is more common in advanced pregnancy when mares contract the infection by inhalation of viral aerosol. The fetus is often autolyzed at the time of abortion but otherwise shows no pathognomonic lesions. Vaccination is protective (see Chapter 11).

Abortion due to the Equine Rhinopneumonitis Herpes Virus (EHVI)

Susceptible mares will abort a well-preserved fetus 1–2 months after exposure to the abortifacient form of EHVI virus. There is usually no evidence of placentitis, but signs of pulmonary edema and fluid accumulation in the thoracic and peritoneal cavities are fairly common. A diagnosis is achieved through histopathology, virus isolation from the peritoneal and pleural fluids and fluorescent antibody examination of the adrenals and other organs. Sometimes abortion storms involving several mares will be encountered, but at the time of abortion the affected mares do not shed significant amounts of virus and need not be isolated from the normal animals. However, the fetuses are a significant source of virus and should be removed immediately. In addition, all the normal mares should be vaccinated against rhinopneumonitis. The general incidence of abortion due to EHVI can be reduced by vaccinating broodmares with a killed vaccine during the 5th, 7th and 9th months of gestation. This strategy is designed to stimulate maximum immunity and achieve protection during the last half of pregnancy, when mares are at maximum risk for abortion. However, protection is never absolute and despite diligent vaccination, mares may still abort due to EHVI. Modified live vaccines may also provide protection against abortion.

It is noteworthy that most foals with the respiratory form of rhinopneumonitis are infected with a subtype of EHVI designated $EHVI_2$. This form of virus rarely causes abortion; therefore, foals with the respiratory syndrome may not be as dangerous in the presence of pregnant mares as was once suspected. Nevertheless, because $EHVI_2$ can cause abortions it is still deemed prudent to keep weanlings separate from broodmares (see Chapter 10).

Abortion due to Progesterone Deficiency

The use of progesterone or progestagens to maintain pregnancy in so-called 'habitual aborters' has been questioned ever since this practice began. It has never been demonstrated in either the human or the mare that primary progesterone deficiency is a cause of abortion. There is also evidence to suggest that embryonal death may sometimes be mediated by chromosomal anomalies or immunointolerance in otherwise normal mares, and that progestagenic supplementation would not save these pregnancies. In the case of mares carrying a donkey conceptus, for example, altrenogest supplementation was of no value in the maintenance of pregnancy. In practice, however, it is difficult to decide whether declining or low serum progesterone levels at the time of abortion are primary or secondary when there are no other obvious causes for the abortion. Therefore, progesterone or progestagen supplementation, and questions as to its value, will be with us for some time to come.

Maintaining Pregnancy

It has recently been demonstrated that pregnancy can be maintained in ovariectomized mares and noncycling mules with 300 mg of progesterone in oil i.m. or 0.044–0.088 mg/kg of altrenogest per os on a daily basis. Because some reports suggest that lower doses of progesterone or altrenogest may not be sufficient to maintain pregnancy in all cases, it is suggested that the higher doses be employed; 1000 mg of repositol progesterone (progesterone in propylene glycol) given i.m. every 4 days will also maintain pregnancy. Some practitioners have employed progestagen supplementation until the end of pregnancy, but it is usually not necessary to continue treatment beyond 100 days because placental progestagen production is sufficient to maintain pregnancy beyond this point.

Progesterone and altrenogest treatments have also been used for routine supplementation of pregnancy in nonovariectomized embryo transfer recipients. However, little information has been generated on the safety of these treatments during pregnancy. Common usage and metabolic studies have shown that there were no obvious detrimental effects of altrenogest after dosing for 3 months or longer. There were also no effects on future cyclicity when this progestagen was fed continuously for up to 2 months. However, no longer-term studies have been conducted on the fertility of offspring derived from pregnancies that have been maintained by progesterone, altrenogest or other progestagens. It is essential that such studies be conducted because some clinical reports in the human have associated progesterone supplementation with masculinization, skeletal defects and other miscellaneous defects of the fetus. Despite these findings, a recent study in over 400 women showed that there was no increased risk in fetal anomalies in subjects whose pregnancy was maintained with either progesterone or 17-OH progesterone during the first trimester of gestation.

Another point of concern about progestagenic support of pregnancies in non-ovariectomzied mares is that of an induced dependency on the progestagenic hormone so that if it were withdrawn prematurely, that is, before day 100 of gestation, abortion would be likely to occur. This concern arises from occasional findings of abbreviated luteal phases in cycling mares treated with altrenogest and a recent similar finding relating to the primary corpus luteum of pregnancy during altrenogest supplementation. It was also shown that serum progesterone fell to baseline within 10–21 days after the onset of altrenogest supplementation in donkey-in-mare embryo transfers that were much earlier in pregnancy than was normally seen in untreated pregnancies of this nature. These data collectively suggest that dependence on exogenous progesterone or progestagens may develop during early pregnancy and that diligent administration of the hormones is necessary if pregnancy is to be maintained.

Other Accidents of Gestation

Uterine torsion, preputial tendon rupture and dystocia can also be interpreted as causes of infertility, but because these conditions are generally regarded as obstetrical matters they are not discussed in this chapter.

Complementary References

Asbury, A. C. (1982) Some observations on the relationship of histologic inflammation in the endometrium of the mare to fertility. *Proc. 28th Ann. Convention of the Amer. Assoc. Equine Pract.*, pp. 401–404.

Baker, C. V. & Kenney, R. M. (1980) Systematic approach to the diagnosis of the infertile or subfertile mare. In *Current Therapy in Theriogenology*, ed. Morrow, D. A. Philadelphia: W. B. Saunders.

Bergman, R. V. & Kenney, R. M. (1975) Representativeness of a uterine biopsy in the mare. *Proc. 21st Ann. Convention of the Amer. Assoc. Equine Pract.*, pp. 355–361.

Dewes, H. F. (1980) Preliminary observations on the use of colostrum as a uterine infusion in thoroughbred mares. *NZ Vet. J.*, **28**, 7.

Ginther, O. J. (1979) *Reproductive Biology of the Mare.* Ann Arbor: McNaughton and Gunn.

Ginther, O. J. (1982) Twinning in mares: A review of recent studies. *Equine Vet. Sci.*, **2**, 127.

Greenhoff, S. R. & Kenney, R. M. (1975) Evaluation of the reproductive status of nonpregnant mares. *J. Amer. Vet. Med. Assoc.*, **167**, 449.

Hughes, J. P., Stahenfeldt, G. H. & Kennedy, P. C. (1980) Estrous cycle and selected functional and pathological ovarian abnormalities in the mare. *Vet. Clin. N. Amer. Large Anim. Pract.*, **2**, 225.

Hyland, J. H. & Bristol, F. (1979) Synchronization of oestrus and timed insemination of mares. *J. Reprod. Fertil. Suppl.*, **27**, 251.

Kenny, R. M., Bergman, R. V., Cooper, W. L. & Morse, G. W. (1975) Minimal contamination techniques for breeding mares: Technique and preliminary findings. *Proc. 21st Ann. Convention of the Amer. Assoc. of Equine Pract.*, pp. 327–336.

Lofstedt, R. M. (1986) Some aspects of manipulative and diagnostic endocrinology of the broodmare. *Proc. Ann. Meet. Soc. Theriogenol.*, pp. 67–93.

Loy, R. G., Pemstein, R., O'Canna, D. & Douglas, R. H. (1981) Control of ovulation in cycling mares with ovarian steroids and prostaglandin. *Theriogenology*, **15**, 191.

Neely, D. P., Liu, I. K. M. & Hillman, R. B. (1983) *Equine Reproduction.* Belvidere: Hoffman-LaRoche Inc., p. 80.

Pascoe, R. R. (1983) Methods for the treatment of twin pregnancy in the mare. *Equine Vet. J.*, **15**, 40.

Sharp, D. C. (1980) Environmental influences on reproduction in horses. *Vet. Clin. N. Amer. Large Anim. Pract.*, **2**, 207.

Swerczek, T. W. (1985) Early fetal death and infectious placental disease in the mare. *Proc. 26th Ann. Convention of Amer. Assoc. Equine Pract.*, pp. 173–179.

Threlfall, W. R. (1980) Broodmare uterine therapy. *Comp. Cont. Ed. Pract. Vet.*, **II**(11), 246.

10

Noninfectious Causes of Infertility in the Dog and Cat

SHIRLEY D. JOHNSTON

Infertility is a clinical sign defined as a state of diminished or absent fertility without implication of whether or not the state is reversible. The goals of the clinician presented with an infertile patient are: first, to define as precisely as possible the problem or problems identified from the infertility problem-specific minimum database (history, physical examination, laboratory evaluation); and second, to determine the cause of the defined problems so as to be able to assess whether or not they are potentially reversible.

THE INFERTILE BITCH AND QUEEN

Elements of the problem-specific minimum database for infertility in the bitch and queen are listed in Table 10.1. The value of accurate records on all previous seasons of the bitch cannot be overemphasized, because of the observation that inappropriate timing of breeding accounts for at least half of female canine conception failures. In the queen which fails to conceive following breeding, the interval from breeding to the next estrus may suggest whether normal copulation, cervical stimulation and induction of ovulation did (interval = 45–60 days) or did not (interval = 14–19 days) occur. In both the dog and cat, history of false pregnancy signs suggests that ovulation did occur. History of previous reproductive disease (dystocia, metritis,

pyometra) may indicate a diagnostic and therapeutic direction. Clients should be questioned carefully about evidence that the male used is fertile and, in the dog, where prostate infection with advancing age is common and may be intermittent, semen from older males should be evaluated and cultured, if possible, as part of the bitch's workup.

Persistent Anestrus

The problem of persistent anestrus should be confirmed by determining whether: (1) the patient is observed adequately to detect estrus; (2) previous ovariohysterectomy (OHE) may have been performed (by history, or abdominal palpation of a suture line and absence of the uterus, or possibly by detecting elevated serum gonadotropin concentrations); and (3) feline patients are exposed to adequate photoperiod (14 h or more light; 10 h dark). If estrus detection or photoperiod are inadequate, these should be corrected and the patient observed carefully for an appropriate period of time (9 months for dogs and 2–3 months from January to August in cats).

Primary anestrus in the bitch and queen is defined as failure to cycle by 2 years of age. Possible causes include gonadal dysgenesis associated with abnormal karyotype (XO monosomy, XXX or XXY trisomy, XX/XY chimerism), thyroid insufficiency, presence of a functional (progesterone-

Table 10.1   Problem-specific minimum database for infertility in the bitch and queen

Component of database	Species*
History	
1. General, nonreproductive history	C,F
2. Cycle information	
(a) Dates of proestrus onsets	C
(b) Dates of estrus onsets	C,F
(c) Days of seasons at which bred	C,F
(d) Method of breeding (ties, AI)	C
(e) Number of breedings observed	C,F
(f) Days of refusal of mating	C,F
(g) Presence and duration (breeding to parturition) of previous pregnancies	C,F
(h) Number of puppies/kittens per pregnancy	C,F
(i) Presence of false pregnancy signs (lactation, nesting) after any seasons	C,F
3. Information on males to which bred (age, whether semen quality has been evaluated, whether he has sired other litters, whether he has failed to sire)	C,F
4. Presence of previous reproductive disorders (such as dystocia, metritis, pyometra, vaginitis, abortion)	C,F
5. Previous drug therapy, if any	C,F
6. Previous pertinent laboratory testing (*Brucella canis* serology, feline leukemia virus testing, thyroid testing, progesterone concentrations in diestrus)	C,F
Physical	
1. General physical examination	C,F
2. Abdominal palpation of uterus (presence and size)	C,F
3. Inspection of vulva (location, size, presence of discharge, if any)	C,F
4. Digital examination of vestibule and vagina	C
5. Inspection and palpation of mammary glands (presence, degree of development, presence of lactation or masses if any)	C,F
Laboratory evaluation	
1. Complete blood count, chemistry profile, urinalysis	C,F
2. *Brucella canis* serology	C
3. Feline leukemia virus test	F
4. Vaginal cytology	C,F
5. Serum concentrations of thyroxine (T4) and triiodothyronine (T3)	C

*C = canine; F = feline.

secreting) luteinized ovarian cyst, glucocorticoid excess (endogenous hyperadrenalism (Cushing's disease) or exogenous glucocorticoid administration), or autoimmune follicular maturation arrest (Figs 10.1, 10.2 and 10.3). Hyperprolactinemia due to a prolactin-secreting pituitary tumor, and depressed serum concentrations of prolactin and LH in patients with insulin-treated diabetes mellitus are conditions associated with amenorrhea in humans that may occur, but have not been described in companion animals.

Diagnostic approach to persistent anestrous patients is to collect blood for karyotype and for serum concentrations of thyroid hormones (thyroxine, triiodothyronine), progesterone, luteinizing hormone (LH) and follicle stimulating hormone (FSH). Karyotypes can be done at a number of

veterinary colleges around the world; sample submission requirements are usually 10 ml heparinized whole blood or a skin biopsy sample in a bath of heparinized blood sent at ambient temperature and at an interval from sample collection to cell culture (the first step in the karyotype procedure) that does not exceed 24 h. Abnormal karyotype indicates irreversibility of the infertile state. Bitches and queens with ovarian dysgenesis due to numerical abnormality of the sex chromosomes usually do not have other abnormalities detected at physical examination.

Thyroid insufficiency, which is common in the bitch and rare in the queen, is usually reversible following replacement therapy with thyroxine (T4) (0.022 mg/kg by mouth twice daily) or triiodothyronine (T3) (4.4 μg/kg by mouth three times daily);

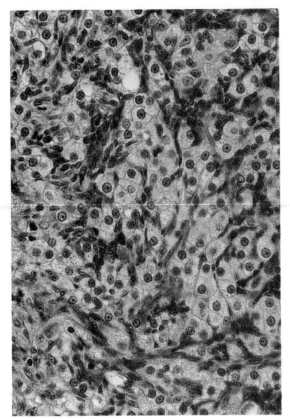

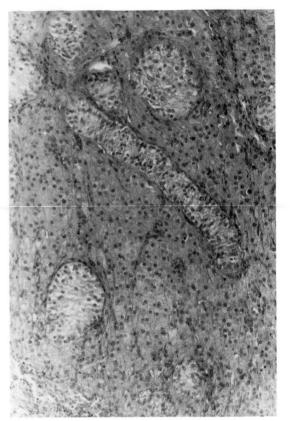

Fig. 10.1 Ovarian histology from a 2½-year-old female sable Burmese cat presented for primary anestrus. The queen had been smaller than littermates since birth; no other physical abnormalities were noted. Chromosome complement was 37,XO (normal female cat karyotype is 38,XX). Ovarian histology revealed inactive germinal epithelium lacking follicles and primordial germ cells; this figure shows interstitial cells of the ovary. H & E stain. Diagnosis: X-chromosome monosomy and ovarian dysgenesis. (From Johnston *et al.* (1983), with kind permission of the authors and editor of *Journal of the American Veterinary Medical Association.*)

Fig. 10.2 Ovarian histology from a 4-year-old female Airedale terrier presented for primary anestrus. No abnormalities were detected at physical examination. Complete blood count, serum chemistry profile, urinalysis, serum thyroxine concentration (2.2 μg/dl) and serum progesterone concentration (0.48 ng/ml) were normal for an anestrous bitch. Chromosome complement was 79,XXX (normal female dog karyotype is 78,XX). Serum LH (670 ng/ml) and FSH (11 210 ng/ml) concentrations were markedly elevated. Ovarian histology revealed presence of large masses of interstitial cells, but no follicles or corpora lutea. This figure shows a solid epithelial cord and large masses of interstitial cells. H & E stain. Diagnosis: X-chromosome trisomy and ovarian dysplasia. (From Johnston *et al.* (1985), with kind permission of the authors and editor of *Theriogenology.*)

estrous cycles resume within 4–5 months following administration of adequate supplementation. Adequacy of treatment should be confirmed by documentation of normal serum concentrations of T3 and T4 3–4 h after medication is administered.

Serum progesterone concentrations exceeding 2 ng/ml are presumptive evidence of luteal function by a normal or persistent corpus luteum; the next step is to repeat serum progesterone measurement 9–10 weeks later to distinguish normal diestrous luteal function (progesterone concentration will have dropped to less than 2 ng/ml) from a luteinized cyst or functional ovarian tumor (progesterone concentration will persist at levels exceeding 2 ng/ml).

Surgical excision is indicated for functional ovarian cysts or neoplasms.

Measurement of serum concentrations of LH and FSH may identify hypogonadotropic states (potentially amenable to therapy), or hypergonadotropic states (suggesting previous OHE or irreversible ovarian failure, such as that observed in gonadal dysgenesis).

In autoimmune ovarian failure, ovarian histology may be necessary to confirm the diagnosis (see Fig. 10.3).

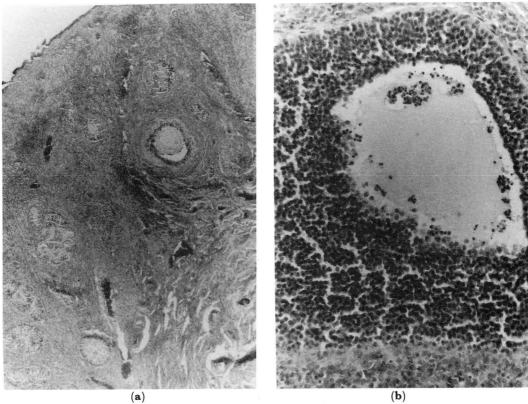

(a) **(b)**

Fig. 10.3 Ovarian histology from a 5-year-old female cocker spaniel bitch presented for primary anestrus. No abnormalities were detected at physical examination except for presence of keratoconjunctivitis sicca. Karyotype (78, XX), and serum concentrations of progesterone (nondetectable), estradiol (20 pg/ml), testosterone (nondetectable), thyroxine (2.6 μg/dl), LH (0.76 ng/ml), and FSH (170 ng/ml) were normal for an anestrous bitch. Fig. 10.3a shows presence of diffuse lymphocytic oophoritis with follicular degeneration and absence of corpora lutea. Fig. 10.3b shows a degenerating follicle with lymphocytic infiltration. H & E stain. Diagnosis: autoimmune follicular maturation arrest.

Inability to Achieve Normal Copulation

Bitches or queens which fail to achieve normal copulation may have a structural abnormality in the vagina or vestibule, may not be in estrus when breeding is attempted, or may have a behavioral objection to copulation with one or all males. Confirmation of this problem is made by observation of breeding in the dog (where the inside tie or coital lock should normally occur, with engorgement and entrapment of the male bulbus glandis inside the female vagina); absence of a tie defines the problem. In the cat, where copulation is brief and difficult to observe completely, the problem is defined by observing queens which do not permit approach by the male or are not induced to ovulate (this occurs only after cervical stimulation in this induced ovulator, and is determined by detecting serum progesterone concentrations exceeding 2 ng/ml for several weeks following mating).

The diagnostic approach to this problem is to examine the bitch or queen when the owner judges her to be in estrus in order to stage her in her cycle (using vaginal cytology to detect cornification and serum estradiol or progesterone concentrations if available) and to perform a digital and/or vaginoscopic examination of the vestibule and caudal vagina to detect any structural abnormality.

Correct staging of the cycle is described below (page 165); in the bitch, inappropriate timing of breeding is corrected by determining ovulation date and using natural or artificial breeding either at or 1–2 days after ovulation. Ovulation may occur as early as 6 days or as late as 26 days following proestrus onset, and is best detected using the diestrous vaginal smear, which occurs 6 days following ovulation, or using serum progesterone concentrations as described on page 165. Alternatively, the client can be counseled to tease the bitch with an intact male starting 2–3 days after proestrus onset and continu-

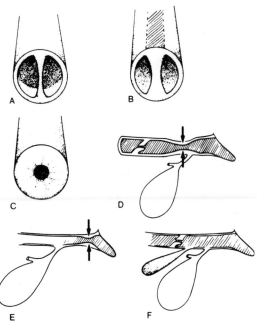

Fig. 10.4 Congenital abnormalities of the vagina and vulva of the bitch. (a) Vertical septum at vestibulovaginal junction. (b) Incomplete fusion of Mullerian ducts partitioning vagina. (c) Annular stricture at vestibulovaginal orifice. (d) Hypoplasia of vestibulovaginal junction. (e) Stenosis at vestibulovulvar junction. (f) Secondary vaginal pouch. (From Wykes & Soderberg (1983), with kind permission of the authors and editor of *Journal of the American Animal Hospital Association.*)

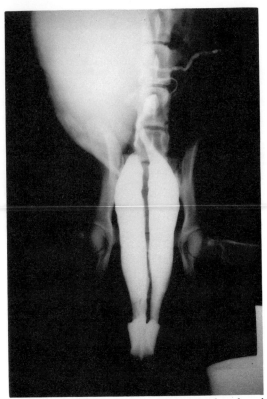

Fig. 10.5 Retrograde vaginogram (ventrodorsal projection) of a 7-year-old female Great Pyrenees presented in early proestrus for vaginal cytology to predict optimal breeding time. Her history was that breeding attempts were made at three previous seasons, and inside ties were never achieved. On digital examination of the vagina a midvaginal obstruction was palpated, which was revealed by retrograde vaginography to be a wall of tissue bifurcating the vagina in a sagittal plane.

ing for 20–30 days in order to detect those bitches which may be normal but not average with regard to onset of sexual receptivity and ovulation time.

Congenital structural abnormalities of the vestibule and vagina are common in the bitch in all breeds; these abnormalities have not been described in the queen (probably due to the small vaginal size and difficulty of adequate examination in this species), but may occur. Annular strictures (vaginovestibular or vestibulolabial) (Fig. 10.4c) are the most common of these abnormalities, accounting for slightly more than half, followed by vertical tags of imperforate hymens (Fig. 10.4a), vertical septa bifurcating the vagina (Figs 10.4b and 10.5) and hypoplasia of the vaginal or vestibular canal (Fig. 10.4d). Detection of one of these abnormalities by digital or vaginoscopic examination of the vagina should be followed by retrograde vaginography to characterize location and extent of the problem (see Fig. 10.5) in order to assess possibility of surgical correction. Most of these abnormalities (except hypoplasia) can be corrected surgically via episiotomy. Alternatively, artificial insemination may

be performed with the understanding that subsequent cesarean section may be necessary.

Vaginal prolapse may also be a structural impediment to copulation in the bitch; although vaginal prolapse has been observed in the queen, it is extremely rare. In type I canine vaginal prolapse the vaginal mass does not protrude through the vulvar cleft, but may obstruct the vagina and prevent normal copulation. Diagnosis is made by digital examination, and treatment is surgical excision of the prolapsed mass late in estrus, or artificial insemination around the mass.

If timing and structural abnormality of the female tract are ruled out as causes of failure to copulate normally, behavioral abnormality is the exclusion diagnosis, and use of a different male or of artificial insemination should be considered.

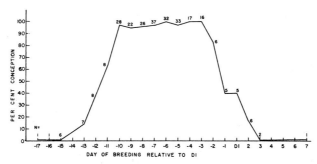

Fig. 10.6 Percentage conception relative to day of breeding. A single breeding was allowed, and charted according to day before or after the first day of the diestrous smear (D1). (From Holst & Phemister (1974), with kind permission of the authors and editor of *American Journal of Veterinary Research*.)

Inappropriate Timing of Breeding During Estrus

Inappropriate timing of breeding is a major cause of conception failure in the canine when owners plan breedings based on a numbered day after proestrus onset (typically around day 12, which is day of ovulation in the average bitch) instead of on a day near ovulation, which can occur many days before or after day 12 of the season in normal bitches. Normal (but not average) bitches may ovulate as soon as 6 days or as late as 26 days after proestrus onset. Although the average bitch ovulates about 2 days following onset of sexual receptivity (estrus), normal bitches may ovulate up to 3 days before to 11 days after estrus onset. Most bitches will ovulate at about the same day of the cycle at every season.

Diagnostic strategy to confirm the problem of inappropriate timing of breeding and to plan breeding management for a future season is based on assessment of previous reproductive history, and on prospective use of daily vaginal cytology with measurement of serial serum progesterone concentrations around suspected time of ovulation. Previous history is most useful in bitches that have had at least one successful pregnancy. In these, day of ovulation is calculated as approximately 63 days prior to parturition. For example, the bitch that whelps 61 days after a day 12 (from proestrus onset) mating is calculated to have ovulated on day 10 after proestrus onset (63−61 = 2; 12−2 = day 10); the bitch that whelps 65 days from a day 17 (from proestrus onset) mating is calculated to have ovulated on day 19 of her season (63−65 = −2; 17−(−2) = day 19). History can also be useful in the absence of previous pregnancy if one can determine that onset of receptivity to mating occurred some time before or after average receptivity (which occurs 10 days after proestrus onset), suggesting that ovulation occurred earlier or later than average.

Daily vaginal cytology can be used to determine approximate day of ovulation by detecting the first day of diestrus (D1), which is the first day after estrus onset (and maximal cornification) that the vaginal smear is composed of more than 50% non-cornified (intermediate and parabasal) cells. D1 occurs approximately 6 days following ovulation, and is a better determinant of ovulation than is day of the cycle from proestrus onset or day of estrus. Clients can be taught to collect daily vaginal cytology samples using saline-moistened cotton-tipped swabs scraped against the ceiling of the vagina cranial to the urethral orifice; these are then submitted for veterinary interpretation and determination of the day of the diestrous smear.

Serum progesterone concentrations may also be used to stage ovulation, as they rise from concentrations during anestrus of less than 2 ng/ml to 2–6 ng/ml on the day of the LH surge (2 days preceding ovulation); thereafter, concentrations of this hormone continue to rise, peaking (at 20–80 ng/ml) about 3–4 weeks following ovulation. Serum progesterone concentrations then decline to baseline, anestrous values by 50–80 days following onset of proestrus. Blood can be collected from clinical patients on several days around the time of suspected ovulation to try and confirm approximate day of ovulation.

Once day of ovulation is determined within the cycle, a breeding management strategy is formulated so that the bitch is inseminated either at or 1–2 days after ovulation. A high conception rate can be achieved in normal bitches bred a single time between 3 and 10 days prior to diestrus onset (or 4 days before to 3 days after ovulation) (Fig. 10.6). Best litter size is achieved when insemination occurs on D4 or D5 (1 or 2 days following ovulation) (Table 10.2). If a breeding strategy must be planned in the absence of information on time of ovulation, best reproductive performance is

Table 10.2 Number of living pups produced per corpus luteum and number of pups per litter (from Holst and Phemister, 1974)

Day of breeding	Number	Total CL	Total living pups	Pups per CL	Pups per litter
D − 11*	3	20	10	0.50	3.3
D − 10	10	74	61	0.82	6.1
D − 9	8	53	46	0.87	5.8
D − 8	7	43	37	0.86	5.3
D − 7	13	92	77	0.84	5.9
D − 6	13	84	69	0.82	5.3
D − 5	6	42	38	0.90	6.3
D − 4	8	57	55	0.96	6.9
D − 3	4	32	20	0.63	5.0

*D refers to time relative to onset of diestrus, determined as the diestrus vaginal smear, or the first day after estrus onset that exfoliated vaginal epithelial cells are predominantly noncornified.

achieved when breeding is started at first receptivity (first day of estrus) and continued every second or third day until the bitch refuses mating by the dog.

Because the queen is an induced ovulator, where the act of copulation and penile stimulation of cervical neurons causes pituitary LH release and ovulation, timing of breeding is usually temporally related to ovulation. Two aspects of the physiology of ovulation of the queen do, however, have clinical implications with regard to infertility. The first is that the queen's ability to release LH in response to coitus may be a function of duration of hypothalamic/pituitary exposure to estrogen, and that sexual receptivity alone does not imply ability to respond to coitus with LH release. This means that breedings early in estrus may not, in some queens, result in ovulation. The second aspect is the observation that magnitude of LH release by the pituitary increases with number of copulations, and that as many as 50% of queens allowed to copulate only a single time fail to release adequate LH to induce ovulation. This means that conception failure following a single breeding may be due to inadequate LH stimulation, which could be treated pharmacologically (with 25 μg GnRH i.m. or 500 u hCG i.m.) or by increasing number of copulations.

Ovulation Failure

Incidence of ovulation failure in the bitch and queen is unknown. In the bitch this disorder (diagnosed by detecting multiple serum progesterone measurements less than 2 ng/ml during the 2 month period following estrus) is associated with short (2–3 months) interestrous intervals. In the queen, ovulation failure is associated with a short (14–19 day) interval to the next estrus, instead of with the 40–45 day (nonpregnant) or 60 day (pregnant) luteal phase which follows ovulation. Bitches which fail to ovulate should be tested for thyroid insufficiency, which may accompany this disorder.

Treatment of ovulation failure is based on administering an ovulation-inducing drug (dogs: 50 μg GnRH i.m. or 1000 u hCG i.m. or 5 mg LH i.m.; cats: 25 μg GnRH i.m. or 500 u hCG i.m.). For canine patients with an inadequate luteal phase (serum progesterone concentrations which decline to baseline prematurely, typically at 4–5 weeks following estrus) progesterone supplementation in pregnancy may be considered.

Abnormal Cycles

Bitches which cycle more frequently than every $4\frac{1}{2}$ months are documented to be less fertile than those that cycle normally; this may be related to failure of their endometrium to slough and regenerate as it does in normal bitches during the long (4 month) anestrus. With the complaint of abnormal cycles the most important first step is to confirm the complaint by characterizing the cycles with vaginal cytology and serial serum progesterone measurements. These data enable the clinician to rule out split heats (where some bloody vaginal discharge and vulvar swelling occur about 1 month prior to a normal season) or receptive behavior at the end of diestrus as manifestations of a true season. Hypothyroidism and uterine infection can be associated with abnormal or irregular cycles, and therefore should be ruled out as well. If short interestrous intervals are present in a euthyroid bitch that ovulates and maintains a normal luteal phase, one may be successful in achieving pregnancy by suppressing estrus with mibolerone for 3–4 months prior to the season at which she is bred.

Diagnosis of abnormal cycles is rare in queens, because the normal range of their cycles is so variable. The queen has estrous periods at 4–30 day intervals (14–19 day modal) when under a constant photoperiod. If photoperiod declines (as it does for outdoor cats in the northern hemisphere in September) the queens become anestrous; if photoperiod is maintained with indoor lighting they will continue to cycle through the winter.

Other Causes of Noninfectious Infertility

Bitches and queens that fail to conceive following good breeding management and mating to a fertile

Table 10.3 Problem-specific minimum database for infertility in the dog and tom

Component of database	Species*
History	
1. General, nonreproductive history	C,F
2. History of litters sired (dates of the female's cycles at which bred, dates litters born)	C,F
3. History of unsuccessful breedings	C,F,
4. Previous drug therapy, if any (glucocorticoids, testosterone, thiacetarsamide, ketaconazole)	C,F
5. Presence of previous reproductive disorders (orchitis, epididymitis, prostatitis)	C,F
6. Previous pertinent laboratory testing (*Brucella canis* serology, feline leukemia virus testing, thyroid testing, semen evaluations)	C,F
Physical	
1. General physical examination	C,F
2. Inspection of prepuce (location, size, presence of discharge, if any)	C,F
3. Extrusion of penis from prepuce and identification of gross anatomy including (androgen-dependent) penile spines in the cat	C,F
4. Palpation of testes and epididymides (for location, size, symmetry, consistency)	C,F
5. Rectal/abdominal palpation of prostate	C
Laboratory evaluation	
1. Complete blood count, chemistry profile, urinalysis	C,F
2. *Brucella canis* serology	C
3. Feline leukemia virus test	F
4. Complete semen evaluation (including determination of semen volume, color, sperm numbers per ejaculate, percentage morphologically normal sperm, cytospin or sediment examination for inflammatory cells)	C,F
5. Quantitative bacterial culture of semen; mycoplasma/ureaplasma culture if possible	C
6. Serum concentrations of thyroxine (T4) and triiodothyronine (T3)	C

*C = canine; F = feline.

male at an ovulatory cycle, should be examined by exploratory laparotomy (1) for patency of the female's tubular tract; (2) for a full-thickness uterine biopsy; and (3) for bacterial (including mycoplasma/ureaplasma) culture of the uterine lumen. Bacterial infection of the uterus (see Chapter 17) is common in the dog and cat and may be a reversible cause of infertility. Segmental aplasia of any part of the Mullerian duct system (female tubular tract, including uterine tubes, uterus, cranial vagina) is uncommon, but has been described, and may prevent sperm from reaching the oocytes. Benign epithelial hyperplasia (at the uterotubal junction) or inflammatory proliferation of uterine or uterine tube tissue may occlude the tubular tract.

Other possible, but poorly documented noninfectious causes of infertility in the female include stress, presence of antisperm antibodies and cervical factors which adversely affect sperm transport. In addition, some data support decreased conception rate and number of puppies whelped in highly inbred dogs (inbreeding coefficients ranging from 0.125 to 0.558) compared to outbred dogs. Infectious causes of reproductive failure in the bitch and

queen (such as canine brucellosis, canine herpesvirus, feline leukemia virus infection, toxoplasmosis; see Chapters 11, 12 and 17) usually occur in females with normal, ovulatory cycles.

THE DOG AND TOM

The problem-specific minimum database for infertility in the dog and tom is listed in Table 10.3 (see also Chapter 5). Semen can be collected from most male dogs into an artificial vagina by masturbation; presence of a proestrous/estrous teaser bitch has been demonstrated to improve quality of the sample collected. Semen collection from the tom is more difficult; although some laboratory cats can be trained to ejaculate into an artificial vagina, for clinical purposes electroejaculation is the most reliable method of collecting a feline semen sample. Electroejaculation is accomplished under ketamine (22 mg/kg i.m.) and valium (2.5 mg i.m.) anesthesia with atropine premedication; a teflon rectal probe is placed over the region of the prostatic urethra, and 180 2–9 volt pulses are applied. In practice, where electroejaculation is usually unavailable, urine collection (by cystocentesis) is recommended following ejaculation to look for sperm, because the cat is known to undergo retrograde as well as antegrade ejaculation. Alternatively, a vaginal wash of the postcoital queen may demonstrate that sperm were present in the ejaculate.

Quantitative semen culture is recommended for all canine semen samples, because bacterial infection of the prostate is a common and reversible cause of infertility in this species. Normal dog semen should have less than 10 000 bacteria per ml, and concentrations exceeding that number are most commonly from the infected prostate gland, where intermittent, recurrent infection in middle-aged to older dogs is common. Normal semen collected by electroejaculation from normal cats may have quantitative bacterial counts exceeding 100 000/ml, so that quantitative bacterial cultures of semen in this species cannot be used to distinguish infection of the genital tract from presence of normal flora. In the dog, bacteria cultured from semen are normal urethral flora (*Escherichia coli*, *Staphylococcus aureus*, *Mycoplasma* spp., *Corynebacterium* spp., *Streptococcus canis*); bacteria cultured from normal cat semen and cat preputial mucosa commonly include *E. coli*, *Staphylococcus* spp., *Streptococcus* spp., *Pseudomonas aeruginosa*, *Proteus mirabilis*, and *Klebsiella oxytoca*. Presence of ureaplasmas on the preputial mucosa has been observed in association with infertility in the male dog, but their precise role in infertility in this species is unknown.

Failure to Achieve Erection and Ejaculation

Males which do not achieve erection in the presence of an estrous teaser bitch or queen should be evaluated for musculoskeletal or genital (testicular, prostatic) pain, for androgen insufficiency states (hypopituitarism, abnormalities of sexual differentiation such as the XXY karyotype, exogenous or endogenous steroid excess, idiopathic testicular atrophy), for neurologic deficit of the parasympathetic innervation which mediates erection, or for behavioral objection to the teaser female or collection procedure. The problem of failure of erection can only be confirmed in dogs in the presence of an estrous teaser bitch, because some normal male dogs will not respond to the artificial vagina and anestrous teaser bitch alone.

Androgen insufficiency states may be evaluated by measuring serum testosterone concentrations before and after stimulation with human chorionic gonadotropin (hCG) (which acts like LH to directly stimulate Leydig cells to secrete testosterone), or

with gonadotropin releasing hormone (GnRH) (which causes pituitary LH release and subsequent elevation in serum testosterone). Resting serum testosterone concentrations in normal male dogs range from 0.5 to 7 ng/ml, and in normal male cats from less than 0.05 to 3.0 ng/ml; 4 h following 44 u/kg hCG i.m., testosterone rises to 4.6–7.5 ng/ml (dogs) or 3.1–9.0 ng/ml (cats), and 1 h following 4.4 μg/kg GnRH i.m., testosterone rises to 3.7–6.2 ng/ml (dogs) or 5.0–12.0 ng/ml (cats) (n = 6). Abnormality of sexual differentiation is diagnosed by karyotype (as was described under persistent anestrus in the female, page 161). Hypopituitarism is diagnosed by measuring decreased serum concentrations of LH and FSH and of other pituitary hormones for which assays may be available, such as adrenocorticotropic hormone (ACTH), thyroid stimulating hormone, and growth hormone. Marked elevation in LH and FSH is an indication that testicular failure (usually irreversible) is present. Steroid excess may be diagnosed based on history, on testing for Cushing's disease (ACTH concentrations, dexamethasone suppression tests) or on serum estradiol and testosterone assays.

Parasympathetic neurologic deficit may be diagnosed by response to parasympathomimetic therapy (bethanechol) in the presence of an estrous female.

Behavioral objection to the female can be diagnosed by attempting semen collection or mating with a different, subordinate female at the male's home; male dogs may respond to the canine pheromone, methyl-*p*-hydroxy-benzoate (1 mg/ml in 70% ethanol) swabbed on the vulva of the teaser bitch.

Failure to Achieve Ejaculation in the Presence of a Normal Erection

In the male with normal erection, thrusting and palpable contractions of the striated smooth muscle surrounding the penile urethra (ischiocavernosus and bulbospongiosus muscles), absence of a fluid ejaculate can be localized to three possible rule-outs: absence of production of seminal plasma; emission failure; or retrograde ejaculation of the sample into the urinary bladder instead of antegrade through the penile urethra.

Absence of seminal fluid production may occur with intersex states (the XXY karyotype or chimeras, diagnosed by karyotype), by premature testicular failure (diagnosed by serum testosterone, LH and FSH assays and testicular biopsy), or by prostatic hypoplasia/aplasia (diagnosed by prostatic ultrasound and biopsy).

Failure of emission (delivery of the ejaculate into

Table 10.4 Causes of infertility in the male

Pretesticular	Hypopituitarism
	Steroid excess (endogenous, exogenous, glucocorticoids, sex steroids)
	Fever
	Thyroid insufficiency
	Diabetes mellitus
	Inguinal/scrotal hernia
	Immotile cilia syndrome
Testicular	Testicular dysgenesis due to abnormal sex chromosome complement (XXY, XX/XY)
	Cryptorchidism
	Testicular infection/inflammation
	Testicular irradiation
	Spermatotoxic drugs (thiacetarsamide, ketaconazole)
	Idiopathic spermatogenic arrest
	Testicular neoplasia
	Hereditary morphologic abnormalities of the sperm (knobbed spermatozoa)
Posttesticular	Segmental aplasia of the Wolffian duct system (epididymides, vasa deferentia)
	Spermatocele
	Prostatic infection/bleeding

the prostatic urethra) may be caused by segmental aplasia or occlusion of the male Wolffian duct system (diagnosed by bilateral prescrotal cannulation of the vasa deferentia with lymphangiography catheters and contrast radiography) or by sympathetic neurologic deficit which responds to sympathomimetic treatment (such as pseudoephedrine HCl, 4–5 mg/kg per os or phenylpropanolamine, 3 mg/kg per os 1 and 3 h preceding semen collection).

Retrograde ejaculation is diagnosed by collecting urine via cystocentesis following ejaculatory behavior and observing presence of sperm cells and alkaline phosphatase, which originates in the epididymides and is present in dog semen in approximate concentrations of 8000–30 000 u/l. Treatment of retrograde ejaculation, like that of emission failure, relies on oral administration of sympathomimetic drugs such as pseudoephedrine or phenylpropanolamine.

Pretesticular Causes of Infertility in the Male

Causes of testicular failure or poor semen quality in the ejaculate can be localized as pretesticular, testicular or posttesticular (Table 10.4). Varied causes from both pretesticular and testicular categories may cause total loss of testicular germinal epithelium, leaving normal to hyperplastic interstitial cells and seminiferous tubules lined only by Sertoli cells (Figs 10.7, 10.8 and 10.9). In these cases testicular histology may confirm irreversibility of the problem, but may not confirm etiology.

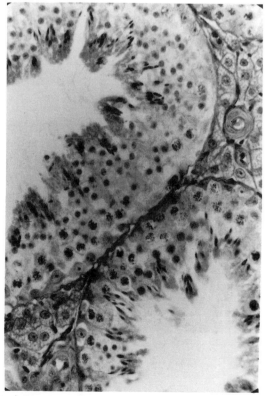

Fig. 10.7 Seminiferous tubules and interstitial cells from a normal dog testis, showing spermatogenic elements of the seminiferous epithelium and elongated spermatocytes imbedded in sertolic cell cytoplasm. H & E stain.

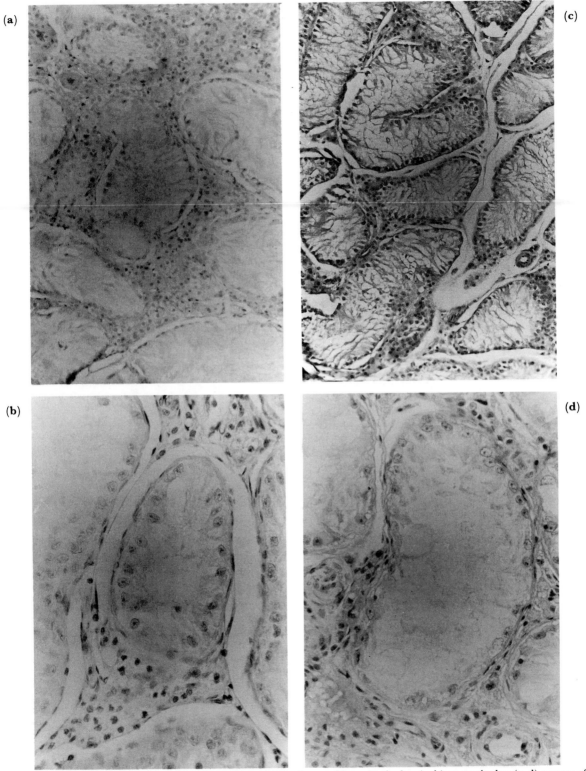

Fig. 10.8 Testicular histology of azoospermic canine patients with pretesticular (a, b) or testicular (c, d) causes of infertility. Seminiferous tubules are lined by Sertoli cells only in patients with diabetes mellitus (a), Cushing's disease (b), bilateral abdominal cryptorchidism (c), and idiopathic spermatogenic arrest (d). H & E stain.

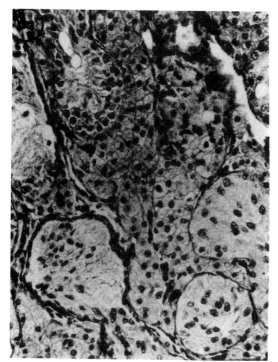

Fig. 10.9 Testicular histology of a sterile male tortoise-shell tabby domestic shorthair cat with a 38,XX/57,XXY diploid-triploid chimeric karyotype. There is no evidence of spermatogonia or their descendents. Only Sertoli cells line the seminiferous tubules. H & E stain. (From Centerwall & Benirschke (1975), with kind permission of the authors and editor of *American Journal of Veterinary Research*.)

Pretesticular causes include decreased gonadotropin secretion (due to spontaneous hypopituitarism or steroid suppression of LH/FSH secretion), fever, thyroid insufficiency, systemic metabolic disease such as diabetes mellitus or chronic renal failure, herniation of omentum or abdominal viscera into the scrotal sac, and immotile cilia syndrome. Diagnosis of many of these is made on history, physical examination and laboratory evaluation of the problem-specific minimum database for infertility in the male (see Table 10.3). In addition, serum LH and FSH concentrations should be measured so as to categorize the patient as hypogonadotropic (potentially treatable), normogonadotropic or hypergonadotropic (probably irreversible testicular failure). Immotile cilia syndrome, where hereditary absence of dynein arms prevents ciliary movement (respiratory tract cilia, sperm tails) is suspected in patients with chronic respiratory disease, bronchiectasis, situs inversus (approximately 50%) and immotile spermatozoa, and confirmed by electron microscopic examination of cross-sections of cilia.

Testicular Causes of Infertility in the Male

Testicular causes of male infertility include congenital causes (such as abnormalities of sexual differentiation, cryptorchidism with abdominal testes, and hereditary morphologic abnormalities of sperm, such as knobbed spermatozoa) and acquired causes (such as infection/inflammation, irradiation, spermatotoxic drugs, testicular neoplasia or idiopathic spermatogenic arrest). These are diagnosed based on history, physical examination, karyotype, semen culture and testicular histology (see Figs 10.7, 10.8 and 10.9). Abnormality of sexual differentiation, such as 39,XXY or chimeric status in the male calico cat, is the only documented cause of infertility or sterility in the male cat. Spermatotoxic drugs include most of the cancer chemotherapeutic agents (such as cyclophosphamide and clorambucil), ketaconazole, amphotericin B and thiacetarsamide.

Idiopathic spermatogenic arrest is a disorder of unknown etiology occurring in young to middleaged (5–7 years) dogs that were once fertile; in these patients testicular atrophy gradually occurs with seminiferous tubules becoming occupied by Sertoli cells only, with total absence of spermatogonia or later stages of germ cells (see Fig. 10.8d). Interstitial cell hyperplasia may occur in response to elevated concentrations of serum gonadotropins which are present with this disorder. There is no known effective treatment. In general, testicular failure due to any of these causes is irreversible.

Posttesticular Causes of Infertility in the Male

Posttesticular reproductive disorders in the male include segmental aplasia of the Wolffian duct system (epididymides, vasa deferentia), bilateral epididymal sperm granulomas or spermatoceles (Fig. 10.10), other inflammatory or neoplastic space-occupying lesions which occlude the outflow tract, and chronic prostatic infection. In these patients, seminal plasma containing low (less than 1000 u/l) alkaline phosphatase is evidence that normal epididymal fluid is not present in the ejaculate. Aplasias or space-occupying obstructions are diagnosed by contrast radiography of the vasa deferentia (via lymphangiography catheters placed into each vas prescrotally) or by gross pathology. Sperm granulomas may be suspected by palpation of epididymal mass(es), and are diagnosed by inspection at time of testicular exploration or castration. Sperm granulomas usually are not surgically correctable.

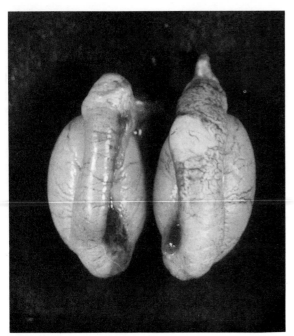

Fig. 10.10 Bilateral spermatoceles (sperm granulomas in the epididymides of a male dog with azoospermia).

Chronic prostate infection is diagnosed by presence of more than 10 000 bacteria per ml and a cytologic inflammatory response in prostatic fluid with radiographic/ultrasonographic confirmation of excessive prostatic reflux of contrast medium and/or cavitating lesions. Prostatic infection (see Chapter 17) is a common cause of infertility in male dogs over age 5, and is one of the few reversible causes of male infertility in this species.

NORMAL FERTILITY IN DOGS AND CATS

With careful management a conception rate of 90% can be achieved in dogs and there is no reliable information on the overall normal level of fertility. In general, the larger the breed the bigger the litter.

Stillbirths can be as frequent as 5%. A 34% mortality rate within 8 weeks of birth has been recorded; most deaths occur in the first week.

Male infertility is not uncommon but there is little accurate information on the actual incidence. The frequency with which animals are discarded because they will not breed is not known.

Complementary References

Allen, W. E. & Renton, J. P. (1982) Infertility in the dog and bitch. *Brit. Vet. J.*, **138**, 185–198.

Centerwall, W. R. & Benirschke, K. (1975) An animal model for the XXY Klinefelter's syndrome in man: tortoiseshell and calico male cats. *Amer. J. Vet. Res.*, **36**, 1275–1280.

Concannon, P. W., Hansel, W. & Visek, W. J. (1975) The ovarian cycle of the bitch. Plasma estrogen, LH and progesterone. *Biol. Reprod.*, **13**, 112–121.

Concannon, P. W., Hodgson, B. & Lein, D. (1980) Reflex LH release in estrous cats following single and multiple copulations. *Biol. Reprod.*, **23**, 111–117.

Holst, P. A. & Phemister, R. D. (1974) Onset of diestrus in the beagle bitch: definition and significance. *Amer. J. Vet. Res.*, **35**, 401–406.

Johnston, S. D., Buoen, L. C., Madl, J. E., Weber, A. F. & Smith, F. O. (1983) X-Chromosome monosomy (37,XO) in a Burmese cat with gonadal dysgenesis. *J. Amer. Vet. Med. Assoc.*, **182**, 986–989.

Johnston, S. D., Buoen, L. C., Weber, A. F. & Madl, J. E. (1985) X Trisomy in an Airedale bitch with ovarian dysplasia and primary anestrus. *Theriogenology*, **24**, 597–607.

Ling, G. V. & Ruby, A. L. (1978) Aerobic bacterial flora of the prepuce, urethra, and vagina of normal dogs. *Amer. J. Vet. Res.*, **39**, 695–698.

Meyers-Wallen, V. N. & Patterson, D. F. (1986) Disorders of sexual development in the dog. In *Current Therapy in Theriogenology*, ed. Morrow, D. A., pp. 567–574. Philadelphia: W. B. Saunders.

Nistal, M. & Paniagua, R. (1984) *Testicular and Epididymal Pathology*. New York: Thieme-Stratton.

Renton, J. P., Munro, C. D., Heathcote, R. H. & Carmichael, S. (1981) Some aspects of the aetiology, diagnosis and treatment of infertility in the bitch. *J. Reprod. Fertil.*, **61**, 289–294.

Shille, V. M., Lundstrom, K. E. & Stabenfeldt, G. H. (1979) Follicular function in the domestic cat as determined by estradiol-17 beta concentrations in plasma: relation to estrous behavior and cornification of exfoliated vaginal epithelium. *Biol. Reprod.*, **21**, 953–963.

Wildt, D. E., Baas, E. J., Chakraborty, P. K., Wolfle, T. L. & Stewart, A. P. (1982) Influence of inbreeding on reproductive performance, ejaculate quality and testicular volume in the dog. *Theriogenology*, **17**, 445–452.

Wykes, P. M. & Soderberg, S. F. (1983) Congenital abnormalities of the canine vagina and vulva. *J. Amer. Anim. Hosp. Assoc.*, **19**, 995–1000.

11

Virus Diseases

J. W. HARKNESS, M. LUCAS, S. EDWARDS and A. E. WRATHALL

CATTLE

Infectious Bovine Rhinotracheitis/Pustular Vulvovaginitis

Infectious bovine rhinotracheitis (IBR) and infectious pustular vulvovaginitis (IPV) are the respiratory and female genital forms of disease caused by bovine herpesvirus type 1 (BHV1). The genital disease in bulls is termed infectious pustular balanoposthitis (IPB). A number of other clinical syndromes are sometimes associated with the virus, including abortion. Subclinical infections also occur. The virus has a worldwide distribution apart from Switzerland and Denmark where there are eradication programs. Its natural host is cattle, and although other species can occasionally be infected, latently infected cattle are the main reservoir.

Serologically, all isolates of the virus are closely related but DNA fingerprinting has indicated that there are at least two main genotypes, and some countries may be free of the more virulent of these. There is strong circumstantial evidence that only one type was present in Britain until the mid-1970s, when a wave of severe respiratory disease swept the country, associated with the other genotype of BHV1. Both are present in North America and continental Europe. Some workers have associated the two types with IPV and IBR respectively but this is not supported by findings in the United Kingdom.

Respiratory Disease and Abortion

IBR can occur in cattle of any age. Epizootic outbreaks in susceptible herds often follow the introduction of new stock (presumably virus carriers). In its most dramatic form, IBR may contribute to the 'shipping fever' complex in feedlots. In enzootically infected herds only sporadic cases may be seen.

The disease is characterized by high fever, ocular and nasal discharges and cough. Intense conjunctivitis (without keratitis), rhinitis and tracheitis are present, sometimes progressing to a pneumonia. The virus denudes the airways of cilia, necrotic ulceration may occur, and in severe cases complete or partial obstruction of the airways by a caseous necrotic plug. Many outbreaks are relatively mild, with complete recovery of all cases. Clinical severity is exacerbated by poor husbandry and intensive housing systems and in such cases there may be a significant mortality from IBR. When adult cows are affected there is a marked but temporary drop in milk yield. In some, but not all, pregnant females the virus reaches the placenta and thence the fetus. It appears that the bovine fetus (except possibly in the final month of gestation) is highly susceptible to BHV1 and if infected undergoes a fulminating, invariably and rapidly fatal, disease characterized by widespread focal necrotic lesions, notably in the liver, kidney and spleen, in which viral antigen can be demonstrated by immunofluorescence. The abortion rate in herds affected by IBR varies from zero, through sporadic cases, to catastrophic epizootics. The reasons for this variability are not known. It is assumed that virus reaches the placenta by hematogenous spread, but viremia during acute IBR is transitory and at low level, and in many individuals may not occur at all. BHV1-induced abortion occurs typically from 2 weeks up to 3 months after the acute phase of IBR infection. It has been postulated that the delay occurs at the placenta, which becomes latently infected and a source of infection for the fetus later in gestation. Experimentally, fetuses inoculated directly in utero die within a few days and exhibit characteristic focal necrotic lesions. Fetuses of all gestational stages are susceptible to BHV1. At some stage during late gestation or the early neonatal period, there is a changeover in susceptibility to the postnatal pattern of respiratory disease. Thus late gestationally infected fetuses may conceivably be born live, and carrying the virus, although there is no evidence that this is a common occurrence. In contrast some newborn calves succumb to acute systemic fatal BHV1 infection and exhibit lesions similar to aborted fetuses.

Genital Disease

A venereally transmitted disease known as *Bläschenausschlag* (IPV) was recognized in Germany in the nineteenth century, and shown in 1928 to be associated with a filtrable agent. It has since been described in many countries in herds with natural mating. The seroprevalence in range cattle may be very high, although the incidence of clinical disease is usually low. In addition, explosive outbreaks of IPB have occurred in bull studs, and although mechanical transmission between bulls by collection apparatus, washing cloths, etc. has sometimes been implicated, the possibility of respiratory shedding and contact or aerosol transmission of the virus should be considered. Outbreaks of concurrent IBR and IPV have been described.

BHV1 may be shed in the semen from infected bulls, or more commonly in the preputial secretions, which can contaminate the semen at collection. The virus survives well the cryopreservation processes used for semen, and can thus be transmitted to susceptible females at artificial insemination.

Acute IPV develops 1–3 days after mating with an infected bull. The cows show evidence of pain by tail swishing and frequent micturition. There is edema and hyperemia of the vulva, with pustular lesions on the mucosal surface and extending into the vagina. Pyrexia (up to 41 °C), anorexia and decreased milk yield may occur in the early acute phase. The lesions heal within 10–14 days but mucopurulent vaginal discharge may persist for several weeks, particularly if there is secondary bacterial infection. A severe form of IPV termed 'epivag' has been described in Africa, in which there is anterior vaginitis and cervicitis in cows and epididymitis in bulls. IPV should be distinguished from granular vulvovaginitis which is a common but low grade infection associated with *Mycoplasma* spp. and in which pustules are not formed.

IPB in bulls may not be apparent until the penis is extruded, although occasionally there is an obvious mucopurulent or even hemorrhagic discharge visible at the preputial orifice. Lesions may occur over the entire mucosal surface of the penis and prepuce and may vary from reddened papules through pustules to frank ulceration, possibly accompanied by hemorrhage. As in cows, the lesions regress in 10–14 days but a mucopurulent discharge may persist for longer, as may shedding of the virus. The acute lesions are painful, but even so libido is often maintained and mating can take place, providing an ideal opportunity for transmission of the virus.

Latency and the Carrier State

Following recovery from the acute phase of infection, cattle become seropositive for antibody to the virus, but also carry the virus (probably for life) in an inactive or 'latent' form in cells of the sensory ganglia in the nervous system. From time to time, particularly in response to stress, the virus becomes active, undergoes a phase of replication, and is shed in the mucus secretions of the respiratory and/or genital tracts. This phenomenon of recrudescence is of particular concern in breeding bulls. Carrier bulls shed the virus only intermittently, so that many of their ejaculates will be safe. However there may be no clinical evidence of recrudescence, and only exhaustive laboratory tests can identify the presence of virus in particular ejaculates.

It has been suggested that bulls which have recovered from respiratory infection with BHV1 are unlikely to shed the virus in the genital tract. This may be so for some individuals, but shedding of recrudescent virus by both respiratory and genital routes in the same animal has been demonstrated and it would be very risky to assume that any seropositive animal is 'safe' for use in breeding programs.

Infertility

The role of BHV1 in bovine infertility remains uncertain. There are reports of poor semen quality from infected bulls although it is not clear whether this was caused by the virus, as others claim it has no effect on semen quality. Natural mating with infected bulls produces IPV in susceptible females but may or may not be associated with subnormal conception rates. Most reports of artificial insemination with BHV1-contaminated semen indicate a low conception rate and shortened estrous cycles following insemination. Recent experimental work offers a possible explanation for this in that the corpus luteum during the luteal phase is highly susceptible to BHV1 given intravenously or by the intrauterine route. Infected corpora lutea were cystic with necrotic foci, together with functional impairment as indicated by low diestral plasma progesterone levels. Intracervical or intrauterine inoculation of BHV1 or BHV1-contaminated semen also induces endometritis.

BHV1 can attach to, but not penetrate, the intact zona pellucida of bovine embryos, so transmission by embryo transfer from infected donors is possible. Trypsinization can remove detectable virus from such embryos. Once hatched from the zona pellucida, the bovine embryo is highly susceptible to BHV1 and is killed within 24–48 h.

BHV1 infertility may be associated with:

1. Reluctance of bulls to mate due to painful IPB lesions.
2. Impaired semen quality.
3. Abnormal hormonal events in females caused by viral infection of the corpus luteum.
4. Failure of implantation due to viral endometritis.
5. Early embryonic death due to viral infection of the embryo.

Diagnosis

BHV1 is readily isolated in cell cultures of bovine origin. Swabs for virus isolation should be of cotton-wool (not alginate), and used to collect a good sample of mucus from the affected site(s) (nose, eyes, vagina, prepuce). Swabs should be protected from drying with liquid transport medium, and kept cool during transit to the laboratory. It is recommended that a number of animals should be sampled during an outbreak, for the best chance of a successful diagnosis. Rapid diagnosis, giving an answer within a few hours, is also possible by immunoassays (notably immunofluorescence) for viral antigens in the samples. The advice of the diagnostic laboratory should be sought for the preferred type of sample. Virus isolation is sometimes possible from aborted fetuses, but antigen detection using immunofluorescence on frozen sections may give better results where autolysis is advanced.

Serology can be used to detect the rising antibody response in paired acute and convalescent serum samples from acute cases. It may be less helpful in abortion cases in that the dam has often seroconverted before the abortion occurs. Serology is also used to detect virus carriers, the assumption being that any seropositive animal (except for young calves which have received colostral antibody) is latently infected. Serum-virus neutralization, passive (indirect) hemagglutination and enzyme-linked immunosorbent assays (ELISA) are all used for BHV1 serology. A recent development of ELISA is the detection of IgM class antibodies as an indicator of recent infection, giving a more rapid serological diagnosis than the traditional reliance on paired samples.

Control

Vaccines are available in many countries. Formulations include inactivated adjuvanted types, and live attenuated strains of the virus which may be designed for intramuscular or intranasal application. Vaccine–virus-induced abortions have been reported with some intramuscular live vaccines used in pregnant cattle; the intranasal preparations (some of which are also 'temperature-sensitive' mutants) are considered safer, with the added advantage of stimulating local immunity. Such vaccines have also been applied intravaginally/preputially to control genital infections. All the live vaccines result in the establishment of latency with the possibility of spontaneous shedding of the vaccine strain on a later occasion. Although many of the vaccines have been shown to provide effective protection against BHV1-induced clinical disease, none of them (inactivated or live attenuated) can totally prevent infection, shedding and the establishment of latency with wild-type virus. Vaccines should therefore be used with caution if the objective is elimination of the virus from a herd.

BHV1 can be eradicated from a herd by a policy of serological testing and culling of reactors. Many bull studs have been cleared by this approach. The result is a fully susceptible herd, and it is important thereafter to maintain a strict control of new entries by a test and quarantine policy.

Bovine Virus Diarrhea (BVD)

The importance of bovine virus diarrhea virus (BVDV) as a cause of reproductive loss has been highlighted by many experimental and field studies of recent years. The virus is very widespread in most cattle populations and antibody prevalences in excess of 70% have been observed in many countries. Nevertheless, wholly susceptible herds exist and in that circumstance spectacular disease outbreaks can result from introduction of the virus. A common means of introduction into clean herds is purchase of, or contact with, an animal which is persistently infected with BVDV. Unlike carrier animals of other diseases, these cattle shed virus continually in high concentration throughout their entire lifetime, spreading infection both vertically and horizontally. Other species, including sheep, goats and deer also harbor the virus and although the biology of BVDV in the latter two species is incompletely known, it is probable that all three can suffer persistent infections in the same way that cattle do.

Most primary infections with BVDV in postnatal life are inapparent, but a few give rise to the clinical condition known as BVD, which is most often a minor illness of a few days duration and negligible mortality characterized by pyrexia, leukopenia and transient viremia, and sometimes accompanied by oculonasal discharge, oral erosions and a brief episode of diarrhea. Milk yield may fall dramatically in dairy cows. Many cows develop antibody to BVDV before they reach breeding age and are immune, but infection of susceptible cattle during pregnancy results in a viremia and spread of the virus to the fetus occurs in most cases. Fetal infection may result in any of a variety of forms of reproductive wastage, and is an essential prerequisite for the development of the normally fatal disease of postnatal life known as mucosal disease (MD). The economic losses associated with prenatal infection far outweigh those following postnatal infection, and recent estimates of the cost of these losses suggest that BVDV infection is one of the most important infectious causes of reproductive inefficiency.

Fetal Infection with BVDV

The bovine fetus which is infected with BVDV transplacentally may suffer any of a number of different sequels. The result may be abortion or stillbirth, a congenitally malformed calf, a weak, undersized calf, or a clinically normal calf. The most important determinant of the outcome is the age of the fetus when infection occurs, but other influences including host genotype and immune status, and the biological characteristics of the virus strain, may also be important.

Fetal age at infection is important principally because the immunological maturity of the fetus is of major significance in the pathogenesis of fetal disease. The ability to mount an immune response to BVDV develops from about 90 days of gestation, and nearly all fetuses are capable of antiBVDV antibody production by 125 days. Infection after this stage in fetal life normally results in the appearance of antibody, the elimination of the virus, and the birth of a clinically normal calf. Infections early in gestation lead to the development of a persistent virus infection in many tissues and organs and, if the fetus survives, the birth of a calf which remains infected with the virus for life. This state seems to result from an inability of the fetus to recognize viral antigens as 'nonself' and a consequent failure to mount an effective immune response. The liveborn calf is serologically negative to the virus, but viremic, and is an efficient transmitter of infection. It also has a high risk of developing mucosal disease. Experimentally, BVDV infections persisting to term have been established by inoculation of the bovine fetus from as early as 45 days and as late as 125 days of gestation.

Some infections result in fetal death and abortion. Diagnostic experience indicates that there are two forms of this sequel, with differing pathogeneses. In the first, an autolyzed fetus is expelled within 5–6 weeks of infection in early and midgestation; infectious virus is not detectable but antibody to BVDV is sometimes present and severe inflammatory pathology may be evident. Fetal mortality in these cases could result from the direct effects of viral replication in tissues, including the placenta, but it seems more likely that it is due to immune-mediated tissue damage.

The second form is distinctly different. It is characterized by the expulsion of a fresh fetus in late gestation, from which it is frequently possible to isolate virus. The pathological lesions and distribution of viral antigen are typical of persistent infections established in early gestation. Expulsion of the fetus may be a result of raised plasma corticosteroid levels in the fetus.

Congenital malformations reported in association with BVDV infection include degenerative cerebellar and cavitating cerebral lesions, cataracts and retinal dysplasia. These abnormalities occur in calves after maternal infection at between approximately 100 and 150 days of gestation and there is an association between their presence and the presence of precolostral antibody, and with the absence of infectious virus. Their pathogenesis may be mediated by the developing fetal immune system. Perinatal mortality is high among calves affected in this way; the degree of locomotor dysfunction varies widely, from complete inability to stand to mild ataxia, and from total blindness to minor visual defects, depending upon the extent of CNS damage.

Growth rates are often markedly depressed. The difficulties of obtaining milk for some individuals may make it essential to provide individual care to ensure survival.

Hypomyelinogenesis, clinically evident at birth as body tremor, appears not to be a common sequel to BVDV infection. Relatively sparse information indicates that it results from infection at before 100 days of gestation. Clinically, this condition usually resolves with time, but the calf is likely to be persistently infected and a source of infection for susceptible in-contact stock.

Persistently infected animals in general are a source of economic loss for the farmer for two reasons. First, mortality rates for these individuals over the first 2 years of life are of the order of 45%, most of the deaths resulting from mucosal disease. Second, many show very poor liveweight gains during this period, and may be markedly stunted by comparison with their normal unaffected peers.

Breeding Abnormalities and BVDV

Some calves persistently infected with BVDV survive to reach breeding age. About 1% of apparently normal cattle going for slaughter are persistently infected with the virus, many of which are well-grown and indistinguishable from unaffected stock. Persistently infected female cattle usually transmit infection to their fetuses, which in turn become persistently infected with the virus and have the potential to repeat the cycle. In this way families of animals which are lifelong carriers and excretors of the virus can appear within herds.

In normal cows and heifers, primary BVDV infection via the oral or intranasal routes does not appear to affect conception rates and is therefore not considered to be a major cause of repeat breeding. A significant reduction in conception rates has been observed experimentally, however, when virus was given by the intrauterine route to seronegative cattle. Infected semen may be derived either from a bull which is persistently infected, or from a bull undergoing acute infection, and can interfere with conception rates, and animals may fail to conceive until they have seroconverted. In one study, this resulted in an average of 2.3 services per conception. Most of the resulting progeny apparently escape infection with the virus, though a persistently infected calf has been observed on one occasion after artificial insemination with BVDV-infected semen experimentally.

The use of semen from persistently infected bulls is often militated against by their poor conformation and poor semen quality, but this may not apply in all cases. Bulls acting as donors at artificial insemination centers should therefore be carefully screened to ensure that they are not persistently infected with BVDV.

The male gametes do not appear to carry infection and provided that proper handling and washing techniques are used, and that the zona pellucida remains intact, the risks of spread of infection during embryo transfer procedures are considered to be minimal. The available evidence suggests that the virus is not taken up by preimplantation embryos, but the use of fetal calf serum in washing fluids must be avoided unless it has been shown to be free from contamination with BVDV. In addition, it is essential that recipient animals are screened for persistent BVDV infection, since the use of such individuals will inevitably result in the birth of persistently infected calves.

Diagnosis

A BVD problem in a herd is usually indicated by the occurrence of cases of mucosal disease, the birth of congenitally abnormal calves, or unexplained abortions. Investigation requires the assembly of as detailed a history as possible of the herd breeding record, clinical disease (including mortality), and illthrift in the previous 2 years. Birthdates of animals affected with mucosal disease usually cluster in time as a consequence of near-simultaneous infection of their dams at 45–125 days gestation. Events such as the introduction of new stock should be viewed as possible sources of infection.

Diagnosis of BVD and MD relies on laboratory tests including serum antibody estimations, virus isolation and virus antigen detection procedures. Persistently infected animals have a constant viremia and are usually detected by virus isolation from blood. Clotted or EDTA blood samples are suitable and the virus, which is non-cytopathic in cell cultures, is demonstrated by immunofluorescence or immunoperoxidase staining. Acute BVDV infections are normally revealed by antibody measurements on blood samples taken not less than 3 weeks apart. Diagnosis of MD is based on the clinical and postmortem picture and the demonstration of cytopathic BVDV in a range of tissues, especially alimentary tract lesions. Congenital abnormalities caused by BVDV are often identified only on clinical grounds, or as part of the general history of disease in the herd. Demonstration of specific antibody in a precolostral serum sample, when available, is useful supporting evidence for the occurrence of transplacental BVDV infection. It is often difficult to confirm that abortion is the result of BVDV infection. The antibody response in the dam is usually complete by the time abortion occurs and rising antibody titers are therefore an inconstant finding. Fresh fetuses expelled late in gestation may yield infectious virus from tissue samples, providing circumstantial evidence of BVDV involvement. Autolyzed fetuses aborted in midgestation are usually negative for virus, but it is sometimes possible to demonstrate antiviral antibody in fetal fluids. A diagnosis of BVDV-induced abortion is often made only after consideration of the full herd history.

Control of BVD

The main objective of schemes for the control of BVD within herds is the prevention of prenatal infections. To achieve this it is essential to ensure that persistently infected heifers and cows do not enter the breeding program; all new additions to the herd must therefore be screened for BVDV viremia and removed if positive.

It is highly desirable to boost levels of immunity in the adult herd and exposure of nonpregnant cows and heifers to contact with identified persistently infected individuals generally results in rapid seroconversion. Where vaccines are available, their use offers a much more controlled means by which to provide satisfactory immunity. Live BVDV vaccines should not be administered during pregnancy, since some vaccinal strains produce fetopathic effects; they must also be used with care in young animals because they may be immunosuppressive and in some cases are apparently capable of precipitating mucosal disease in persistently infected animals. Killed vaccines are thus inherently safer.

An alternative approach employed in some circumstances has been to test all animals over 6 months of age for persistent infection, and remove the positive individuals from the herd. This strategy incurs substantial costs in blood sampling and laboratory testing fees and results in a herd which is without immunity and vulnerable to large losses in the future. Maintaining this expensively attained infection-free status may be difficult and time-consuming in practice, and by comparison with a vaccination-based strategy represents a less satisfactory option.

Fibropapillomata of the Genitalia

Fibropapillomata (warts) are caused by a virus of the papilloma group. They occur sporadically on the penis in bulls and less frequently on the vulvovaginal epithelium of cows.

Transmission may be by direct contact with infected animals. Where direct genital contact does not occur, infection may be transmitted indirectly by the muzzle or lips during licking of the perineal area.

The genital tumors have a grayish-white surface. Older lesions may show a necrotic center. Unlike papillomata of the integument which show a cauliflower-like appearance with a rough, dry, horny, gray, hairless surface, those of the genitalia are smooth-surfaced and moist.

The lesion essentially consists of fibrous tissue covered with epithelium. Young lesions are cellular with numerous mitotic fibroblasts and little collagen, but as the age of the tumor increases, the interwoven bundles of collagen predominate with fewer mitotic figures. Secondary changes include mucoid degeneration, edema and necrosis. In exceptional cases tumors may show focal calcification. The epithelium covering the growth is relatively thick and consists of 10–50 cell layers with finger-like processes extending into the fibrous tissue.

Symptoms

In bulls with lesions on the penis the first sign of disease is often hemorrhage from the preputial cavity after service. In severe cases, a bull may refuse to serve, and occasionally a wart may be visible at the preputial orifice. However, in many cases, the penis must be extruded to disclose the warts on the epithelium of the preputial cavity.

In the vulvovaginal cavity, single or multiple warts up to a few centimeters in diameter occur in the epithelium. They are not normally visible externally, although occasionally one may protrude from the vulva after calving. Systemic disturbance is not characteristic of the disease.

Diagnosis

Clinical findings are normally sufficient for diagnosis. If necessary, biopsy and histological examination of the lesion will confirm the diagnosis.

Treatment and Control

Formalized tissue vaccines give a durable, but not absolute, immunity. Some immunized animals respond to reinfection by producing small lesions which persist only a short time.

Vaccination can also be used therapeutically. Results are variable but the use of vaccine can cause rapid regression of warts. The results of other methods of treatment are also variable. Topical application of a solution of podophyllin has been used successfully. Lithium antimony thiomalate repeatedly injected intramuscularly causes rapid regression in many cases. Iodine, formalin, arsenic and bismuth have all been used locally with varying results. In the case of larger growths, surgical removal is indicated.

Other Viral Infections of Cattle

A number of viruses are known to be capable of crossing the placenta to infect the bovine fetus, but in many cases their causative role in infertility and reproductive loss is uncertain. For some, including enzootic bovine leukosis and bovine syncytial viruses, there is general agreement that they do not cause significant fetal pathology. In other cases insufficient information is yet available to establish their importance. Little is known about fetal infections with bovine respiratory syncytial virus, polyoma virus or bovine rotavirus beyond the fact that antibodies have sometimes been found in fetal fluids or sera. Their association with abortion is unproven. There is evidence which suggests that parainfluenza type 3 virus, bovine adenoviruses and bovine parvovirus may be involved in bovine reproductive losses. These agents are very common in the cattle population and are more often associated with symptoms other than abortion and infertility; this makes it more difficult to establish cause–effect relationships satisfactorily. Three viruses require special comment.

Bovine Enterovirus

A single serotype of bovine enterovirus (F266a) has been associated in the past with catarrhal vaginocervicitis accompanied by infertility, with irregular estrous cycles and lowered conception rates. Abortions also occurred in affected herds, but there is no evidence from experimental studies that enteroviruses cause abortion. The disease is afebrile and characterized by a postcoital vaginal discharge and congestion of the mucosa of vagina and cervix. A yellow gelatinous exudate may be present. The disease lasts for several days, or occasionally for some weeks, but normally few animals are affected and recovery is rapid. Diagnosis depends upon demonstration of rising antibody titers. The success rate for virus isolation is low. No specific treatment or prophylaxis is available.

Two enterovirus serotypes have also been occasionally associated with orchitis and vesiculitis, in naturally diseased bulls. The virus appears to arrest spermatogenesis and adversely affects mature spermatozoa, and infection is accompanied by marked fall in semen quality. Motility may be severely depressed, and sperm concentration can fall to 25% of normal values. Recovery is spontaneous and complete by about 3 months postinfection. There is no specific treatment or vaccine.

Parainfluenza Virus Type 3

Parainfluenza type 3 (PI3) virus is an RNA virus in the Paramyxovirus group and is an important respiratory pathogen in calves and possibly sheep. From time to time it is isolated from aborted bovine fetuses, whilst a number of surveys have found antibodies to the virus in both normal and aborted fetuses with prevalence rates varying from 0 to 18%. The virus has also been isolated from the testis of an infertile bull.

Experimentally, when inoculated directly into midgestational bovine or ovine fetuses, PI3 virus was fetopathic, producing bronchiolitis and interstitial pneumonia, followed by either abortion or growth retardation. A fetal antibody response was demonstrable from the 20th day after inoculation. There was no evidence of transplacental infection following the inoculation of seropositive pregnant heifers or ewes. There are no reports of experimental studies in seronegative dams. As a high proportion of adult animals are seropositive it is generally considered that, although a potential fetopathogen, PI3 virus is not a major cause of reproductive loss.

Bovine Herpesvirus Type 4

Bovine herpesvirus type 4 (BHV4), also known as bovine cytomegalovirus, is a slow-growing virus which has been isolated from cattle with a variety of disease syndromes, including metritis, vulvovaginitis, orchitis, respiratory disease and lymphosarcoma, as well as from healthy cattle. It is uncertain whether it plays any significant role in the pathogenesis of these conditions. Specific diagnosis is difficult and the virus has usually been isolated incidentally in the course of routine virological investigations. Cattle do not develop neutralizing antibodies but indirect immunofluorescence or ELISA techniques can be used for serology. No specific control measures are possible.

In addition to the above, several viruses have been isolated from aborted fetuses or named as occasional causes of abortion. In areas where these agents are widely distributed their possible involvement in reproductive failure must be considered. They include bluetongue virus, akabane virus, Rift Valley fever virus, Wesselsbron disease virus, foot-

and-mouth disease virus, rinderpest virus, and the virus of malignant catarrhal fever.

SHEEP

Border Disease

Border disease (BD) or 'B' disease was first described as a distinct clinical entity in lambs born in the area along the border between England and Wales. It is a congenital viral infection of sheep and goats characterized by embryonic and fetal death, which may result in abortion, mummification or stillbirth, and by the birth of small lambs of low viability with nervous symptoms and abnormally hairy pigmented birth coats. The disease has been reported in many European countries and from Australasia, North America and the Near East.

BD is caused by a pestivirus which is closely related to the virus of bovine virus diarrhea (BVD) of cattle, and more distantly to that of classical swine fever (hog cholera). Significant antigenic differences may exist between BD and BVD viruses but experimentally BD virus in cattle causes abortion and fetal pathology resembling that produced by BVD virus, and BVD virus can cause BD in sheep. Fetal infection occurs following BD replication in the placentome of a susceptible ewe and, as in BVD, the outcome depends principally on the developmental age of the fetus when infection occurs. Virus strain variation and host genotype are less important influences.

Persistent virus infection, myelin dysgenesis, hairy birth coat and growth retardation are associated with infection of the fetus at earlier than 60 days of gestation. Classically affected newborn lambs show a marked tremor, which may be severe enough to interfere with suckling, and a hairy, rough fleece, often with patches of pigment. They are small, with short legs and domed heads, and rarely there may be congenital articular rigidity. After fetal infection at between 61 and 78 days, when the fetal immune response is at an early stage of development, the sequelae observed are hydranencephaly and cerebellar dysplasia. The newborn lamb lacks the stigmata of classical BD; it has eliminated the virus and usually possesses precolostral antibody. Clinically, the lamb with cerebral cavitation may show nervous signs such as head tilt and circling.

From approximately 80 days of gestation, the ovine fetus is able to mount an effective immune response, resulting in the elimination of infection and the production of antibody before birth. Pathological changes are minimal and most of these lambs appear normal at birth.

Adult sheep which become infected with BD virus show only a mild transient malaise but the fetus may be fatally damaged. Embryonic and fetal death account for about 30% of losses due to BD virus infection. It is likely that the most important routes of transmission in natural cases are via oral and nasal secretions. Persistently infected ewes transmit the virus to the fetus in successive pregnancies. Transmission by infected semen may also occur. In some countries outbreaks of disease have followed the use of live vaccines contaminated with BD or BVD virus. Interspecies spread occurs easily and infected cattle can be a source of infection for sheep, and vice versa. Persistently viremic lambs shed virus in all body excretions and secretions. Placentas are a source of infection following abortion.

Diagnosis

A clinical diagnosis can be made on a flock basis when there is a history of stillbirth, abortion and the birth of weak, hairy lambs with nervous signs. However, the variable pattern of natural disease makes clinical diagnosis of individual cases difficult. Diagnosis may be established by the demonstration of central nervous system hypomyelinogenesis and isolation of virus in cell culture. Virus is readily isolated from excretions, secretions and various organs of persistently viremic lambs. Virus is detected by immunofluorescence or immunoperoxidase staining of infected cell cultures.

Seroconversion of BD susceptible sheep occurs following natural infection, and is detected using a serum neutralization test.

Treatment and Control

No entirely effective or safe vaccine is yet available for the prevention of disease. Preventive measures include purchase of replacement stock from flocks with a history of freedom from clinical disease. Ewes of uncertain origin should be mixed with the existing flock at least 6 weeks before mating. Following disease outbreaks lambs should be reared only for slaughter and ewes producing affected progeny in more than one season should be culled.

Contagious Pustular Dermatitis

A venereal form of this disease has been recognized in England since 1903, and has been reported from continental Europe and North America. The disease manifests itself as ulcers on the vulva of the ewe, and the preputial orifice and occasionally the penis of the ram. It appears soon after the rams are turned out and spreads rapidly within the flock. In the ewe the early lesion is a small pustule, often at the junction of the vulval skin and vaginal mucosa. Later it spreads to form a shallow ulcer which may become infected with secondary bacteria. The ram quickly becomes reluctant to give service and the sequel may be a prolonged lambing period.

Diagnosis may be made on clinical grounds alone, but confirmation whenever necessary is best made by examination of moist active scab material by direct electron microscopy. Treatment is largely confined to control of secondary bacterial infections using emollient preparations containing broad spectrum antibiotics. Use of live vaccines to control disease in the face of an outbreak is not recommended. Measures to minimize the effects of the disease by segregation of affected and in-contact sheep are to be preferred. This form of CPD does not tend to recur in subsequent years in traditional flocks.

Other Virus Diseases

As in cattle, several virus diseases of sheep have been associated with abortion and other forms of reproductive loss. In areas of the world where the agents are prevalent, Rift Valley fever, Nairobi sheep disease, rinderpest and Wesselsbron disease should be considered as possible causes of abortion.

HORSES

Equine Viral Arteritis

Equine arteritis virus has been classified as the only member of the genus *Arterivirus* in the family of nonarthropod-borne togaviruses. This family also includes bovine virus diarrhea virus and swine fever virus. However, this classification may only be temporary.

Clinical Signs and Epidemiology

The disease probably existed long before the first report of virus isolation from fetuses during an outbreak in standardbred horses in the United States in 1957. Since then outbreaks have been described in other parts of America and in Europe. Antibodies to the virus have been found in horses from most countries where studies have been carried out. From serological evidence the virus in the United States appears to be endemic in the standardbred breed but rare in thoroughbreds, although an outbreak in

thoroughbreds occurred in 1984 in Kentucky, United States. In Europe, thoroughbreds and riding horses have been affected by the disease and there is serological evidence of infection in standardbreds. The disease has so far not been recognized in Britain, though a survey of a selected population of horses in the United Kingdom showed a low prevalence of antibodies.

The incubation period is about 7 days. A range of clinical signs can be observed in infected horses, although some fail to show these signs and the disease may go unnoticed. Typically there is a fever, edema of legs and dependent parts of the body and under the jaw, discharges from eyes and nose, cough, inflammation of the conjunctival and mucous membranes, periorbital edema, depression, loss of appetite and a skin rash most commonly on the neck. Death is not usual in natural disease outbreaks but is more common after experimental infections with some strains of the virus.

In animals that die, postmortem examination may reveal edema and congestion of lymph nodes and viscera of the peritoneal and pleural cavities. There may be parenchymal degeneration of the liver, kidney and heart muscle, pneumonia and inflammation of the intestinal tract. Microscopically there is a generalized vasculitis.

Abortion has been seen in some outbreaks but not all. The percentage of aborted or stillborn foals can be as high as 80%.

Experimental infections of pregnant mares resulted in abortions and lesions were present in the uterus of the mare. Abortions or fetal deaths occurred within 7–10 days of infection. Mares sometimes showed no clinical signs of infection themselves. In some cases there were no lesions attributable to the virus in the fetus or placenta, though virus was isolated from both sites. Lesions in the fetuses included edema of the inguinal, pectoral, mediastinal and sublumbar tissue, excess peritoneal fluid and slight edema of the lungs. Hemorrhages were seen in the conjunctiva and mucous membranes of the respiratory and digestive tracts. Lesions were much less severe and less characteristic than the changes that accompany fetal infection with equine herpesvirus. It has been concluded that abortion occurs primarily as a result of damage to the uterus of the mare rather than as a consequence of infection of the fetus.

Virus can be isolated from infected horses from nasopharynx, blood, urine and semen for 1–2 weeks and is then eliminated in most cases. In experimental infections virus persisted in the kidneys for up to 19 days and was isolated from the urine 16 days after infection. In some cases virus persists in the urogenital tract; virus has been found in the urine of one mare 5 months after infection, and currently available evidence suggests that the duration of the carrier state in the stallion can vary from several months or weeks to a period of years during which time virus can be demonstrated in the semen. During the 1984 outbreak in Kentucky there was evidence that mares bred to infected stallions were infected via the genital tract. However the most common route of transmission is probably the respiratory tract. The role of the virus in early fetal death has yet to be clarified.

Diagnosis

The isolation of the virus and the demonstration of rising serum antibody titers are useful in the diagnosis of active infection. The virus can be isolated in a variety of cells of equine, rabbit and monkey origin. The serological test probably most commonly used is a virus neutralization test with added complement, but other tests have also been described. It is thought that serum antibody titers can last for several years after initial infection, and titers have been found in horses known to be persistently infected.

Control

Control is effected by the detection and isolation of infected animals. A vaccine has been used in the United States.

Equine Herpesvirus Type 1 (EHV1)

Clinical Signs and Epidemiology

EHV1 infection can cause abortions. Infection with the virus is common in horses worldwide and horses in the United Kingdom often experience infection in the first year of life. Abortion may occur in only one or two mares in a herd but can occur in 50% or more. The route of infection is probably via the respiratory tract, followed by virus spread via the blood across the placenta to infect the fetus, resulting in abortion. Pregnant mares may abort 14–20 days after exposure without necessarily showing clinical signs of disease. Most mares abort at 6–11 months of gestation. Fetuses aborted before the 6th month of gestation are usually decomposed but fetuses after 7 months of age are expelled fresh. Infected foals may be born live but die soon after

birth. Changes seen postmortem are jaundice, hemorrhages on mucosal surfaces, excess pleural fluid, pulmonary edema, enlargement of the spleen (splenomegaly) and necrosis of the liver. In all cases where lesions occur typical intranuclear inclusions are seen when tissue sections are examined microscopically.

There are two subtypes of the virus: subtype 1, which is most commonly associated with abortion, but also with respiratory disease in the United Kingdom; and subtype 2 which is primarily a respiratory pathogen but is sometimes associated with abortion. Subtype 2 has been considered by some workers to vary sufficiently from subtype 1 to be classified as a different type, EHV4. Monoclonal antibodies and restriction endonuclease DNA fingerprinting have been used successfully to classify strains.

It has been shown that virus persists in some animals for years and can be reactivated by subjecting the animals to such stresses as weaning, castrating and moving. These carrier animals act as continuing sources of virus within the horse population.

Diagnosis

Abortion due to EHV1 can be diagnosed on the basis of histopathology of the fetus and by rising antibody titers detected by complement fixation, virus neutralization and ELISA tests. Serum neutralizing titers persist and are widespread in the horse population, but complement fixing titers last for a shorter time and are more use as an indication of recent infection. Rising titers do not invariably occur following recrudescence of a latent infection. Tissue cultures of equine origin have been used successfully for virus isolation and cells of calf, lamb, guinea-pig and rabbit are also susceptible.

Control

Immunity to reinfection is shortlived, which is probably the main reason why, although live and killed virus vaccines have been produced, these have often been of doubtful efficacy. Safety has also been a problem especially with certain live vaccine strains which have caused abortion.

It is recommended that animals should not be introduced from an outside source into a group of pregnant mares because of the risk of introducing the virus. Stress should be avoided in order to minimize the probability of recrudescence of virus in carrier animals.

Equine Infectious Anemia

Clinical Signs and Epidemiology

Equine infectious anemia has been recognized as a disease in horses for more than a century but the virus has only recently been classified as a retrovirus. In common with other retroviruses it produces persistent infections where antibody and virus coexist in the blood throughout the life of the host. Clinical symptoms in the horse may be absent or may occur in sequential episodes separated by several weeks or months. Transmission is by biting flies and by any procedure that results in the transfer of blood from an infected to a susceptible horse, for example by use of a hypodermic needle.

The disease is especially common in some parts of the world (such as Central America) but exists in many countries. The United Kingdom is free of the disease.

Fetal infections can occur in pregnant mares infected with the virus. Placental transfer is most likely to occur if the mare shows clinical signs during pregnancy; carrier mares that remain healthy infect their foals less commonly. Abortion has been described in association with a fetal infection, but whether abortion was due to infection is not known. Infected foals may show clinical signs after birth and may die.

Diagnosis

In 1970 Coggins and Norcross reported on the use of an agar gel immunodiffusion test which has since formed the basis of many testing and control programs. Since then other serological tests such as complement fixation, serum neutralization, hemagglutination inhibition, ELISA, radioimmunoassay and indirect immunofluorescence have been used successfully to detect antibodies.

Control

The disease can probably be eradicated by removal of serological reactors. It is rare to find a horse that is infected while being consistently serologically negative.

Venezuelan Equine Encephalitis

Infection of pregnant mares with epizootic strains of Venezuelan equine encephalitis can result in abortion. This virus does not exist in the United Kingdom.

Parvovirus

A parvovirus was isolated from aborted equine fetuses in Canada during an outbreak of abortion in mares on a single farm. Further evidence is needed to clarify the role of this virus in abortion.

PIGS

Many viruses have been associated with reproductive disorders in pigs, but pragmatically it is useful to consider them in two broad categories: those in the so-called 'SMEDI' group (such as porcine parvovirus) which are very widespread and common in the majority of pig herds; and those (like swine fever virus and Aujeszky's disease virus) which are becoming increasingly rare in developed countries where control schemes are in operation.

'SMEDI' Viruses, Swine Fever Virus and Aujeszky's Disease

Over the past two decades the acronym 'SMEDI' (derived from stillbirth, mummification, embryonic death, infertility) has been widely used to denote a common disease syndrome originally thought to be caused by transplacental infection with enteroviruses. It has now become clear that the syndrome is almost invariably the result of porcine parvovirus (PPV) infection. Epidemiologically the different viruses in the SMEDI group seem to behave similarly: they are contagious and spread rather easily by direct or indirect contact to susceptible (nonimmune) pigs. They may also be transmitted via semen. They rarely, if ever, cause any illness in adult or even in young pigs, immediately after birth, and their significance depends on the fact that if gilts or sows are infected when pregnant their embryos are liable to be damaged or killed by transplacental infection. Once infected, sows usually develop lifelong immunity.

Probably because it is a pantropic virus which infects lymphoid as well as many other tissues, antibody titers following PPV infection can be very high. Colostral titers in pigs born to seropositive sows are often high too, and consequently such pigs may take up to 6–9 months before they will pick up wild virus infection naturally and develop an active immunity. Even in herds where PPV infection is endemic, therefore, the prolonged life of colostral antibody can mean that breeding females run the risk of viral infection during pregnancy and are thus liable to experience reproductive failure. With the enteroviruses, although the reproductive failure manifestations are similar to those of PPV, once these viruses become endemic in a herd they seldom cause trouble because colostral immunity is comparatively shortlived. This means that young breeding stock have ample opportunity to be infected before they are mated. There are, however, several different serotypes of porcine enterovirus, so in theory problems could arise whenever a new one with a potential for crossing the placenta gets into the herd.

Reproductive Manifestations

Manifestations of the milder, SMEDI-type of virus infections in affected herds include returns to service, often at irregular intervals, small litters, mummified fetuses and, if the whole litter dies in utero, failures to farrow.

Abortion, however, is rarely if ever a feature with this virus group, although it is common with the more virulent virus diseases such as swine fever, African swine fever, Aujeszky disease and foot-and-mouth disease. The reason for this difference is that the latter diseases commonly cause systemic effects in the mother of sufficient severity to disturb or terminate the hormonal control mechanisms of pregnancy. Transplacental infection leading either to fetal disease or death, with production of mummified fetuses, stillbirths, and weak or deformed piglets which die in the early postnatal period, may also be a feature in those sows which do not abort. Certain attenuated vaccinal strains, and some mild field strains, of swine fever virus cause mainly prenatal disease, deformity and death rather than maternal failure. In addition there are a number of other viruses which have on occasion been associated with reproductive disorders, especially fetal death with mummification, and production of congenitally diseased piglets. These include Japanese encephalitis (this occurs throughout much of the Far East and is transmitted by mosquitoes), porcine cytomegalovirus, encephalomyocarditis (EMC) virus (normally carried by and associated with disease of rats and mice), infectious bovine rhinotracheitis (IBR) virus and swinepox virus.

The outcome of virus infections during pregnancy in sows depends on the stage of gestation, the virulence of the virus involved and the immune status of the host. As inferred above, infection of fully susceptible pregnant sows with virulent strains of swine fever virus frequently leads to severe clinical illness with abortion. Infection of inadequately immunized pregnant animals with virulent or attenuated swine fever virus, on the other hand, often results in mummified fetuses, stillbirths and neonatal deaths. The latter syndrome is, therefore, similar to that caused by other viruses which cause little or no ab-

normality in maternal health (for example, the SMEDI group), so there may be no clinical indication of the presence of swine fever infection in the adult herd other than the reproductive manifestations.

Symptoms

In affected individual sows, depending on the type of virus, reproductive symptoms may or may not be preceded by systemic disturbances, and these may only be slight when they do occur. The proportion of sows affected varies depending on the proportion of susceptible sows present at the time. Japanese encephalitis virus infections have affected 70% of litters in some outbreaks; mainly those farrowed in late summer. There may be a total loss of all piglets farrowed, or alternatively litters may contain combinations of mummified fetuses, stillbirths, neonatal deaths, weak piglets born alive and normal healthy piglets. Some of the surviving piglets may have chronic symptoms such as trembling. Experimental inoculation of pregnant sows with attenuated, lapinized swine fever virus affected up to 40% of the piglets. With other strains of swine fever virus, and with the congenital tremor agent, almost 100% may be affected. The relatively high proportion of piglets affected by viruses helps to differentiate viral disorders from most hereditary congenital disorders where the proportion of piglets affected is usually much lower, often 25%.

Fetal Pathology

Calcification of the fetal skeleton begins at about 35 days of gestation, and before this time and if fetal death occurs, there may be complete resorption of all the fetuses but the sow may or may not return to estrus. If she does not return she becomes what is colloquially known as 'pseudopregnant'. Death of only some fetuses leads to reduced litter size. Fetuses which die later in pregnancy tend to undergo incomplete resorption with the result that mummified fetuses may be expelled along with live piglets at term or, if all have died, they may be retained for a prolonged period so that at full term farrowing does not occur.

After about the 70th day of gestation the fetal immune system may resist virus infection and sometimes enables the virus to be thrown off successfully, with recovery. Specific virus antibody may then be detected in the blood and other body fluids of such fetuses, and this provides valuable diagnostic evidence.

The gross appearance of fetuses with many types

of prenatal virus infections are similar: they present themselves as small, dying, or dead fetuses in various stages of mummification. Mummified fetuses vary from small, brown or black objects of 1 cm or less which are tightly enveloped in the dried membranes, to gray-brown, more or less dehydrated, but well-formed fetuses. The size of mummified fetuses in a single litter may vary greatly because death can occur at different stages. Spread from fetus to fetus is often a feature of in utero virus infections, and this can help to distinguish them from other transplacental agents (for example, toxins) which tend to strike all members of the litter simultaneously. Stillborn piglets are those which are fully developed but born dead at full term, indicating uterine death just before or during parturition.

Ascites and subcutaneous edema are commonly reported in association with all types of prenatal virus infection, and edema of the mesentery, mesocolon, and perirenal tissues may be noticed in fresh cases. When autolysis and hemolysis have proceeded further, excessive reddish fluids are frequently found in the pleural and peritoneal cavities. The thoracic and mesenteric lymph nodes are sometimes severely congested, and petechiae may occur on serous membranes. In some fetal virus infections additional lesions may be seen; for example, with Aujeszky's disease, necrotic foci may be seen in the livers and spleens. Deformed heads, brains and noses have been observed following infections with attenuated, lapinized swine fever virus, and congenital hydrocephalus has been reported with Japanese encephalitis virus. Occasionally malformed kidneys, lungs, eyes or limbs occur, notably with swine fever. Myocardial lesions may be seen in fetuses dying with encephalomyocarditis, and skin lesions in those with congenital swinepox.

In piglets with congenital trembling caused by swine fever infection (CT type AI) cerebellar hypoplasia is a fairly constant finding, usually in association with hypomyelinogenesis throughout the central nervous system. Another, as yet unidentified agent, probably a virus, causes congenital tremor of a less severe type (CT type AII) without cerebellar hypoplasia but usually with hypomyelinogenesis. Two other forms of congenital tremor (CT types AIII and IV) in pigs are caused by recessive genes (CIAIII is a sex-linked recessive), and another form (CT type AV) is caused by trichlorphon, an organophosphorus compound used to treat parasitic conditions such as mange.

Histological lesions characteristic of a viral encephalitis are sometimes present in fetuses affected by viruses such as swine fever and parvovirus, and such lesions are usually diffusely distributed throughout the brain. Vessels may show perivascular cuffing with round cells and, occasionally, focal gliosis can be observed in the gray and white matter.

Virus Transmission

Epidemiologically, most viruses involved in porcine reproductive disorders are transmitted by direct contact with other pigs. Japanese encephalitis virus which is transmitted by mosquitoes is a notable exception. Other types of infection spread through contact with a contaminated environment or indirectly via personnel, infected food or vermin. Infection may also be transmitted in semen. PPV is a particularly resistant virus and can persist for several weeks in empty pig accommodation if the conditions are right.

Although often asymptomatic, enteroviruses and PPV are widespread in pig populations, and are present sporadically if not continuously in most herds. Symptomless carriers of Aujeszky virus are also common. It is possible that congenital virus infections, by reducing viability, may contribute or predispose to some of the high levels of piglet mortality, the immediate cause of which is overlaying at birth; they may also contribute to mortality in the early weeks of life. It is, however, unlikely that infection commonly spreads from infected stillbirths to the healthy piglets because of colostral protection of the latter. Such protection will not, of course, occur if the interval between exposure to infection and parturition is insufficient to allow antibody production by the mother.

Diagnosis

Herd records provide the essential foundation for early detection of reproductive failure and may reveal distinctive patterns attributable to virus infection. A tentative diagnosis can often be made on clinical grounds too. For example, the history of the herd may indicate the presence of swine fever in young, nonpregnant pigs, and there may be tremblers and neonatal deaths in litters. Usually, however, a firm diagnosis can only be established by laboratory tests.

In the case of the common endemic porcine viruses such as PPV and enteroviruses of the SMEDI group, the results of such laboratory tests must be interpreted with great care. Demonstration of virus in fetuses or piglets, and positive precolostral fetal sera are usually valid indicators of infection but antibody titers in sows may often be meaningless because, unless the herd status has been regularly monitored, recent infections cannot easily be distinguished from those which occurred months or years ago. Because the principal manifestation is mummification (as distinct from abortion), by the time this is observed, weeks may have elapsed since the sow became infected; it will then be futile to look for rising titers.

Less common diseases like swine fever, Aujeszky's disease, encephalomyocarditis and Japanese encephalitis virus can be identified by virus isolation and specific serological tests; gross pathology (for example, the cerebellum:brain weight ratio), histopathology and fluorescent antibody tests are also applicable in some cases.

Treatment and Control

Although no treatment of individual animals is possible with any of these viral diseases, steps can sometimes be taken at the herd level to curtail the effects of an outbreak on reproductive performance. With enterovirus and PPV infections, disease may not be recognized clinically until the fetopathic effects have been produced and the virus has spread to all susceptible animals. By this time the scope for ameliorative measures is naturally very limited. It is only possible to facilitate the development of immunity amongst nonpregnant and prepubertal animals, either by direct contact with the infected sows or by deliberately feeding them with mummified fetuses, placentas, etc. All pregnant animals, on the other hand, should be isolated until after parturition, and only then exposed to infection. Such improvised 'vaccination' produces an adequate resistance in many cases because this type of infection tends to become established and persist, especially in large herds. The recent advent of injectable killed and live virus vaccines for porcine parvovirus is providing more precise methods of control, although prolonged persistence of colostral antibody and low antigenicity of some commercial killed vaccines does mean that vaccination may have to be repeated prior to each successive pregnancy to give prolonged protection.

Ideally, home-reared gilts and purchased nonpregnant females should be managed so that they encounter natural infection and develop immunity to the viral flora of the herd before mating. Pregnant animals, on the other hand, should not be brought in.

In so-called minimal-disease herds attempts have been made to overcome infectious disease problems by initially stocking with pigs delivered by hysterectomy. However, even if this is successful at first, the difficulties associated with subsequent introduction of new genetic lines remain. Purchased boars, for example, could be infected, and introduction of further hysterectomy-delivered piglets might bring in viruses. The use of artificial insemination should provide an answer, though it must be remembered that some viruses can be carried in semen. Proper management of stud boars in AI centers will overcome this risk. Embryo transfer is one method whereby the whole genetic complement can be imported with negligible disease risk.

In countries where severe epidemic diseases like swine fever still exist, control of their effects on reproduction can be obtained only by control of the diseases as a whole. This depends on local conditions. With swine fever, where there is no eradication program, a suitable killed virus vaccine, such as killed crystal violet vaccine, presents no direct reproductive problems, but is unsatisfactory in that in later pregnancies it can result in hemolytic disease of the newborn. Live attenuated vaccines are now available which are safe and effective.

The control of Japanese encephalitis depends principally on the use of vaccines because mosquito control is rarely practicable. This virus, however, is only a problem in the Far East. So far encephalomyocarditis in pigs seems to have occurred only in Australia, and its prevention entails the control of rats and mice.

Where Aujeszky's disease occurs sporadically, an outbreak is often followed by normal reproductive performance, and once the disease has become endemic in a herd no special management is required. Some aid might be given during the acute phase of an outbreak by the use of hyperimmune serum or immunoglobulin in pregnant sows, which confers protection for 1 or 2 weeks. Vaccination is widely used in some countries but no product is yet available which is entirely satisfactory from the point of view of preventing circulation of field strains.

Complementary References

Allen, G. P. & Bryans, I. T. (1986) Molecular epizootiology, pathogenesis, and prophylaxis of equine herpesvirus-1 infections. *Prog. Vet. Microbiol. Immunol.*, **2**, 78–144.

Barlow, R. M. (1983) Some interactions of virus and maternal/foetal immune mechanisms in Border Disease of sheep. *Prog. Brain Res.*, **59**, 255–268.

Barlow, R. M. & Patterson, D. S. P. (1982) Border disease of sheep: a virus induced teratogenic disorder. *Fortschr. Vet. med.*, **36**.

Bolin, C. A., Bolin, S. R., Kluge, J. P. & Mengeling, W. L. (1985) Pathologic effects of intrauterine deposition of pseudorabies virus on the reproductive tract of swine in early pregnancy. *Amer. J. Vet. Res.*, **46**, 1039–1042.

Bowen, R. A., Elsden, R. P. & Seidel, G. E. (1985) Infection of early bovine embryos with bovine herpesvirus-1. *Amer. J. Vet. Res.*, **46**, 1095.

Brownlie, J., Clarke, M. C. & Howard, C. J. (1984) *Vet. Rec.*, **114**, 535.

Castrucci, G., Frigeri, F., Cilli, V., Donelli, G., Ferrari, M., Chicchini, U. & Bordoni, E. (1986) A study of a herpesvirus isolated from dairy cattle with a history of reproductive disorders. *Comp. Immun. Microbiol. Infect. Dis.*, **9**, 13–21.

Coggins, L. & Norcross, N. L. (1970) Immunodiffusion reaction in equine infectious anaemia. *Cornell Vet.*, **60**, 330–335.

Coignoul, E. L. & Cheville, N. F. (1984) Pathology of maternal genital tract, placenta, and fetus in equine viral arteritis. *Vet. Pathol.*, **21**, 333–340.

Dennett, D. P., Barasa, J. O. & Johnson, R. H. (1976) Infectious bovine rhinotracheitis virus: studies on the veneral carrier status in range cattle. *Res. Vet. Sci.*, **20**, 77.

Doll, E. R., Bryans, J. T., McCollum, W. H. & Crower, M. E. W. (1957) Isolation of a filterable agent causing arteritis of horses and abortion by mares. Its differentiation from the equine abortion (influenza) virus. *Cornell Vet.*, **47**, 3–41.

Dunne, H. W., Wang, J. T. & Huang, C. M. (1974) Early in utero infection of porcine embryos and fetuses with SMEDI (entero-) viruses: mortality, antibody development, and viral persistence. *Amer. J. Vet. Res.*, **35**, 1479–1481.

Edington, M., Watt, R. G., Plowright, W., Wrathall, A. E. & Done, J. T. (1977) Experimental transplacental transmission of porcine cytomegalovirus. *J. Hyg. Cambridge*, **78**, 243–251.

Gibb, E. P. J. & Rweyemamu, M. M. (1977) Bovine herpesviruses. Part I. Bovine herpesvirus 1. *Vet. Bull.*, **47**, 317.

Harkness, J. W., Wood, L. & Drew, T. (1984) Mucosal disease in cattle. *Vet. Rec.*, **115**, 283.

Huang, J., Gentry, R. F. & Zarkower, A. (1980) Experimental infection of pregnant sows with porcine enteroviruses. *Amer. J. Vet. Res.*, **41**, 469–473.

Joo, H. S., Donaldson-Wood, C. R., Johnson, R. H. & Campbell, R. S. F. (1977) Pathogenesis of porcine parvovirus infection: pathology and immunofluorescence in the foetus. *J. Comp. Pathol.*, **87**, 383–391.

Joo, H. S., Dee, S. A., Molitor, T. W. & Thacker, B. J. (1984) In utero infection of swine fetuses with infectious bovine rhinotracheitis virus (bovine herpesvirus-1). *Amer. J. Vet. Res.*, **45**, 1924–1927.

Kirkbride, C. A. & McAdaragh, J. P. (1978) Infectious agents associated with fetal and early neonatal death and abortion in swine. *J. Amer. Vet. Med. Assoc.*, **172**, 480–483.

Kluge, J. P. & Mare, C. J. (1974) Swine pseudorabies: abortion, clinical disease, and lesions in pregnant gilts infected with pseudorabies virus (Aujeszky's disease). *Amer. J. Vet. Res.*, **35**, 911–915.

Liess, B., Frey, H.-R., Orban, S. & Hafez, S. M. (1983) *Deut. Tierarzl. Wochenschr.*, **90**. 261.

Liess, B., Orban, S., Frey, H.-R., Trautwein, G., Wiefel, W. & Blindow, H. (1984) *Zentralbl. Vet. med. B*, **31**, 669.

Links, I. J., Whittington, R. J., Kennedy, D. J., Grewal, A. & Sharrock, A. J. (1986) An association between encephalomyocarditis virus infection and reproductive failure in pigs. *Aust. Vet. J.*, **63**, 150–152.

McClurkin, A. W., Coria, M. F. & Cutlip, R. C. (1979) *J. Amer. Vet. Med. Assoc.*, **174**, 1116.

McClurkin, A. W., Littledike, E. T., Cutlip, R. C., Frank, G. H., Coria, M. F. & Bolin, S. R. (1984) *Can. J. Comp. Med.*, **48**, 156.

McCollum, W. H., Prickett, M. E. & Bryans, J. T. (1971) Temporal distribution of equine arteritis virus in respiratory mucosa, tissues and body fluids of horses infected by inhalation. *Res. Vet. Sci.*, **12**, 459–464.

Mengeling, W. L. & Paul, P. S. (1986) Interepizootic survival of porcine parvovirus. *J. Amer. Vet. Med. Assoc.*, **188**, 1293–1295.

Miller, J. M. & Van der Maaten, M. J. (1984) Reproductive tract lesions in heifers after intrauterine inoculation with infectious bovine rhinotracheitis virus. *Amer. J. Vet. Res.*, **45**, 790.

Mumford, J. A. & Bates, J. (1984) Trials of an inactivated equine herpesvirus 1 vaccine: challenge with a subtype 2 virus. *Vet. Rec.*, **114**, 375–381.

Neufeld, J. L. (1981) Spontaneous pustular dermatitis in a newborn piglet associated with a poxvirus. *Can. Vet. J.*, **22**, 156–158.

Parsons, T. D., Smith, G. & Calligan, D. T. (1986) Economics of porcine parvovirus vaccination assessed by decision analysis. *Prevent. Vet. Med.*, **4**, 199–204.

Parsonson, I. M. & Snowdon, W. A. (1975) The effect of natural and artificial breeding using bulls infected with, or semen contaminated with, infectious bovine rhinotracheitis virus. *Aust. Vet. J.*, **51**, 365.

Paul, P. S. & Mengeling, W. L. (1986) Vaccination of swine with an inactivated porcine parvovirus vaccine in the presence of passive immunity. *J. Amer. Vet. Med. Assoc.*, **188**, 410–413.

Pensaert, M. & De Meurichy, W. (1973) A porcine enterovirus causing fetal death and mummification. II. Experimental infection of pregnant sows. *Zentralbl. Vet. Med. B*, **20** 760–772.

Peter, C. P., Tyler, D. E. & Ramsey, F. K. (1967) Characteristics of a condition following vaccination with bovine virus diarrhea vaccine. *J. Amer. Vet. Med. Assoc.*, **150**, 46.

Pointon, A. M., Surman, P. G., McCloud, P. I. & Whyte, P. B. D. (1983) The pattern of endemic parvovirus infection in four pig herds. *Aust. Vet. J.*, **60**.

Prozesky, L., Thomson, G. R., Gainaru, M. D., Herr, S. & Kritzinger, L. J. (1980) Lesions resulting from inoculation of porcine foetuses with parvovirus. *Onderspoort J. Vet. Res.*, **47**, 269–274.

Roeder, P. L. & Drew, T. W. (1984) Mucosal disease of cattle: a late sequel to fetal infection. *Vet. Rec.*, **114**, 309.

Saxegaard, F. (1970) Infectious bovine rhinotracheitis/infectious pustular vulvovaginitis (IBR/IPV) virus infection of cattle with particular reference to genital infections. *Vet. Bull.*, **40**, 605.

Schlafer, D. H. & Mebus, C. A. (1981) African swine fever in pregnant sows. *Proc. U.S. Anim. Health Assoc.*, **85**, 281–288.

Singh, E. L., Thomas, F. C., Papp-Vid, G., Eaglesome, M. D. & Hare, W. C. D. (1982) Embryo transfer as a means of controlling the transmission of viral infections. *Theriogenology*, **18**, 133.

Steck, F., Lazary, S., Fey, H., Wandeler, A., Huggler, C. H., Oppliger, G., Baumberger, H., Kaderli, R. & Martig, J. (1980) Immune responsiveness in cattle fatally affected by bovine virus diarrhea–mucosal disease. *Zentralbl. Vet. med. B*, **27**, 429.

Sweasey, D. & Patterson, D. S. P. (1979) Congenital hypomyelinogenesis (border disease) of lambs: postnatal neurochemical recovery in the central nervous system. *J. Neurochem.*, **33**, 705–711.

Swift, B. L. & Trueblood, M. S. (1974) The present status of the role of the parainfluenza-3 (PI-3) virus in fetal disease of cattle and sheep. *Theriogenology*, **2**, 101.

Terpstra, C. (1981) Border disease: virus persistence, antibody response and transmission studies. *Res. Vet. Sci.*, **3**, 185–191.

Timoney, P. J. (1985) Epidemiological features of the 1984 outbreak of equine viral arteritis in the thoroughbred population in Kentucky, USA. *Proc. Soc. Vet. Epidemiol. Prevent. Med.*, pp. 84–89.

Timoney, P. J., McCollum, W. H., Roberts, A. W. & Murphy, T. W. (1986) Demonstration of the carrier state in naturally acquired equine arteritis virus infection in the stallion. *Res. Vet. Sci.*, **41**, 279–280.

Thorsen, J. & Kahrs, R. (1984) Serological diagnosis of virus-induced abortions, stillbirths and congenital anomalies in cattle. *Vet. Med. Small Anim. Clin.*, **5**, 18.

Van Oirschot, J. T. (1983) Congenital infections with non-arbo togaviruses. *Vet. Microbiol.*, **8** 321–361.

Westaway, E. G., Brinton, M. A., Gaidamovich, S. Y. A. *et al.* (1985) Togaviridae. *Intervirol.*, **24**, 125–139.

Wittman, G., Gaskell, R. M. & Rziha, H. J., eds (1984) Latent herpes virus infections in veterinary medicine, pp. 161–256. The Hague: *Martinus Nijhoff*. Publisher for the CEC.

Wong, F. C., Spearman, U. G., Smolenski, M. A. & Loewen, P. C. (1985) Equine parvovirus: initial isolation and partial characterization. *Can. J. Comp. Med.*, **49**, 50–54.

Wrathall, A. E. (1975) *Reproductive Disorders in Pigs.* (Review Series No. 11, Commonwealth Bureau of Animal Health) Farnham Royal, UK: Commonwealth Agricultural Bureaux.

Wrathall, A. E., Wells, D. E., Cartwright, S. R. & Frerichs, G. N. (1984) An inactivated oil-emulsion vaccine for the prevention of porcine parvovirus-induced reproductive failure. *Res. Vet. Sci.*, **36**, 136–143.

Wyler, R. (1985) European isolates of bovine herpesvirus 1: a comparison of restriction endonuclease sites, polypeptides, and reactivity with monoclonal antibodies. *Arch. Virol.*, **85**, 57.

12

Brucellosis

M. J. CORBEL

BRUCELLA SPECIES

Brucellosis is an infectious disease of animals transmissible to man and caused by bacteria of the genus *Brucella*. It is a major cause of reproductive failure in domestic animals in many parts of the world producing abortion and sometimes infertility in cattle, sheep, goats, dogs, swine and species of more localized economic importance such as buffalo, camels, reindeer and yaks.

Currently six species of *Brucella* are recognized: *Brucella abortus*, *B. melitensis*, *B. suis*, *B. neotomae*, *B. ovis* and *B. canis*. These vary in the frequency with which they infect particular host species. Thus *B. abortus* infects cattle and other Bovidae preferentially but is sometimes transmitted to other hosts including deer, dogs, horses, sheep, goats and man. *B. melitensis* primarily infects sheep and goats but can be transmitted to many other host species and is the most important cause of brucellosis in man. *B. suis* varies in host range according to biovar. *B. suis* biovars 1, 2 and 3 have the pig as their principal host, although hares also act as an important natural reservoir of biovar 2. *B. suis* biovar 4 primarily causes infection in reindeer but is sometimes transmitted to predators. *B. suis* biovar 5 has only been found as a natural infection of murine and cricetine rodents in the Caucasus. All *B. suis* biovars have the capacity to cause serious infection in man.

The other *Brucella* species show a much greater degree of host specificity than *B. abortus*, *B. melitensis* and *B. suis*. *B. neotomae* has been isolated only from the desert wood rat (*Neotoma lepida* Thomas) on a few occasions and no verified cases of natural infection in other species, including man, have been reported. *B. ovis* also displays a high degree of host specificity and natural infections have been found only in sheep though other ruminant species can be infected under experimental conditions. Although it can produce abortion in pregnant ewes its major impact is on the male reproductive tract, infection often resulting in infertility. *B. canis* has the dog as its primary host, producing placentitis and abortion in the pregnant female and infertility in the male. The infection is occasionally transmitted to man.

All *Brucella* species have the ability to grow intracellularly and can survive and multiply within a variety of cell types, including the polymorphonuclear and mononuclear phagocytes of non-immune animals. By this means the organisms can establish persistent infection in the reticuloendothelial system. They also tend to localize in the reproductive tract and mammary glands. Infection in the male may result in frank orchitis or epididymitis resulting in impaired fertility, but is often asymptomatic in the nonpregnant female. During the course of gestation, brucellas tend to invade the developing placentomes and thence the fetal fluids and tissues. Growth in the placental cotyledons in particular may be profuse, causing extensive loss of placental function, and usually resulting in abortion during the last third of gestation.

With the exception of infection caused by *B. ovis* and to a lesser extent, *B. canis* and *B. suis*, where the

Table 12.1

Taxonomic designation	Nomen species and biovar		CO_2 requirement	H_2S production	Growth on media containing	
					Thionin*	Fuchsin*
B. melitensis biovar melitensis	1 B. melitensis	1	—	—	+	+
	2	2	—	—	+	+
	3	3	—	—	+	+
B. melitensis biovar abortus	1 B. abortus	1	(+)	+	—	+
	2	2	(+)	+	—	—
	3	3**	(+)	+	+	+
	4	4	(+)	+	—	+†
	5	5	—	—	+	+
	6	6**	—	—	+	+
	7	9	—	+	+	+
B. melitensis biovar suis	1 B. suis	1	—	+	+	—††
	2	2	—	—	+	—
	3	3	—	—	+	+
	4	4	—	—	+	(—)
	5	5	—	—	+	—
B. melitensis biovar ovis	B. ovis		+	—	+	(+)
B. melitensis biovar canis	B. canis		—	—	+	—
B. melitensis biovar neotomae	B. neotomae		—	+	—	—

L = Confluent lysis; PL = partial lysis; NL = no lysis.

*Concentration = 1/50 000 w/v.

(+) = Most strains positive; (−) = most strains negative.

**For more certain differentiation of *B. abortus* biovar 3 and biovar 6, thionin at 1/25 000 (w/v) is used in addition; biovar 3 = +, biovar 6 = −.

impact on the male reproductive tract is considerable, the most important effect of brucellosis is abortion with its resultant economic consequences.

BACTERIOLOGY

Taxonomy

The six currently recognized nomen species of *Brucella* are differentiated on the basis of their preferred natural host, their pattern of utilization of amino acid and carbohydrate substrates in oxidative metabolism tests and their susceptibility to lysis by brucella-phages. Within the three major species, *B. abortus*, *B. melitensis* and *B. suis*, a number of biovars have been defined on the basis of requirement for supplementary CO_2, H_2S production, growth in the presence of the dyes thionin and basic fuchsin and agglutination reaction with antisera monospecific for the A and M epitopes of the major surface antigens.

Recently, as a result of DNA–DNA hybridization studies, which have failed to disclose significant differences between the polynucleotide sequences of DNA from the six currently recognized nomen species, it has been proposed that the genus comprises a single species. On the basis of taxonomic convention, this would be designated *Brucella melitensis*. The currently recognized nomen species would then be reclassified as biovars of *B. melitensis*. The proposed nomenclature, together with the current usage are shown in Table 12.1. To avoid confusion, it has been recommended that the new nomenclature should be reserved for taxonomic purposes and that the current nomenclature should be retained for other purposes. This convention has been followed in this chapter.

In the past, phenotypically similar organisms now classified in the genera *Bordetella* and *Francisella* have been included in the *Brucella* genus. Genetic studies have shown that there is no relationship between these organisms and *Brucella*. Recent observations using ribosomal RNA–DNA hybridization have indicated that the *Brucella* genus is genetically related to *Agrobacterium*, *Rhizobium*, *Mycoplana*, *Phyllobacterium* and the unnamed Centers for Disease Control group Vd. This implies that *Brucella* and

Characteristics used in classification of the genus *Brucella*

Agglutination with monospecific antisera			Lysis by phage at RTD							Substrates metabolized oxidatively												
A	M	R	Tb	Wb	Bk$_2$	Iz$_1$	R	R/O	R/C	L-alanine	L-asparagine	L-glutamic acid	L-arabinose	D-galactose	D-ribose	D-glucose	i-erythritol	D-xylose	L-arginine	DL-ornithine	L-citruline	L-lysine
−	+	−				PL																
+	−	−	NL	NL	L	or	NL	NL	NL	+	+	+	−	−	−	+	+	−	−	−	−	−
+	+	−				L																
+	−	−																				
+	−	−					*R strains only*															
+	−	−																				
−	+	−	L	L	L	L	L	L	L	+	+	+	+	+	+	+	+	−	−	−	−	−
−	+	−																				
+	−	−																				
−	+	−																				
+	−	−								−	−	+	+	+	+	+	+	+	+	+	+	+
+	−	−								−	−	+	+	+	+	+	+	+	+	+	+	+
+	−	−	NL	L	L	PL	NL	NL	NL	−	−	+	−	−	+	+	+	+	+	+	+	+
+	+	−				or				−	−	+	−	−	+	+	+	+	+	+	+	+
−	+	−				L				−	+	+	−	−	+	+	+	+	+	+	+	+
−	−	+	NL	NL	NL	NL	NL	L	L	−	+	+	−	−	−	−	−	−	−	−	−	−
−	−	+	NL	NL	NL	NL	NL	NL	L	−	−	+	−	−	+	+	+	−	+	+	+	−
			NL																			
+	−	−	or	L	L	L	NL	NL	NL	−	−	+	+	+	+	+	+	−	−	−	−	+
			PL																			

†Some strains of this biotype are inhibited by basic fuchsin.
††Some isolates may be resistant to basic fuchsin, pyronin and safranin 0.

these other organisms evolved from common precursors probably existing as freeliving soil bacteria.

Definition

The genus is defined as follows: small nonmotile, nonspore-forming gram-negative cocci, coccobacilli or short rods with rounded ends, 0.5–0.7 μm wide by 0.5–1.5 μm long, occurring singly, in pairs or short chains. They are not acid-fast but the organisms resist decolorization by weakly acid or alkaline solutions as in the Stamp modification of the Ziehl–Neelsen stain or the modified Köster method. The organisms are chemo-organotrophs and grow best in complex media containing multiple amino acids, thiamine, nicotinamide, biotin and pantothenic acid. X factor (hemin) and V factor (nicotinamide adenine dinucleotide) are not essential for growth. The growth of many strains is improved by blood or serum.

Energy-yielding processes are oxidative and fermentation of carbohydrates does not occur in peptone media. Oxygen is essential although nitrate can be used as an electron donor. Some strains have an obligatory requirement for a CO_2-enriched atmosphere. All strains are catalase-positive and most are oxidase-positive. Most strains will reduce nitrates to nitrites. Citrate is not utilized as sole carbon source and indole and acetyl methylcarbinol (Voges–Proskauer reaction) are not produced. The methyl red reaction is negative, *o*-nitrophenol-β-D-galactoside is not usually hydrolyzed. Litmus milk is unchanged or rendered alkaline, urea is hydrolyzed to a variable extent and H_2S production is also variable. Gelatin is not liquified and blood cells are not lyzed. Optimum growth occurs at 37 °C, range 20–40 °C. Optimum pH for growth is between 6.6 and 7.4. Guanine + cytosine content of DNA is 55–59 mol%. The average genome size is between 2.37 and 2.82 × 10⁹ daltons (D). DNA polynucleotide homology for all members of the genus is >90%. Internal protein antigens are specific to the genus.

The organisms are mammalian parasites with a broad host range and can survive and replicate in mononuclear phagocytes.

Genetics

All members of the genus *Brucella* are very closely

related genetically and show almost complete homology of nucleotide sequences in DNA–DNA hybridization tests. The genetic differences between the various nomen species are too small to justify their recognition as true species although they can be differentiated on the basis of phenotypic properties.

Little is known about the detailed genetics of *Brucella*. Conjugation has not been detected and structures functionally associated with this, such as pili, have not been demonstrated. Similarly, attempts to produce transformation with homologous or heterologous DNA have been unsuccessful. Various attempts to detect plasmids or other forms of extrachromosomal DNA have also given negative results. However, evidence of transduction has been reported and some *Brucella* strains appear to be lysogenic.

Various lytic phages have been isolated from *Brucella* strains and occasionally from environmental sources. These phages are genus-specific and their precise pattern of lysis shows a close correlation with the nomen species. Phage typing plays a useful role in the routine identification of *Brucella* isolates and the reactions given by the more important phage strains are summarized in Table 12.1. Spontaneous variations in the genetically determined properties of *Brucella* occur fairly frequently. Probably the commonest is the dissociation of smooth phase cultures to the rough phase or various intermediate forms. This is associated with loss or reduction of virulence, changes in antigenic structure and phage lysis pattern and alteration of colonial morphology and related properties. Variations in other properties such as CO_2 requirement, H_2S production, dye and antibiotic sensitivity occur with varying frequency.

Other types of variation, including the production of cell wall-defective forms, are more readily reversible and may involve mainly phenotypic changes.

Nutrition and Metabolism

Laboratory adapted strains of *Brucella* can grow on chemically defined basal media containing ammonium ion as the sole nitrogen source. However, the majority of strains, particularly fresh isolates, require more complex media containing multiple amino acids and vitamins, especially thiamine, biotin, nicotinamide and pantothenic acid, as well as iron, magnesium and manganese ions.

Growth is best in the presence of blood or serum and strains of *B. abortus* biovar 2 and some of biovars 3 and 4 and *B. ovis* will not grow in serum-free media. Serum dextrose agar is a suitable medium for the growth of all species and biovars although many strains will grow on good quality peptone media such as trypticase soy or tryptone soya agar without serum supplementation. Culture media can be made selective for *Brucella* by the incorporation of antibiotics. Farrell's serum dextrose agar containing bacitracin, cycloheximide, nalidixic acid, nystatin, polymyxin B and vancomycin is suitable for isolation of most strains. The less inhibitory vancomycin, colistin, furadantin, nystatin formulation is more suitable for the more antibiotic-sensitive strains such as those of *B. ovis*.

Many strains of *B. abortus* and those of *B. ovis* require supplementary CO_2 for growth. This does not serve simply to lower oxygen tension but is utilized as a nutrient and incorporated into nucleotides and amino acids. Brucellas are aerobic and metabolism is essentially oxidative. The organisms have a complex electron transport system involving cytochromes a, a_3, b, c, and o, flavoproteins and ubiquinone.

Although most strains, with the exception of *B. ovis*, can utilize glucose as an energy source many, especially those of *B. abortus*, will oxidize *i*-erythritol preferentially. This carbohydrate derivative is present in the placental cotyledons and fetal fluids of cattle, sheep, goats and swine and in the male genital tracts of these species and is probably at least partly responsible for the localization and prolific growth of brucellas in these animals.

Apart from glucose and *i*-erythritol, a wide range of amino acid and carbohydrate substrates is oxidized. The pattern of utilization of these varies with the preferred host species and shows a close correspondence with phage lysis patterns. Oxidative metabolism patterns have therefore been employed for the identification and classification of *Brucella* strains. They can be determined quantitatively by manometric methods or semiquantitatively by thin layer chromatography.

In general, strains of *B. abortus* and *B. neotomae* will oxidize amino acids and carbohydrates but not urea cycle intermediates; strains of *B. melitensis* will oxidize amino acids but few carbohydrates other than glucose and *i*-erythritol, strains of *B. ovis* follow a similar pattern but do not utilize glucose or *i*-erythritol whereas strains of *B. suis* and *B. canis* oxidize the full range of substrates including amino acids, carbohydrates and urea cycle intermediates.

Oxidative metabolism tests tend to be hazardous and inconvenient to perform on highly pathogenic organisms such as *Brucella*, so for routine identification purposes they have been largely replaced by phage lysis tests. Nevertheless, they may still offer the only means of identifying atypical or phage resistant strains at nomen species level.

Resistance and Survival

Under appropriate conditions brucellas can persist in the environment for very long periods. The organisms resist drying, especially in an organic substrate, and can remain viable in dust or soil for up to 10 weeks. They can also survive in water for up to 70 days and when frozen can survive for much longer periods. At temperatures just above freezing point the organisms have survived in aborted fetuses and uterine exudates for at least 6 months, in bovine feces for at least 1 year and in liquid manure for up to $2\frac{1}{2}$ years. They can survive in frozen tissues for many years.

Their resistance to inactivation by heat or ionizing radiations is comparable with that of other vegetative gram-negative bacteria. Thus dilute suspensions are killed by exposure at 60 °C for 10 min and by all of the pasteurization procedures designed to kill *Mycobacterium tuberculosis*. Dense suspensions of *Brucella* strains may not be inactivated by moderate heat and repeated exposures or boiling may be necessary.

Brucellas are sensitive to a wide range of disinfectants including strong acids and alkalis, hypochlorite, iodophors, phenolics (for example 1% Lysol), formaldehyde, ethylene oxide. The presence of organic matter and exposure to low temperatures drastically reduce the efficacy of chemical disinfectants and allowance must be made for this when disinfecting grossly contaminated articles or premises. Xylene at a final concentration of 1 ml/l or calcium cyanamide at 20 kg/m³ have been recommended for killing brucellas in slurry but exposure times of up to 1 month may be needed.

For decontamination of skin following accidental or occupational exposures, concentrated soap solutions containing substituted phenols have been recommended but ethanol, isopropanol, dilute hypochlorite or iodophors are suitable alternatives.

Antibiotic Sensitivity

Brucellas show high sensitivity *in vitro* to a wide range of antibiotics and chemotherapeutic agents including some penicillins, many aminoglycosides, chloramphenicol, tetracyclines, ansamycins and aminocyclitols. Sensitivity to macrolides, sulphonamides and trimethoprim and their combination, co-trimoxazole, is variable. Most strains are resistant to vancomycin, lincosamides, peptides such as bacitracin and the polymyxins, metronidazole, nalidixic

acid, oxolinic acid and antifungal agents. Some of these agents have been employed in selective media for the isolation of *Brucella* from contaminated materials.

Tetracyclines, with or without streptomycin, have been the agents of choice for the therapy of human brucellosis, with co-trimoxazole as an alternative. However, tetracyclines alone are less effective than rifampicin. The currently recommended regimen employs rifampicin at 600–900 mg, together with doxycline 200 mg, taken together as a single daily dose for a minimum of 6 weeks. Rifampicin alone is recommended for the treatment of young children. Therapy is not recommended for brucellosis in farm animals. It may be justified in the case of pedigree stock being used as embryo donors but the suppression of infection is likely to be temporary. It has been tried, with very limited success, in *B. canis* infection in dogs.

Antigenic Structure

All *Brucella* strains in the smooth phase show extensive crossreactions in agglutination tests with unabsorbed polyclonal antisera. This occurs because the surface antigens reacting in these tests possess structural features which are common to all smooth strains. The main surface antigen detected by serological tests such as agglutination, complement fixation or immunospecific staining, is the smooth lipopolysaccharide (S-LPS) complex. This consists of a core region, probably similar for all *Brucella* strains, composed of lipid A and a core polysaccharide containing glucose, mannose and quinovosamine and the linking glycose 2-keto-3-deoxyoctulosonic acid. Attached to the core polysaccharide is the O chain which determines the major serological specificity of the S-LPS. It comprises a homopolymer of about 100 residues of *N*-formylated perosamine (4-formamido, 4, 6-dideoxy D-mannose).

In the case of strains typified by *B. abortus* biovar 1 (A epitope dominant) the *N*-formylated perosamine residues are linked by the 1 and 2 carbon atoms to give a straight chain, whereas in strains typified by *B. melitensis* biovar 1 (M epitope dominant) the first four residues of every five are linked in this way but every fifth residue is linked by its 1 and 3 carbon atoms to produce a 'kinked' chain. These differences can be detected in serological tests with monoclonal antibodies to the A and M epitopes or by polyclonal antisera made specific for the A and M epitopes by crossabsorption.

Brucella strains in the rough phase do not crossreact with smooth strains in agglutination tests and do not possess the A and M epitopes. The rough lipopolysaccharide (R-LPS) complex lacks the smooth O chain and probably consists of lipid A and a modified core polysaccharide.

Other antigens located on or near the surface of rough or smooth *Brucella* strains are the outer membrane proteins and the peptidoglycan of the cell wall. These, together with the LPS are the main components involved in stimulating protective immunity to *Brucella* infection.

Other antigens are located intracellularly and consist of proteins, glycoproteins, peptides and polysaccharides. The protein antigens are diagnostically significant because they are specific to the *Brucella* genus and do not crossreact with antibodies evoked by other bacteria. They are also the main components of brucellin preparations used in intradermal tests for delayed hypersensitivity to *Brucella*.

Crossreactions

An antigenic relationship exists between smooth *Brucella* strains and *Escherichia coli* 0:116 and 0:157, *Francisella tularensis*, *Salmonella* group N (0:30 antigen), *Pseudomonas maltophilia*, *Vibrio cholerae* and *Yersinia enterocolitica* 0:9. Exposure to these organisms can result in the development of diagnostically significant titers of antibodies reacting in serological tests for brucellosis. Where chemical characterization of the crossreacting antigen has been performed, substituted perosamine residues have been identified as the structures responsible for the crossreaction. In the case of *Y. enterocolitica* 0:9 the O chain of the S-LPS is identical with that of A-dominant strains of *Brucella*. This results in the most extensive crossreaction and the most difficult to resolve by diagnostic tests. Fortunately, *Y. enterocolitica* 0:9 seems to be rare in the United Kingdom, and from the veterinary point of view *E. coli* 0:157 is the organism most frequently implicated in crossreactions with *Brucella* in the small proportion of cases where an agent can be identified.

Crossreactions probably account for less than a quarter of the total number of false-positive serological reactions to *Brucella* given by bovine sera in the United Kingdom. The majority of such reactions, which occur mainly to the serum agglutination and Rose Bengal plate tests, are attributable to EDTA-labile agglutinins.

Pathogenicity

Strains of *B. abortus*, *B. melitensis* and *B. suis* are pathogenic for a wide variety of animal species, usually producing generalized infections with a bacteremic phase followed by localization in the reticuloendothelial system and frequently the genital tract. Infection in the pregnant animal is quite likely to result in placentitis and abortion. Localization may also occur in mammary tissue with excretion in the milk. The organisms can survive and multiply in polymorphonuclear and mononuclear phagocytes as well as other cell types.

The more host-specific species *B. neotomae*, *B. ovis* and *B. canis* produce similar effects in their natural hosts but are difficult to transmit to other species.

Laboratory animals, including mice, guinea-pigs and rabbits can be infected with the various *Brucella* nomen species, the severity of infection depending upon the virulence of the strain. For typical strains, the order of pathogenicity is usually *B. melitensis* > *B. suis* > *B. abortus* > *B. neotomae* > *B. canis* > *B. ovis*. Infection is rarely fatal except when heavy inocula of highly virulent strains of *B. melitensis* or *B. suis* are used. The only obvious effect of infection may be reticuloendothelial hyperplasia, especially of the spleen. In more severe infections local lesions of liver, spleen, testes, epididymides and joints may develop.

Ecology

Brucellas are facultative intracellular parasites and are not known to pursue a life cycle independent of their natural host species. Although the organisms can survive for quite long periods in the environment, in dust, soil and water, there is no evidence that they multiply in these situations. They have been isolated from ticks and hematophagous insects from time to time in the USSR and some other countries but the role of arthropods in transmitting and maintaining the infection is unclear. The indications from areas in which brucellosis has been eradicated from the farm animal population are that the disease does not reestablish itself from environmental sources.

Usually, the infection in secondary hosts undergoes limited lateral transmission. An exception to this is *B. suis* biovar 2 which can cycle between wild hares and domestic swine. It is also possible for *B. abortus* and *B. melitensis* infections to be maintained in wild ruminants with transmission to domesticated species. In practice, this seems to happen infrequently.

Immunology

Infection with *Brucella* or immunization with vaccines usually results in the development of both antibody and cell-mediated immune responses to the antigens of the organism. However, both types of response are not invariably produced, nor do they necessarily develop simultaneously. The development, magnitude and persistence of these responses is affected by many factors.

In the case of infection, the virulence of the strain, size of inoculum, route of entry, age, sex, pregnancy status, species and resistance of the host will all influence the nature of the immune response. In the case of vaccines, the type of preparation used, in other words whether an attenuated live vaccine or killed vaccine with or without adjuvant, whether prepared from a smooth or nonsmooth strain, the dose, route and immunization schedule, will all interact with individual host factors to determine the type of response, its magnitude and duration.

Both antibody and cell-mediated immune responses are diagnostically useful but the former are much easier to standardize and quantify than the latter. The immune responses induced by vaccination with some type of preparation can be difficult, and in some cases impossible, to differentiate from those resulting from infection with virulent strains.

Cell-mediated Immunity

Brucellas are facultative intracellular parasites and can survive and multiply within both polymorphonuclear and mononuclear phagocytes as well as other types of cell. During the acute, bacteremic phase of infection only a minority of organisms may be located within cells. As infection progresses into the chronic phase, probably most of the persisting brucellas are intracellular. Phagocytosis, particularly by polymorphonuclear leukocytes, is promoted by antibodies. The role of antibody-directed cytotoxicity in immunity to brucellosis is not clear but recent studies with monoclonal antibodies can be interpreted in terms of it contributing to the control of the infection. Nevertheless, most of the available evidence suggests that recovery from brucellosis is largely, if not entirely, dependent upon the acquisition of increased intracellular bactericidal activity by differentiated mononuclear phagocytes. This process of activation occurs in mononuclear phagocytes stimulated by interleukins released by T-lymphocytes responding specifically to antigens. This type of T-lymphocyte response is subject to regulation by class II immunoregulator molecules of the major histocompatibility complex (MHC).

Cell-mediated immunity is associated with delayed (type IV) hypersensitivity which can often be revealed by intradermal injection of appropriate antigen preparations. Delayed hypersensitivity to *Brucella* antigens can be induced by infection with virulent strains, vaccination with attenuated strains, or immunization with nonliving antigen preparations especially if incorporated in an oily adjuvant. Although its development usually parallels the development of the increased intracellular bactericidal activity associated with cell-mediated immunity, delayed hypersensitivity may be directed towards nonprotective antigens and does not necessarily correlate with protective immunity. However, in the form of the intradermal or intrapalpebral test it offers a convenient procedure for detecting animals previously exposed to *Brucella* antigens under sensitizing conditions. In the absence of vaccination, such sensitization is only likely to result from infection.

Provided that antigens free of S-LPS are used, the intradermal test can be useful in differentiating *Brucella*-infected animals from those giving serological crossreactions as a result of exposure to other bacteria.

Humoral Immunity

The sera of cattle, sheep, goats and pigs contain immunoglobulins of the IgA, IgG_1, IgG_2 and IgM isotypes. Although the nomenclature is similar for the four species, the immunoglobulin isotypes do not necessarily have identical properties. In relation to their role in the immune response to *Brucella* antigens, detailed information is available only for the bovine isotypes.

Following exposure to a heavy inoculum of a virulent field strain or parenteral vaccination with a smooth attenuated strain such as *B. abortus* S19, initially antibodies of the IgM isotype are produced. They can usually be detected in the 1st or 2nd week after exposure, normally from the 4th or 5th day onward. They are rapidly followed by antibodies of the IgG_1 isotype. Production of IgG_2 antibodies may also occur, particularly following infection or repeated exposure through vaccination. Serum IgA antibodies are usually produced in low concentrations. In the case of persistent infection caused by a virulent strain, the IgG response is sustained and persists at a high level, often for years. Some IgM production may also be sustained but is greatly overshadowed by the IgG response.

The response to vaccination with an attenuated strain depends upon the age of the animal and the dose and route used. Usually, in young animals given the full dose of strain 19 vaccine (8×10^{10} organisms) at 6 months old or less, the IgG antibody responses decline to diagnostically insignificant levels within 3–6 months. Any residual antibody persisting after this time is usually of the IgM isotype.

Following exposure to small doses of virulent

Brucella strains, antibodies may not appear until 1–3 months later or even longer depending upon the size and route of the inoculum and the pregnancy status of the animal. Under these conditions the IgM response may not be observed to precede the IgG response and antibody titers tend to show a slow increase rather than the dramatic rise seen after exposure to a large antigenic mass. Many animals exposed to very small inocula may develop self-limiting infection accompanied by a transient low grade antibody response, others may not develop a detectable response. A significant proportion of animals do not develop antibodies of the IgG isotypes until one or more weeks after abortion or parturition. Some of these animals may have low titers of IgM antibodies a few weeks earlier but these may fail to be detected by screening tests or may be attributed to residual vaccinal titers or nonspecific reactions.

The role of the various isotypes in the antibody response of sheep and goats to infection with *B. melitensis* has received limited study. The overall pattern of response is similar to that observed in cattle exposed to *B. abortus*, but the relative contributions of the IgG_1 and IgG_2 isotypes have not been determined. Even less information is available on the role of the various immunoglobulin isotypes in the response of pigs to *B. suis* infection.

The identity of the immunoglobulin classes involved in the antibody response to *Brucella* antigens is of practical importance as the various serological tests used in diagnosis differ in their capacity to detect different isotypes. Thus bovine antibodies of the IgA, IgG_1, IgG_2 and IgM isotypes can all react in the standard serum agglutination test (SAT) but those of the IgM class are the most efficient. The activity of IgG_1 antibodies in this test can vary and in some circumstances they can block the agglutinating activity of other isotypes. The agglutinating and precipitating activity of IgG_1 antibodies is promoted by high salt concentrations or acid conditions and this isotype is particularly active in the Rose Bengal plate test (RBPT) and the radial immunodiffusion test.

The agglutinating activity of IgM but not IgG is reduced or eliminated by disulfide bond disrupting agents such as 2-mercaptoethanol or dithiothreitol, by selective precipitation with the dye Rivanol (6,9-diamino-2-ethoxyacridine lactate) and by exposure to moderate heat. This has been exploited in various modified agglutination procedures designed to differentiate residual vaccinal IgM antibodies from the IgG agglutinins more likely to be associated with active infection.

In effect, only antibodies of the IgG_1 isotype are detected when the complement fixation test (CFT) is performed by the warm fixation method after serum inactivation at 58 °C for 30 min. IgA and IgG_2 are inactive in this test and IgM is largely inactivated by the heating procedure. IgM may be detected by other modifications of the CFT. IgG_2 antibodies in sufficient concentration can block complement fixation by IgG_1 and produce prozones, incomplete fixation patterns and false-negative reactions. This effect is avoided if the indirect hemolysis test is used instead of the conventional complement fixation procedure.

Antibodies of all isotypes except IgM can react in the Coombs antiglobulin test but the precise specificity of this, as in the case of enzyme immunoassay or radioimmunoassay procedures depends upon the nature of the antiglobulin reagent used to detect antibody binding. IgM and IgA antibodies participate in the milk ring test. IgG_1 and IgG_2 antibodies, if present in high concentration, can interfere with ring formation and form a precipitate or agglutinate which settles out instead of rising into the cream layer of the milk.

In all of the tests described, with the exception of immunodiffusion or enzyme immunoassay or radioimmunoassay procedures using specially purified antigens, the antibodies detected, irrespective of isotype, are directed mainly towards the O chain of the S-LPS antigen.

Nonspecific Agglutinins

Crossreacting antibodies resulting from exposure to bacteria possessing surface antigens structurally related to those of *Brucella* are predominantly of the IgM isotype. However, *Y. enterocolitica* 0:9, and to a lesser extent *E. coli* 0:157, can evoke detectable IgG antibody responses in cattle and pigs.

The nonspecific agglutinins present in a high proportion of uninfected cattle which react to the SAT or RBPT are independent of antibody activity but result from the interaction of the Fc portion of certain IgM, and rarely also IgG_1, molecules with undefined receptors on the *Brucella* cell surface. This interaction can be blocked by ethylene diamine tetra acetic acid (EDTA) and ethylene glycol *bis* (β-amino-ethyl) ether N,N,N^1,N^1 tetra acetic acid (EGTA) and some structurally related chelating agents. It is not blocked by structurally related components without chelating activity nor by chelating agents of unrelated structures. The blocking effect probably depends upon structural analogy between the immunoglobulin Fc binding site and EDTA or EGTA and not on the sequestering of divalent cations.

It has been suggested that partially degraded IgM molecules are involved in this type of reaction, which may account for 70–80% of agglutination reactions given by bovine sera with negative CFT titers to *B. abortus*. False-positive reactions caused by these agglutinins can be avoided by performing the SAT in a diluent containing 0.01 molar EDTA or EGTA disodium salt in phosphate buffered saline at pH 7.2 instead of the conventional phenol-saline diluent.

VACCINES

These may consist of live attenuated strains which are intended to undergo limited replication in the host, stimulating an effective immune response before being eliminated, or they may consist of preparations containing killed cells of virulent or attenuated strains or even cell fractions usually incorporated in an adjuvant to increase the immune response. In either case the protection conferred is not absolute and is dependent upon many factors such as: species, breed, age, sex and pregnancy status of the vaccinated animal; the nature of the vaccine and the dose and route by which it is administered; and the virulence, dose and route of infection of the challenging strain. In general, vaccines can play a useful role in controlling brucellosis, by limiting its spread and reducing its economic impact. They are most unlikely to succeed in eradicating the disease, however, and in any control program should be supplemented by the application of hygienic measures and the elimination of known infected stock.

The choice of vaccine depends upon the local circumstances including the nature of the infecting strain, the prevalence of the disease, the presence of reservoirs of infection in other species including wildlife, systems of management and geographic and economic factors. These factors may change during the course of a control program and this will influence vaccination strategy. For example, in the early stages of a control program when the disease is highly prevalent, the degree of immunity produced and its duration are more important than the effect on diagnostic tests. In the later stages of a control campaign it may be advantageous to use vaccination schedules or vaccines which produce less persistent immune responses. Therefore when devising a control strategy the following factors have to be taken into account:

1. The extent to which vaccination is to be part of the control program.

2. Which vaccine or vaccines are to be used and to which populations they are to be applied.
3. The manner in which the vaccines are to be applied to ensure adequate coverage of the susceptible population. To achieve an effective coverage and to break the chain of infection in areas at risk, a coverage of at least 70% of susceptible animals will probably need to be achieved. Low or erratic use of vaccines is likely to introduce diagnostic complications while contributing little to the control of the disease.
4. The means of monitoring progress of the vaccination campaign and whether any modifications of vaccination policy are to be introduced as the situation changes.
5. The stage at which to stop vaccination bearing in mind the cost of diagnostic complications in the face of a low prevalence of the disease and the costs of manufacture and administration of the vaccine itself.
6. Regulations governing international trade in animals may be relevant. For example countries free of *B. melitensis* may not permit importation of animals vaccinated with *B. melitensis* vaccine even if they are from brucellosis-free areas. The effect of persistent vaccinal antibody titers on export–import tests may also be significant.
7. Possible hazards to personnel and the population at large arising from the use of the vaccine.

In addition to problems relating directly to the vaccination strategy the vaccines themselves have to fulfil certain minimum criteria.

Safety

1. In the case of live attenuated vaccines, the strain must be stable and not revert to full virulence even after repeated passages *in vivo*.
2. It should not cause any adverse reaction, either local or general in the target animal.
3. It should persist in the animal only for the minimum period required to establish an adequate immune response.
4. It must not produce a carrier state.
5. It should not be transmitted between animals and should not be excreted, particularly in consumable products such as milk.
6. It should not interfere with the interpretation of diagnostic tests.

Efficacy

Ideally, the vaccine should protect all animals against all levels of infection likely to be encountered under field conditions and the protection should be lifelong.

Quality Control

It is essential that the properties of each batch of vaccine should be monitored to ensure adequate safety of the product and uniformity of quality. For live vaccines, freeze-drying probably offers the best means of achieving an adequate shelf-life. However, the best conditions have to be determined for each vaccine.

It is important that each batch of vaccine should be subjected to an adequate potency test. The product should also be subjected to comprehensive re-evaluation if any significant changes are introduced in the source of seed material or the method of manufacture.

For killed vaccines, apart from safety and potency tests, the quantity and quality of the adjuvant should be controlled, as should the quantity of antigenic material incorporated into each dose. Adjuvant preparations need monitoring to control efficacy and freedom from adverse reactions.

Live Vaccines

B. abortus *Strain 19 Vaccine*

B. abortus strain 19 was developed for the immunization of cattle but has also been applied to other species including sheep, goats, reindeer and yaks. It gives relatively poor protection against *B. melitensis* and *B. suis* and is now only recommended for protection of cattle against *B. abortus* infection. The strain is a stable smooth-intermediate variant of *B. abortus* biovar 1 which does not require CO_2 for growth but is inhibited by penicillin and thionin blue. The growth of some seed sources but not all is inhibited by *i*-erythritol. The strain also shows an unusually high oxidation rate with L-glutamic acid.

There is ample evidence that the strain is stable and does not revert to virulence even after repeated passage in pregnant animals. It causes a slight reaction at the inoculation site and a brief febrile response may follow. In lactating cattle it causes a sharp but temporary fall in milk yield. Persisting infection is rare but the organism has occasionally been recovered from lymph nodes or other sites months or years after vaccination. It has also been associated with the 'lame persistent reactor syndrome', an arthropathy usually involving one or both femorotibial joints and accompanied by a high antibody response to *B. abortus* up to several years after vaccination. This syndrome has been found in

about 0.5% of vaccinated cattle in Britain. A similar syndrome has also been reported from Australia.

The recommended dose of strain 19 vaccine used in Britain until the end of 1979 was 8×10^{10} live cells given subcutaneously to female calves between 4 and 6 months old. In some countries this interval has been extended up to 8 months. In the United States, the official dosage has been reduced to between 3×10^8 and 3×10^9 live organisms given subcutaneously between 4 and 12 months of age to both beef and dairy cattle. It is claimed that under these circumstances most of the female cattle lose their antibody titers within 16–18 months. However, some studies have shown that 5–10% of animals may retain substantial titers for 12 months or longer. These antibodies are very difficult to differentiate from those resulting from natural infection. The complement fixation test, the IgG enzyme immunoassay and the radial immunodiffusion test all assist in achieving differentiation but this is not possible in every case.

An alternative immunization schedule is to give two doses of $5–10 \times 10^9$ live organisms by the intraconjunctival route 4–8 months apart. This has produced good immunity to challenge with negligible serological reactions. Oral administration of the vaccine has also been claimed to give similar results in limited studies.

Strain 19 vaccine gives a relatively good immunity but some doubts still exist over its duration especially with reduced dose schedules or unusual routes of administration. The use of the vaccine was prohibited in Britain after 1979 following the success of the Brucellosis Eradication Scheme in reducing the prevalence of the disease to a very low level.

B. melitensis *Rev 1 Vaccine*

This is a live attenuated nonstreptomycin dependent revertant derived from a streptomycin dependent derivative of a virulent strain of *B. melitensis*. The strain has stable low virulence for sheep and goats and induces very good immunity to *B. melitensis*. It can produce persistent infections however and may be excreted in the milk. This has not been identified with any public health hazard however, although the strain retains some residual virulence for man.

In goats and sheep, the vaccine is usually given by the subcutaneous route at a recommended dose of 10^9 live cells when the animals are 4–6 months old. A lower dose of $5–10 \times 10^4$ live cells has been suggested for the vaccination of adult sheep and goats when it is necessary to provide protection as soon as possible. Lambs can also be immunized by intraconjunctival instillation of 10^4 live cells in a 0.1 ml dose. This produces effective protection but with little serological response.

Rev 1 vaccine will also protect cattle against *B. abortus* as well as *B. melitensis* and has been used in areas where the latter infection is present in small ruminants. It will also protect sheep against *B. ovis* infection.

B. suis *Strain 2 Vaccine*

This is an attenuated strain of *B. suis* biovar 1 and was developed in China for the immunization of sheep and goats against *B. melitensis*. The vaccine has been used effectively for the control of ovine and caprine brucellosis in Inner Mongolia. Its residual pathogenicity is comparable with that of *B. abortus* strain 19. It does not produce abortion in pregnant cattle, sheep, goats or pigs nor does it persist in the tissues of immunized animals. If given by the oral route it does not result in persistent antibody responses. The vaccine is normally given in drinking water, 10^{10} live organisms are used for protecting sheep and goats against *B. melitensis*. A dose of 5×10^9 live organisms is recommended for cattle and two doses of 2×10^{10} live organisms will give pigs some protection against infection by *B. suis* by most routes except by natural service. The duration of protection is up to 4–5 years for sheep and goats but is less certain for cattle and pigs.

Killed Vaccines

B. abortus *Strain 45/20 Vaccines*

These contain killed cells of *B. abortus* strain 45/20 incorporated in an oil emulsion adjuvant. Originally the vaccine strain, a rough variant of *B. abortus* biovar 1, was used as a live vaccine but reverted to virulence *in vivo*. In principle, the vaccine should not induce antibodies reacting with smooth *B. abortus* antigens. In practice this has not been found the case and studies with monoclonal antibodies have confirmed the presence of epitopes common to rough and smooth *B. abortus* strains on the surface of strain 45/20.

Many commercially produced preparations have been in use in various countries. Experience with these has produced conflicting results. In some, good protection has been reported, in others the level of protection has been poor and adverse reactions have been common. Much of the controversy arises from the difficulty of controlling the quality of the vaccine. Usually, two doses of 45/20 vaccine given 6–12 weeks apart are recommended, often with annual booster doses thereafter. The vaccine can be used on animals of any age, whether pregnant or not, and therefore can be used to supplement other vaccines in a control campaign.

Single doses of 45/20 vaccine have been reported to give good protection. In Australia, the effect of the vaccine in stimulating an anamnestic antibody response to smooth *B. abortus* antigen in animals incubating the infection has been exploited to eradicate the disease from herds of range cattle.

The duration of immunity given by 45/20 vaccine is uncertain and problems of batch variation make quality control difficult. The use of vaccines of this type is to be recommended only in exceptional circumstances.

B. melitensis *H38 Vaccine*

This consists of killed cells of smooth virulent *B. melitensis* strain 53 H38 incorporated in an oil emulsion adjuvant. It can give effective immunity against *B. abortus* or *B. melitensis* and can be used in animals of any age or pregnancy status. However, it provokes severe local reactions and stimulates unacceptably persistent antibody responses which cannot be differentiated from active infection by serological tests. This vaccine is obsolescent and there are few indications for its use.

Zoonotic Importance *B. melitensis* was originally isolated from fatal human cases of Malta fever, and it was the occurrence of this disease which eventually drew attention to the existence of the infection in goats. *B. abortus* and *B. suis* on the other hand, were isolated from animal cases before their association with human disease was recognized. Indeed, for a considerable time, it was believed that *B. abortus* was not pathogenic for man. Now of course the importance of these three species, together with *B. canis*, as the cause of substantial morbidity and even mortality in human populations is widely recognized. Indeed, on a worldwide basis brucellosis is probably one of the most prevalent zoonoses.

B. melitensis is probably the most frequent cause of severe acute infection in man although *B. suis* can cause severe chronic disease with complications involving the skeletal, central nervous and other systems. *B. abortus* infection is usually less severe but can be disabling and fatal cases occur occasionally. *B. canis* usually causes a relatively mild infection in man and in some countries a high prevalence of seropositive but asymptomatic individuals has been observed among the population. No human infections caused by *B. neotomae* or *B. ovis* have been recorded although individuals seropositive to the latter organism have been detected in some sheep-raising areas.

Infections caused by *B. abortus* or *B. melitensis* are often acquired by contact with infected animals, especially after abortion or parturition, or by exposure to dust or fomites contaminated by such animals. Such infections tend to be occupational affecting most frequently farmers and their families, abattoir workers and veterinarians. Infections in the general population usually result from ingestion of contaminated dairy produce, especially unpasteurized milk, cream, soft cheeses and ice cream. Strongly acidified cheeses, butter and yoghurt pose a minimal risk as their processing tends to eliminate viable brucella organisms. Infections caused by *B. suis* biovars 1, 2 and 3 usually result from contact with infected pigs or their meat products. Abattoir workers are especially at risk as persistent bacteremia is quite common in infected pigs and the numbers of organisms in their solid tissues can also be high. *B. suis* biovar 2 is the least dangerous of these to man and recorded incidents of infection have been few. *B. suis* biovar 4 is associated with disease in reindeer and human infection is acquired by contact with these animals or their secretions. Infected meat and milk also present a substantial hazard and in some subarctic populations outbreaks of brucellosis have been attributed to the consumption of uncooked reindeer bone marrow. *B. suis* biovar 5 has not be reported to cause natural infection in man but has produced severe laboratory-acquired brucellosis.

Laboratory workers are also at risk of infection from the other *Brucella* nomen species and biovars and special precautions should always be taken when handling the organism or specimens likely to contain it in large numbers. Brucella vaccines also present a significant hazard. The live vaccine strains can produce infection and severe hypersensitivity reactions in man; killed vaccines, especially those containing an oil emulsion adjuvant, can provoke severe local reactions if accidentally injected. Veterinarians and others involved in handling these materials should always take precautions designed to minimize exposure to them.

Human-to-human transmission of infection has been reported on rare occasions. Circumstantial evidence implicated sexual contact as the route of infection and *B. melitensis* was involved in each case. However, such incidents are extremely rare and for practical purposes animals are the only significant source of human infection. The eradication of the disease from domestic animals would eliminate the risk of transmission to man quite apart from improving animal health and productivity.

CATTLE

Bovine brucellosis is a worldwide problem except for the limited number of countries from which the disease has been eradicated. In most developed countries it has been brought under control, if not finally eliminated, and many, including Britain, have now become 'officially brucellosis-free'. In others, for example the United States, Australia, New Zealand, the western USSR, bovine brucellosis has been eradicated from most areas but persistent foci remain in some localities.

In many developing countries, brucellosis has emerged as an increasing economic and public health problem as these countries have attempted to develop their dairy industries. In some parts of the Middle East and Mediterranean region, *B. melitensis* derived from local sheep and goat populations has infected imported and highly susceptible cattle.

Epidemiology

Bovine brucellosis is usually caused by biovars of *B. abortus*, but infections caused by *B. melitensis* are common in those parts of the world where the organism is prevalent in sheep and goat populations. *B. suis* biovars can also infect cattle and isolations have been reported from China and several South American countries. In the latter situation, dye-resistant variants of *B. suis* biovar 1 were the predominant type isolated. When the disease was prevalent in the United Kingdom, *B. abortus* biovars 1, 5, 9, 2, 4, 3 and 6 were isolated in that order of frequency; biovar 1 was by far the most common, accounting for >80% of isolations. Currently, the number of isolations is small and only *B. abortus* biovar 1 has been found in recent years. The other nomen species of *Brucella* have never been indigenous to Britain.

Worldwide, *B. abortus* biovar 1 is usually the predominant biovar in cattle kept under intensive conditions. Exceptions to this were formerly Belgium and The Netherlands where *B. abortus* biovar 3 used to be the predominant type. This biovar is usually predominant in tropical countries among the indigenous cattle. *B. abortus* biovar 6 is usually the next commonest type in this situation but is often difficult to distinguish from biovar 3. The other biovars are much less common and their identification can be useful in studying the epidemiology of brucellosis within an area. Unfortunately, the tendency for one or two biovars, usually *B. abortus* biovars 1 and 3, to predominate within an area limits the value of biotyping for tracing the sources of outbreaks. Recent studies have shown that a limited number of antibiotic sensitivity profiles exist within individual biovars. As these are genetically stable they could be useful for tracing the sources of infection.

Details of the nature of the infecting organism and its likely sources are relevant to control programs. However much more extensive information is also needed on the prevalence of infected herds and of infection within herds as well as details of the geographical distribution, methods of management, size of farms, use of vaccines, availability of technical support and infrastructure and possible sources of reinfection in wild animal populations, before a program can be developed to control and ultimately eradicate the disease.

Information on prevalence can be obtained from herd tests. For dairy herds, the milk ring test gives a good indication of the distribution of infected animals and can often be followed up by cultural examination of the positive samples. This, however, is less effective when bulk tank samples from large herds are used. Serological tests on blood samples can give more useful information. The Rose Bengal plate test or the plasma ring test are very useful for screening purposes and for identifying infected herds. However, the results of these need to be confirmed by more specific tests on individual samples, such as the complement fixation test, or isolation of the organism from milk, vaginal discharges or the lymph nodes of animals sent for slaughter. The routine examination of all diagnostic material submitted for investigation of abortion in adult animals also provides a good opportunity for monitoring the prevalence of brucellosis. In beef herds the situation can be monitored by examining serum samples collected from animals in markets, using rapid tests such as the Card test or Rose Bengal plate test. A traceback system can also be employed on animals going for slaughter if these are identified at the point of origin by a tag or brand. Sera collected at slaughter can then be tested, positively reacting samples traced to the herd of origin and further testing carried out on the remainder of the herd.

Any survey to determine the prevalence of brucellosis must be carefully planned. The sample of herds examined should be representative of aspects such as herd size, breed of animals, management system and vaccine usage so that the results can be analyzed statistically. An example of such a study was that conducted in Britain by Leech and colleagues before the eradication scheme was begun.

Where relevant, attempts should also be made to assess the prevalence of the disease in other possible reservoirs of infection, including wild animals such as bison, deer, hares, foxes and rodents and in other domestic species such as sheep, goats, horses and dogs.

Sources of Infection

By far the commonest reservoir of *B. abortus* infection is cattle, which also form the commonest source of infection to clean herds. Infection is most frequently introduced into a clean herd by the purchase of an infected animal which is either pregnant, recently aborted or recently calved.

Contamination of water and food supplies is also a source of infection, for example, by discharges from infected animals and/or by spreading infected slurry on clean pasture. The practice of sharing equipment between various farms is also a potential danger, as well as vehicles proceeding from an infected farm to a clean farm. In many cases, however, it is not possible to identify the source of infection in spite of extensive enquiries.

There have been numerous reports concerning the part played by the bull in the introduction of disease into a clean herd. Following initial success in reproducing the disease experimentally in cattle by intravaginal inoculation of cultures or of infected material, it was believed that the disease could be spread by sexual transmission and that the bull was an important vector. However, subsequent studies found that the disease was not transmitted when heifers were served naturally by infected bulls. Recent work has also shown that while bulls can become infected in early life and retain the infection into adult life they are rarely responsible for the introduction or spread of the disease in cows by natural service.

While there is considerable evidence that the bull is not an important transmitter of the disease by natural service, there is also evidence that infection can be spread by means of artificial insemination using semen from an infected bull. This occurs particularly when infected semen is deposited directly into the uterus. It has been estimated that semen from an infected bull may contain between 100 and 50 000 organisms/ml, and in many cases the numbers of organisms present may not be sufficient to establish infection.

Routes of Infection

Probably the commonest route of infection is by ingestion although much of the early literature records failure to transmit the disease by this route. This may have been because the organisms become nonviable during the feeding or possibly because young calves were often used and fed on milk of reactor cows with no bacteriological proof of excretion. The use of young calves in much of this experimental work raises the whole question of the susceptibility of young calves to brucellosis and the different response which they give compared with adult animals.

Animals can be readily infected experimentally via the conjunctival sac and extensive evaluations of vaccines in cattle have been made using this route of infection. Reports indicate that more than 90% of susceptible cattle can be regularly infected in this way. *Brucella* can also penetrate both the unbroken and scarified skin.

Transmission via the teat canal has also been suggested as a route of infection but laboratory results and extensive field experience have not confirmed this as an important route. While animals can be experimentally infected following intravaginal inoculation, experimental studies and extensive field investigations using known infected bulls have shown that this is not an efficient or common route of infection. The consequences of congenital or neonatal infection of calves by *B. abortus* has received attention in recent years. It has been known for many years that newborn live calves from infected dams can contain viable brucellas in their tissues and that this could be associated with a pneumonitis. There has been controversy over the duration of infection in such calves. Extensive field experience in the control of the disease as well as smaller and more detailed investigations have shown that calves can clear themselves of infection. It has also been observed that calves fed on infected milk can excrete brucellas in their feces for up to 4 weeks after the cessation of feeding.

Recent studies in both Britain and France have confirmed that a proportion of calves born to infected dams can harbor infection and retain it into adult life. Such animals often become negative to serological tests and remain so until parturition. In at least one such case, infection was retained for at least 10 years, apparently without seroconversion.

These observations are clearly relevant to the control of the disease, and underlie the importance of undertaking repeated tests when eradicating the disease from a herd, especially when using replacement heifers born to reactor dams. The extent to which congenitally or neonatally acquired infections persist into adult life is still not known.

Bacteriological studies conducted postmortem following recent oral challenge or natural infection have often revealed infection especially in the lymph nodes draining the head and neck. When the organisms enter by the oral route they are taken up in the mandibulopharyngeal region, enter the draining lymph nodes and are then distributed throughout the rest of the body.

When the disease is introduced into a previously clean and susceptible herd it can spread rapidly, producing numerous abortions. However, not all animals become infected and this may be due, in part, to variations in the size and virulence of the challenge dose and to the greater natural resistance of some individuals. It is also possible that various strains within biovars of *B. abortus* may vary in their pathogenicity although various studies have failed to establish any connection between the biovar involved and specific herd problems. Other factors such as stocking density, management system, the introduction of new stock purchased from outside the herd, the use of vaccines and antibiotics, hygienic practices and the rate of infection, probably play the most important roles in determining the spread of brucellosis within the herd.

Course of the Disease

When brucellosis is introduced into a 'clean' herd of susceptible animals the disease may run an acute course with 50% or more of the animals aborting. The percentage of animals which abort depends in part on the percentage that are pregnant and the stage of pregnancy at the time of infection. Non-pregnant animals can also acquire the infection and in these cases the organism tends to localize in the supramammary and other lymph nodes. If these cows subsequently become pregnant, the periodic bacteremia that occurs can lead to infection of the uterus and the placenta. In these cases, therefore, a longer interval will elapse between the time of infection and subsequent abortion.

The majority of cows abort once, though some may abort twice or even three times but this is exceptional. Large numbers of organisms are excreted in the placenta and vaginal discharge after abortion and excretion may persist for some weeks although the numbers are usually much reduced at that stage. In exceptional cases, excretion may persist for 6 months or even 2 years. At the next parturition excretion may also occur in the placenta and vaginal discharge irrespective of whether parturition occurred at full term or earlier. Such animals are a serious source of danger to other animals as, having calved to term, they do not arouse suspicion.

Retention of the placenta commonly follows abortion and may lead to secondary bacterial infection. A catarrhal or purulent endometritis may occur, possibly accompanied by extensive damage to the uterus and Fallopian tubes and the formation of sterilizing adhesions. Whether or not the placenta is retained, abortion is followed by the discharge from the uterus of a brownish yellow mucopurulent material for 1 or 2 weeks.

The subsequent abortion history depends on the method of management. Where heifers are normally kept apart from the main herd, infection will only occur when they join it and abortion will take place during the second gestation. Where heifers are allowed to run with the main herd, abortions will occur in pregnant heifers. Thereafter, abortions occur as fresh susceptible animals are brought into the herd either by purchase or rearing.

Experience gained in the eradication of the disease in Britain has shown that in some cases the first evidence of infection or of breakdown occurs among the heifers. There is evidence that in some cases this has arisen from the practice of retaining and rearing heifers born of infected dams.

Some animals appear to recover from the disease as judged by the failure to recover the organism from either milk or vaginal discharges at parturition. This may also be accompanied by a decline in serum antibody titers. It is, however, impossible to predict which animals will recover and how long recovery will take, nor is it possible to guarantee that such animals will not have a subsequent recrudescence of infection.

Pathogenesis

In natural infections, *Brucella* cells enter the animal body either through the skin or through the mucosal surface of the conjunctivae, gastrointestinal, genital or respiratory tract. Precisely how penetration of these natural barriers is achieved is not known. However, once entry is gained to the tissues, the organisms are rapidly phagocytosed by various cell types. Attachment to these may be facilitated by a lectin-like substance identified on the surface of *B. abortus*. Phagocytosis is also promoted by antibodies but these will not be present in animals not previously exposed to the organism or its antigens. The subsequent fate of the brucella cells depends on the virulence of the infecting strain and the resistance of the host. Fully virulent *Brucella* strains can survive and multiply in both mononuclear and polymorphonuclear phagocytes of susceptible hosts.

Within phagocytic cells, the organisms are transported to regional lymph nodes where they produce lymphoid hyperplasia and an acute inflammatory response. From these foci of infection in lymph nodes, the infection spreads via the hematogenous route to other lymph nodes and to reticuloendothelial cells in the liver, lungs and spleen and, in the

pregnant animal, to the uterus, placenta and mammary gland. During the course of the disease, repeated incidents of bacteremia may result from release of the organisms from foci within the reticuloendothelial system. The factors promoting such incidents are not fully understood but stress and changes in hormonal status resulting from reproductive activity for example are likely to be involved.

During hematogenous dissemination, extracellular organisms are exposed to the normal antibacterial defence mechanisms of the host and probably many are trapped and killed within the organs of the reticuloendothelial system. The bactericidal action occurs in two phases, before and after phagocytosis. The prephagocytic phase involves exposure to serum factors including both specific antibodies and a nonimmunoglobulin brucellacidal protein found in normal bovine serum and the sera of normal guinea-pigs, rabbits, sheep and man but not in mouse, rat, hamster, dog or pig sera. This factor is heat and acid-labile and can be absorbed by heat-killed brucella cells or cell walls. In the immunized animal, antibodies may also play a role in removing brucella organisms from the circulation, mainly by provoking their phagocytosis. Recent studies with monoclonal antibodies have also shown that those directed towards certain epitopes can kill brucella cells directly in the presence of complement. The relevance of this to natural infection is not yet clear, however.

Following phagocytosis, the organisms may then be exposed to intracellular bactericidal processes including hydrogen peroxide and superoxide formation and halogenation by the myeloperoxidase–hydrogen peroxide–halide system, cationic proteins and digestive enzymes. However, in the case of virulent strains of *B. abortus* the initiation of intracellular bactericidal processes can be prevented by the release of bacterial virulence factors. One of these has been identified as a high molecular weight cell wall component, probably lipopolysaccharide, which can prevent the degranulation of neutrophil polymorphonuclear leukocytes. Another has been identified as a cyclic nucleotide. This also prevents degranulation of neutrophil polymorphonuclear leukocytes and activation of the myeloperoxidase system. Similar bactericidal processes occur in mononuclear phagocytes but it has yet to be shown if the same factors are involved in their inhibition by brucella cells.

While brucellosis is essentially a disease of sexually mature animals, it would be wrong to ignore the evidence that young animals are susceptible to infection although in a milder form than pregnant animals. Both the degree of dissemination in the body and the bacterial counts in various tissues have been shown to be lower after inoculation of non-pregnant ones and the degree of inflammation was also milder.

There has been much speculation as to the reasons for the predilection of *B. abortus* for the pregnant uterus and placenta. It has been estimated that the fulminating infection following experimental inoculation of pregnant heifers is confined almost entirely to the fetal cotyledons, chorion, and the purulent fetal fluids, which contain an estimated 90% of the total number of organisms found in both the maternal and the fetal tissues. This special predilection has been attributed to the presence in the placenta of *i*-erythritol which has been shown to stimulate the growth of *Brucella* both *in vitro* and *in vivo*; *i*-erythritol is preferentially utilized by *B. abortus* as an energy source and trace amounts can stimulate its intracellular growth. Parenteral administration of *i*-erythritol to guinea-pigs and calves also increases the severity of infection; *i*-erythritol is present in both the normal and infected placenta of cattle, sheep, goats and swine as well as in the seminal vesicles and testis of the males of these species. It has not been found in the human placenta or in that of rabbit, guinea pig or rat. *i*-Erythritol has also been shown to stimulate the growth of virulent strains of *B. abortus* more than that of avirulent strains.

Following abortion there is a further heavy invasion of the blood stream with organisms which is then followed by a rising blood titer. This preferential growth in the placenta leading to eventual abortion and at the same time the much more limited multiplication at other sites within the body may explain the cases where brucella organisms can be recovered from the placenta whilst maternal serum is serologically negative. Practical field experience in the diagnosis and control of the disease testifies to the need for a second serological test 14 days after abortion in order to establish a diagnosis in these cases.

The much milder nature of the disease in sexually immature heifers together with its known intracellular habitat may also explain the low or even absent serological response of these animals. During pregnancy, however, the disease is much more acute and the tremendous multiplication not only in the placenta but also in the lymph nodes leads to a more vigorous antibody response.

Although in most young animals infection is eliminated before the animal has reached sexual maturity and pregnancy, once mature animals do become infected the disease persists in most cases for the remainder of the productive life of the animal even in the face of high levels of circulating antibody.

The dissemination of *Brucella* throughout the body is indicated by the range of lymph nodes and other tissues found to be culturally positive. The udder and the supramammary, iliac and retro-pharyngeal lymph nodes are the sites most commonly infected. There seems to be no essential difference either in the persistence or the localization of infection between animals naturally or artificially infected. The rate of isolation of the organism seems to be more or less constant for a period of at least 4 years after exposure. After this period the rate of isolation declines somewhat but organisms have been observed to persist for up to 11 years.

Isolation of the organism from the uterus of infected but nonpregnant animals is unusual except in recently parturient animals; shedding of organisms in vaginal discharges can last for up to a month after parturition, although there are records of shedding for at least 2 years. Although the isolation of the organism before calving has been reported to occur infrequently, recent studies on experimental infections in pregnant and nonpregnant animals have shown that the organism could be recovered from vaginal swabs 39 days after exposure in the case of nonpregnant animals and 11 days after exposure in pregnant animals.

The high rate of isolation of the organism from the udder and the supramammary lymph nodes is reflected in the numbers excreted in milk which can vary from a few hundreds up to 200 000 organisms/ml. The numbers are said to be highest in the immediate postcalving phase and then to decline or become intermittent, although a more consistent and abundant excretion has been reported towards the end of the lactation when the milk yield was reduced. Generally, excretion appears to be less abundant in vaccinated animals that become infected and in some cases may be absent. Not all quarters of the udder excrete the organism and it is therefore essential to examine a sample of milk obtained from each of the four quarters. It has been observed that the hindquarters and especially the right hindquarter is the one most frequently infected. The organism may also be isolated from udder secretions of infected but unbred heifers.

Intermittent bacteremia is a feature of brucellosis although attempted isolation from blood is not routinely practiced partly because of the low numbers of organisms present and the intermittency of bacteremia.

Hygromas affecting both the hind and the fore-limbs are often reported especially in older infected animals and the organism has been isolated from such fluids. Hygromas seem to be especially common in tropical countries among native breeds of cattle and are usually caused by *B. abortus* biovar 3. It is not known whether their formation is a consequence of environmental conditions, peculiarities of the host or to specific properties of the infecting strain.

The pathogenesis of the disease in bulls is similar to that in the female except that the seminal vesicles and the testes are involved; the reason for the predilection in bulls is similar to that in the female, namely the presence of *i*-erythritol. Because they reach sexual maturity at an earlier age than heifers, younger bulls are believed to be more susceptible to the infection. Field experience confirms that infection can be acquired at an early age and retained into adult life. Neonatal infection can take place in bulls in the same way as in heifers.

Experimental infection of bulls has been produced by instilling large numbers of organisms into the preputial cavity but the success rate has been low. It is possible that bulls can become infected by serving cows that are still excreting the organism via the genital tract but this probably happens infrequently.

The number of organisms excreted in the semen of infected bulls varies greatly not only between bulls but between various ejaculates of the same bull; figures varying from 100 to 50 000 organisms/ml have been reported. The greatest numbers are believed to occur in the early stage of the disease, with the numbers decreasing or ceasing altogether in the later, chronic phase when the foci of infection become walled off. It is during the chronic phase that the serum titers may fall below diagnostically significant levels. In some cases, animals seem to stop excreting the organism and the serological titers may even decline to pass levels. However, the time taken for this to occur varies greatly and it is impossible to forecast.

If administered to young bulls strain 19 vaccine can persist and cause lesions both in the testicles and seminal vesicles. It is therefore inadvisable to use this vaccine on bulls. However, in circumstances in which the risk of exposure to infection is high and there is no other means available for controlling the disease, the benefits of vaccination may outweigh the risks of complications.

Pathology

In the pregnant cow the disease is essentially a necrotizing placentitis and ulcerative endometritis. The placental cotyledons are swollen, necrosed and covered with a yellowish or brownish sticky exudate which often extends into the depths of the crypts. The degree of change varies from one cotyledon to another and a minority of cotyledons may be normal. The intercotyledonary areas are frequently thickened and opaque, presenting a leathery appearance (Fig. 12.1). Large numbers of brucellas are present in the endothelial cells and chorion. Histologically, the disease is characterized by a marked leukocytic infiltration, especially with lymphocytes and plasma cells, congestion and cellular proliferation leading to necrosis. In the uterus there is an interstitial inflammation leading to a severe ulcerative endometritis.

Brucellosis does not give rise to clinical mastitis although excretion in the milk is often associated with the presence of other infections such as those caused by streptococci and staphylococci which makes studies of cell-associated changes difficult to interpret. Macroscopic changes and cell count change are not specific although an increase in mononuclear cells, limited to the infected quarters and related to a subclinical mastitis, has been reported. There are no obvious changes in the appearance of the milk although the cell counts may be increased. Histologically there may be a mild diffuse interstitial mastitis with accumulation of lymphocytes and plasma cells.

After experimental challenge there is an acute lymphadenitis in the nodes draining the site of infection. The infection spreads to the spleen and more remote lymph nodes, especially the supramammary and iliac. Infection is accompanied by considerable proliferative activity leading to hyperplasia and acute inflammation. Later, large numbers of plasma cells are formed in the medullary cords and the adjacent sinuses undergo severe catarrhal change. The picture in nonpregnant heifers is similar but milder.

The infection in the fetal lungs produces bronchopneumonia with congestion, fibrinous exudation and cellular infiltration.

Lesions in the bull are largely confined to the genital organs. The seminal vesicles and epididymines may be enlarged with areas of chronic interstitial inflammation and necrosis of the tubular epithelium of the vesicles. The epididymines contain multiple granulomas with infiltration of lymphoid, plasma and epithelioid cells surrounding giant cells; some granulomas may be calcified. In the early stages of the disease the testes may be enlarged but later they become smaller than usual because of contraction of the fibrous tissue. Basement membranes of many tubules may be thickened with evidence of suppressed spermatogenesis.

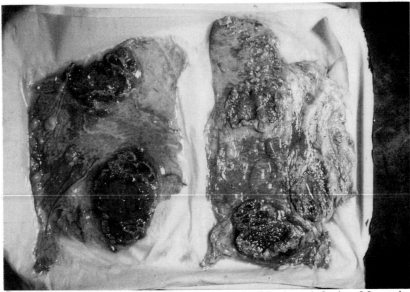

Fig. 12.1 Placenta from a cow aborting in late gestation as a result of *B. abortus* infection. Many placentomes are necrotic and partially autolyzed and the intercotyledonary membranes show areas of thickening and congestion.

Diagnosis

Often the only clinical sign of brucellosis is the occurrence of abortion and retained placenta in the pregnant female, usually during the last third of the gestation period. Disease in the male may manifest itself as orchitis, epididymitis and inflammation of the seminal vesicles. Rarely, other localizing lesions such as hygromas of large joints may develop. None of these signs is pathognomic for brucellosis, however and diagnosis has to be based on the demonstration of the causative organism or on the immune response to its antigens. In the latter case serological procedures are commonly used but methods for the demonstration of cell-mediated immunity, most frequently the intradermal test for delayed hypersensitivity are also available.

All of these procedures have their specific advantages and disadvantages and should be used complementarily to each other to overcome their limitations.

Demonstration of the Causative Organism

Cultural Examination All brucella strains are slow-growing organisms requiring a rich medium to support good growth. The products from which isolations are sought are often contaminated with fast-growing organisms which make the isolation of brucella difficult.

A number of selective media have been developed which support the growth of even fastidious strains of *B. abortus* (for example, *B. abortus* biovar 2) from a small inoculum and which control and suppress the growth of contaminating organisms. The formulae of such media are given in Appendix I (page 22).

The following principles should be observed when culturing brucellas:

1. Appropriate safety precautions should be taken. This will include the use of an efficient biohazard cabinet for handling infectious material, especially cultures. Adequately trained staff should carry out all manipulations involving infectious material. Facilities must be available for the disinfection of the working environment and for disposing of contaminated material once examination is completed.
2. The starting material should be as fresh and clean as possible.
3. Adequate numbers of plates should be inoculated.
4. The surface of the medium should be dry and therefore all plates should be incubated for 1 h with the lids partially open before use.
5. Plates should be incubated at 37 °C in an atmosphere containing 10% added CO_2. Purpose-built CO_2 incubators are now available and provide suitable conditions for growth which often occurs earlier than with the traditional methods.
6. Plates should be examined for brucella colonies after 2 or 3 days of incubation. Any suspicious-looking colonies should be preliminarily identified on the basis of their appearance, serology

Table 12.2 Staining methods for *Brucella*

Modified Ziehl–Neelsen stain	*Modified Köster stain*
1. Dry and fix smear	1. Dry and fix smear
2. Flood with dilute 3% carbol fuchsin for 10 min	2. Stain with a freshly prepared mixture of 2 parts saturated safranin* solution and 5 parts normal KOH solution, for 1 min
3. Decolorize with 0.5% acetic acid for 1–10 s	3. Wash carefully in tap water
4. Wash and counterstain with 1% methylene blue for 2 min	4. Decolorize with 0.1% solution of sulfuric acid for about 10 s
5. Wash and dry in air	5. Wash thoroughly in tap water
	6. Counterstain with 1% methylene blue solution for 2–3 s
	7. Dry in air or blot carefully
Brucella organisms stain red	Brucella organisms stain pink or red and are often in clumps within cells

*Safranin: Mix powder in distilled water and leave overnight at 37 °C to dissolve.
Saturation point 6.25 g/100 ml at 26 °C.
Potassium hydroxide (normal) 56 g/l distilled water.

and gram-staining. Subcultures can then be made for transmission to specialized laboratories for more detailed classification.

Brucella can be isolated from the following materials:

1. Fetal stomach contents collected under sterile and safe conditions, for example, with a sterile syringe and needle or evacuated blood sampling tube.
2. Other fetal tissues including the lungs, liver, spleen and, in the case of gross contamination, the brain.
3. Pieces of placental cotyledon; these should be chosen with care to avoid grossly contaminated areas and yet to choose obviously diseased ones.
4. Vaginal discharges collected with a sterile swab.
5. Colostrum or milk samples, collected as aseptically as possible and including a sample from each quarter of the udder; boric acid may be added to the sample to control the multiplication of contaminants especially if there is any delay during transit.
6. Semen samples collected as aseptically as possible.
7. Samples of tissues collected during postmortem examination, for example, pieces of udder tissue and the supramammary, iliac and retropharyngeal lymph nodes. In more detailed examinations other lymphoid tissue and samples from testes and seminal vesicles can also be examined. The collected material should be as uncontaminated as possible and is homogenized either by a mechanical homogenizer or by grinding in a mortar with sterile sand.

Biological Examination Guinea-pigs may be inoculated with suitably prepared specimens, usually either tissue homogenates, the combined cream layers and deposits from centrifuged milk samples, or semen. The inoculations are usually made by the subcutaneous route but where grossly contaminated material is to be used, it can be applied by skin scarification or by the oral route. Gas gangrene antiserum is sometimes given in an attempt to reduce mortality in guinea-pigs inoculated with contaminated samples. It is desirable to use at least pairs of guinea-pigs for each specimen. One guinea-pig of each pair is then killed 3 weeks and the other at 6 weeks after inoculation. The spleen is cultured and the serum examined for antibodies to brucella. A positive result in either case is indicative of brucellosis.

As an alternative to guinea-pigs, mice can be inoculated either intravenously or subcutaneously with samples. The mice are killed 7 days after inoculation and the spleen and liver cultured.

Examination of Stained Preparations Members of the genus *Brucella* besides being gram-negative also resist decolorization by weak acids. This observation is made use of in special staining techniques such as the modified Köster and Ziehl–Neelsen methods (Table 12.2). It should be stressed that neither method is specific for *Brucella*; the modified Ziehl–Neelsen method also gives a positive result for Q fever or chlamydial infection. Consequently a positive smear is not proof of brucella infection, neither is a negative smear proof of absence of infection. However, these techniques can be very useful in screening products of abortion and normal calving, such as placentas and stomach contents, for presumptive evidence of infection.

The presence of the organism may also be revealed by immunospecific staining with antibody labelled with an enzyme or a fluorescent dye. The organism is seen in infected cells as characteristic intracellular clumps. Numerous extracellular organisms released from disrupted cells may also be seen in smears. They often appear different morphologically from those seen in smears stained with tinctorial stains. Although immunospecific staining enables brucella organisms to be distinguished from other infectious agents, the results have to be interpreted with considerable expertise. The method therefore has few advantages over tinctorial stains for routine examination.

Serological Examination

Serological tests have been very widely used in the diagnosis of brucellosis using such diverse materials as serum, milk, whey, vaginal mucus and semen samples. These materials can be subjected to a wide variety of tests, including the agglutination test in tubes or on plates, the complement fixation test, antiglobulin test, the fluorescent antibody test, indirect hemagglutination or hemolysis tests, immunodiffusion tests, enzyme immunoassays and radioimmunoassays. Other treatments, such as heating, acidification or disulfide bond reduction may be performed in conjunction with agglutination tests to make them more specific.

Brucellosis is a disease with a long and variable incubation period and a chronic stage; furthermore the use of vaccines can affect the interpretation of tests. Therefore, numerous studies have been made to evolve tests or testing schedules that are satisfactory under all conditions, that is in the early incubative stage of the disease, in the silent chronic carrier, in vaccinated animals and those that have succumbed to field infection. Additionally, and ideally, a test should also be cheap, easy to perform, easy to interpret and capable of automation.

No serological test will detect specific antibodies if they are not present; increasing the sensitivity of a test or devising a new one of increased sensitivity while helping to solve one problem is likely to introduce others.

During eradication campaigns, when large numbers of blood samples are collected, dispatched to the laboratory and recorded, there are many opportunities for error, particularly when repeated or supplementary tests are included. The urgency of the test results must be balanced against the increased possibility of error.

In the course of the natural disease animals which have been correctly vaccinated, as well as others that have not been vaccinated, will be exposed to challenge of varying size and virulence. The different stages of gestation will particularly affect the incubation period. Some animals with a high degree of resistance exposed early in pregnancy to a low challenge dose may not show any change until parturition when cultural and smear examinations of the placenta may be positive for *Brucella* but serological tests negative. Titers may develop after parturition.

Animals exposed to infection late in pregnancy may also have an infective calving at term with titers only developing after calving. Vaccinated animals may resist infection completely although they may show an anamnestic serological response with consequent fluctuations in titers.

The use of syringes contaminated with either living or killed strain 19 vaccine may also introduce sufficient antigenic material to lead to an anamnestic response which then wanes after an interval depending on the size of the challenge dose. In some cases it has been reported that vaccination against other unrelated diseases such as leptospirosis or pasteurellosis may cause fluctuations in the titer. It has been postulated that various unidentified stress factors may also influence titers.

During the chronic stage of the disease titers demonstrated by some tests may decline. In an unknown proportion of animals it is claimed that natural clearance of the infection may occur and with the passage of time titers may reach pass levels. Lastly the use of unstandardized antigens or those standardized without reference to international preparations may give rise to apparent differences in titers.

The magnitude of the antibody response is thus not a static affair; it is influenced by both external and internal factors. Titers are almost certain to fluctuate from physiological factors and also because of the imprecision of the tests themselves.

The Serum Agglutination Test   This has been the most widely used of all available serological tests. Provided that the antigen is properly standardized against the international standard anti-*Brucella abortus* serum the serum agglutination test can play a useful part in diagnosis. As a definitive test on the infective status of an animal it has some serious shortcomings, however:

1. The test detects nonspecific agglutinins and crossreacting antibodies as well as specific antibodies arising from brucella infection and vaccination.
2. In the incubative stage of the disease the test may be the last of all the available tests to detect diagnostically significant titers.
3. After abortion the test may be the last to detect diagnostically significant titers.
4. In the chronic stage of the disease the agglutinin titers tend to wane, often becoming negative when those of some other tests remain positive.

For these reasons numerous supplementary tests have been introduced. These are often based on empirical observations and are aimed at increasing the specificity of tests during the early and late stages of the disease and differentiating reactions following vaccination from those arising from field infection. These supplementary procedures consist of subjecting serum to heat, to disulfide bond reducing agents such as mercaptoethanol, or to treatment with acid or with the acridine dye Rivanol.

An important recent modification includes the addition of EDTA disodium salt to the diluent to eliminate nonspecific agglutination caused by Fc binding reactions.

Although the serum agglutination test has the advantages of technical simplicity, reproducibility and a recognized system of international units for standardization, the disadvantages of the procedure mean that it can no longer be recommended as a primary test for brucellosis diagnosis.

The Complement Fixation Test In terms of specificity and sensitivity, this test is regarded as the most reliable of the routine diagnostic tests available for the serological diagnosis of brucellosis. It has the disadvantage of technical complexity and hence imposes a demand for skilled operatives.

It is available in numerous modifications and can be performed in tubes, perspex trays or in microtitration equipment. Automated or semiautomated procedures based on continuous flow or mechanized diluting methods are also in use. Cold or warm fixation can be used for the primary reaction between serum, antigen and complement. In the warm fixation method, the reaction mixture is usually incubated at 37 °C for 30 min. In cold fixation, the mixture is held at 4–8 °C overnight. Both types of fixation have their advantages and disadvantages:

1. Cold fixation is more sensitive, especially to IgM antibodies but is also more prone to anticomplementary activity in poor serum samples.
2. Cold fixation produces higher titers in positive samples and may give a higher overall detection rate.
3. Cold fixation is slower, inconvenient and reduces the working week by 1 day, hence fewer samples can be processed with the same resources.
4. Warm fixation is much more liable to produce prozones than cold fixation, hence several dilutions of each serum have to be tested.
5. Warm fixation is much more adaptable to a rapid turnover of samples than cold fixation.

A system of international complement fixation test units based on the second international standard for anti-*Brucella abortus* serum has been developed. In principle, this should allow greater ease of standardization of the complement fixation test and thus greater uniformity in the results obtained by different laboratories. In practice, mainly because of the numerous variables which can be introduced into the test by its many technical modifications, this has been difficult to achieve.

The complement fixation test is much more effective at detecting specific antibodies to *Brucella* than antibodies resulting from vaccination or from crossreactions induced by other organisms. It is well established that in calves vaccinated with standard doses of strain 19 the titers detected by the serum agglutination test reach their maximum in about 14–21 days and then decline, reaching pass levels (less than 100 i.u.) in most cases by 18 months of age. The titers detected by the complement fixation test however become negative much sooner, in most cases within 6 months of calfhood vaccination.

The position in adult animals exposed to field infection is somewhat the reverse in that reactions to both tests develop at approximately the same time although the complement fixation test may detect diagnostically significant levels before the serum agglutination test. As the disease becomes chronic the titers detected by the serum agglutination test tend to fall, and may even reach values less than 100 i.u. whereas titers detected by complement fixation persist at diagnostically significant levels, rarely dropping to suspect or pass levels.

The complement fixation test has therefore been accepted as a definitive test of greater value than the serum agglutination test in the early and late stages of the disease. Provided that calves are vaccinated with strain 19 between 90 and 120 days of age and tested at and beyond 18 months of age, the test can also play a useful part in differentiating vaccinal from infection titers.

Plate Agglutination Tests Following the observation that the agglutinins produced by vaccination were

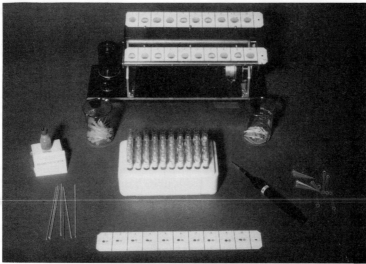

Fig. 12.2 Apparatus used for the manual Rose Bengal plate test.

more acid-labile than those following field infection, an acid antigen plate agglutination test was developed by using the antigens routinely used for the plate test but adjusting the pH to 3.6 just before use. A further development of this was the buffered brucella antigen plate test or the Rose Bengal plate test in which cells stained by the dye Rose Bengal are incorporated at a certain density in a buffer of pH 3.65 ± 0.05. At this pH the activity of IgM is much reduced and it has been shown that the immunoglobulin responsible for the greater part of the activity in the Rose Bengal plate test is IgG_1 which is also the isotype largely responsible for mediating the complement fixation test. IgG_2 also is active in the direct agglutination test but not in the complement fixation test.

In the standard procedure drops of 0.03 ml of serum are mixed with equal volumes of antigen on an enamel plate and then rocked for 4 min before reading (Fig. 12.2).

The Rose Bengal Plate Test This was introduced in Britain as an official screening test in 1970 both for the Brucellosis Incentives Scheme and for compulsory area eradication testing. Sera are initially screened with the Rose Bengal plate test. Negative sera are not normally tested further; but positive sera are then subjected to serum agglutination and complement fixation tests and the results interpreted depending on the strain 19 vaccination status of the animal. These further tests are necessary because the Rose Bengal plate test alone is believed to be oversensitive, even in herds where no infection is believed to exist. Subsequently an automated

Rose Bengal agglutination test for brucellosis was described. In this so-called ADAM system, the tests are conducted on 35 mm transparent plastic tape. The tape moves at a constant speed with the sample tubes moving in a chain alongside it. Metered volumes of antigen are dispensed from a reservoir onto the tape in discrete droplets of specific shape and size. A rotating sampling device transfers a similar volume of serum from the sample tube onto the antigen already on the tape. The section of nylon tube used for the sampling procedure is automatically discarded and a new section is used for each successive sample. This procedure eliminates any danger of carryover from one sample to another. The discrete droplets of combined serum and antigen move into an enclosed section where they are incubated and thoroughly mixed by fine jets of humidified air; so crosscontamination of samples cannot occur during the mixing procedure (Fig. 12.3).

After a predetermined period of incubation each test is scanned by a fixed optical reading system for the presence of agglutination. A narrow beam of light is passed through the center of each test and the emergent light is collected by a photomultiplier. This converts the light signal into an electrical signal which is then analyzed electronically to detect and count agglutinates larger than $10 \mu m$.

Each result is recorded on either a teletape or printer unit and includes the following information: a sample reference number, a total count of detected particles or agglutinates, the validity of the test and a colored indication as to the positive or negative status of the sample as determined by a preset

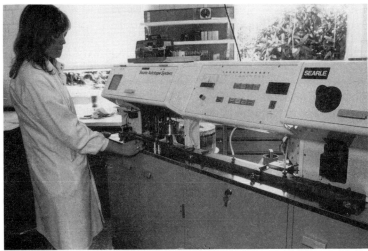

Fig. 12.3 ADAM system used at the Central Veterinary Laboratory, Weybridge for automated testing of blood samples in the Rose Bengal plate test. This system can process up to 1200 samples/h.

threshold value. A viewing screen is mounted to enable visual observation of the tests and agglutinates may be seen clearly within the penned profile. An automatic tube marking system identifies all positive samples. On completion of the test the used tape is wound up in a plastic cassette containing a suitable bactericidal agent to minimize infective risk. The system has a normal throughput rate of up to 1200 samples/h.

Disulfide Bond Reduction Tests The reducing agents mercaptoethanol or dithiothreitol are used especially when sera show anticomplementary effects to the complement fixation test. In these tests any IgM activity is destroyed by adding the disulfide bond reducing agent to the serum which is then subjected to a routine tube agglutination test. The test therefore provides presumptive evidence for the presence of IgG by comparing titers before and after treatment.

Rivanol Precipitation Tests These involve the mixing of serum diluted in distilled water with aqueous Rivanol solution to precipitate the more strongly negatively charged proteins, including IgM. IgG is largely unaffected by the procedure and after removal of excess Rivanol by absorption on activated charcoal, agglutinins of this isotype are detected by the conventional agglutination procedure. This test has been widely used in the United States and found particularly valuable for examining sera that are not suitable or accessible for testing by the complement fixation test.

Indirect Hemolysis Test An indirect hemolysis test

for bovine brucellosis has also been developed based on the observation that alkali-treated brucella lipopolysaccharide antigen can attach itself to erythrocytes. If the coated erythrocytes come into contact with the specific brucella antibody in the presence of complement then they are lysed. All the reagents can be added at the same time and prozones are said not to occur. The necessity for coating the erythrocytes daily is a disadvantage. The test is said to be unaffected by vaccination with strain 19 since animals so vaccinated would be completely negative by 8 weeks at the most after vaccination. However, titers following 45/20 vaccination remain positive longer than those from the serum agglutination or complement fixation tests.

Enzyme Immunoassay These tests generally use an antiglobulin reagent linked to an enzyme, usually peroxidase, phosphatase or urease, to detect binding of antibodies to antigen adsorbed to an immobile support—frequently a plastic microtitration tray—but tubes, beads or sheets of suitable material can be used. The binding of enzyme-labelled antiglobulin to the support via the antibody and antigen is detected by addition of a chromogenic enzyme substrate. Variations on this procedure include using an antibody adsorbed to the support to capture antigen which is then available for reaction with antibody in the test serum. An alternative approach assesses competition between antibodies in the test serum with enzyme labelled antibodies in binding to the immobilized antigen.

In all of these procedures the number of intermediate steps and hence the sensitivity and technical difficulties can be multiplied by introducing intermediate antiglobulin reagents, biotin-avidin or protein A immunoglobulin detection reagents. Enzyme immunoassays lend themselves to automation and to microvolume procedures and once developed to an adequate degree of reliability can prove at least as sensitive and specific as the complement fixation test but more economical in labor and reagents. Such an immunoassay has been adopted for routine testing of bovine serum samples in Canada in the place of the complement fixation test. Similar procedures have also received extensive evaluation in some Australian states with favorable results.

Like the radioimmunoassay, enzyme immunoassays can be readily tailored to detect specific immunoglobulin isotypes or antibodies to a range of different antigens. An alternative procedure has been used to detect *Brucella* antigen in suspected infected material and found to compare favorably with cultural methods.

Enzyme immunoassays are not entirely trouble-free, however, and they need to be applied by staff who are fully conversant with their peculiarities. *Radioimmunoassay* has been developed for diagnosis of bovine brucellosis. One test system used in Australia was specific for IgG_1 and IgG_2 but not IgM antibodies to *B. abortus*. As in the case of enzyme immunoassay the nature of the immunoglobulin isotypes detected or the specificity of the antigens used can be easily changed at will. Because of the need for radioisotope handling facilities and radiation counting equipment, radioimmunoassay has tended to be displaced by enzyme immunoassay. It does have the advantage of giving more precise quantitative assessments of antibody binding than is usually the case with enzyme based systems, however.

The radial immunodiffusion test employs an agarose gel containing brucella polysaccharide B hapten in 10% w/v sodium chloride solution to detect precipitating antibodies of the IgG_1 isotype. The test is rapid and has been claimed to differentiate animals infected with virulent strains of *B. abortus* from those vaccinated with strain 19. Subsequent studies have indicated that recently vaccinated animals may give positive reactions to this test. There is also some doubt as to the precise nature of the antigen involved in the reaction. According to one study polysaccharide B consists of a cylic polymer of 20 glucose residues and is poorly antigenic. It has been suggested that the activity of the preparations used in the radial immunodiffusion test is attributable to the presence of about 10–20% of degraded S-LPS antigen.

Differential Tests for Use on B. abortus *Strain 45/20 Vaccinates*

Immunization with *B. abortus* strain 45/20 adjuvant vaccine is likely to result in persisting, if low grade, titers of complement fixing antibodies to *B. abortus*. These antibodies cannot be distinguished from those resulting from infection in tests employing smooth *B. abortus* antigen. To overcome this problem, agglutination, complement fixation and immunodiffusion tests using antigens prepared from *B. abortus* strain 45/20 or other rough brucella strains have been devised. Several studies have shown that these tests are effective in identifying animals of unknown status which have been immunized with 45/20 vaccine. Unfortunately they do not permit the conclusion to be drawn that an animal is not also infected with virulent brucella.

The Anamnestic Test   This test is based on the principle that an animal previously exposed to smooth brucella antigens will produce an accelerated reaction, that is, an anamnestic response, on reexposure to small amounts of these antigens. As *B. abortus* strain 45/20 contains reduced proportions of antigens present in smooth strains this is generally used as the provoking antigen. The animals are blood tested before vaccination, then again about 6 weeks later, and any showing a substantial rise in titer to smooth *B. abortus* are identified as reactors and removed from the herd. This test has been used successfully in the Republic of Ireland and in some Australian states. It cannot be employed if the animals have been vaccinated with *B. abortus* S19 or other vaccine based on a smooth strain. It is essential to ensure that the batch of vaccine used does not itself contain substantial amounts of smooth antigen.

Blood Tests   Because of the cost of collecting blood samples specifically for brucellosis surveillance tests, samples collected for other purposes can be used; for example, blood plasma collected for enzootic bovine leukosis testing can be subjected to a modified ring test for the presence of brucella antibodies. In this, one drop of milk ring test antigen is added to 1 ml of known brucellosis-negative milk and 0.2 ml of blood plasma added. After mixing and incubation at 37 °C for 1 h, the test is read in the usual way. A negative result is taken to indicate freedom from infection; if a reaction occurs, a blood sample is collected and subjected to standard tests.

Another variation is to dilute the blood plasma 1/20 in phenol saline, add standard agglutinating antigen and read after overnight incubation. If agglutination occurs at this single dilution, a blood sample is collected and subjected to standard tests.

In both cases the status of the animals is determined on the results of standard serum tests.

Milk Tests The most widely used milk test for brucellosis is the milk ring test which detects brucella antibodies in milk. It is a valuable screening procedure both in the periodic testing of brucellosis-free dairy herds and in locating potentially infected herds. Churn or bulk tank samples of milk from all milking animals are tested regularly in some countries. In Britain a representative sample from all dairy herds that sell their milk to the milk marketing boards is tested every month.

The test depends on the presence of fat globule agglutinin, which causes fat globules to cluster and rise to the surface of the sample, and lipophilic brucella antibodies, belonging to the IgA and IgM isotypes. When a brucella antigen, suitably stained with, for example, hematoxylin, is added to the milk a stained antibody–antigen complex is formed. The complex adheres to the fat globules which rise to form a colored cream layer seen as a ring at the top of the tube. The following factors can affect the validity of the test:

1. Incorrect sampling causing excessive cream or insufficient cream to be present in the sample; this can be a particular problem with certain breeds and individual cows.
2. Excessive shaking which can adversely affect the creaming ability of the sample.
3. Excessive heating, for example, temperatures above 43 °C for over 5 min will lead to a marked reduction in the brucella antibody content.
4. Storage at high temperatures for long periods causes a serious loss of antibody, while samples stored at 4 °C are suitable for testing without much loss of titer for up to 2 weeks.
5. The proportion of antigen added to the milk: the standard procedure is to add one drop of stained antigen to 1 ml of milk; increasing the volume of antigen decreases the sensitivity of the test.
6. False-positive reactions may be given when milk is tested on the day of collection or by milk from cows with mastitis; the presence of colostrum or milk from cows in the drying-off period may also give a false-positive reaction.

The milk ring test can also be done on milk from individual animals using either a composite sample for each animal or a separate sample from each quarter of the udder. The samples are often screened by the test before further cultural and biological tests. A variation is the milk ring dilution test in which the test milk is diluted in samples negative to the milk ring test. Reactions occurring at dilutions of over 1/10 are likely to be caused by infection; reactions due to vaccination tend to disappear at dilutions of 1/10 or over. Crossreactions caused by antibodies to other bacteria such as *E. coli* 0:157 or *Y. enterocolitica* 0:9 can occur at high dilutions but usually will not exceed 1/10.

Milk and whey samples can be subjected to other tests such as the complement fixation, enzyme immunoassay and whey agglutination tests. The latter is less influenced than the milk ring test by nonspecific factors but is also much less sensitive. Brucella is more likely to be isolated from milk samples that are positive to the whey agglutination test but may also be recovered when this test is negative. The whey agglutination test is used as an adjunct to other tests or in cases of mastitis where a milk ring test is not possible.

Enzyme immunoassay can be employed on whole milk samples as well as whey and is now regarded as the most useful test for checking samples reacting to the milk ring test. Indeed there are indications that this test is superior to the milk ring test for herd surveillance. An IgM-specific immunoassay tends to give results closely parallel with those of the milk ring test, but an IgG_1-specific immunoassay is more sensitive at detecting infected animals and gives fewer false-positive reactions.

Tests on Vaginal Mucus Vaginal mucus may be subjected to an agglutination test to detect locally produced antibodies that are strongly indicative of infection. However, false positive reactions may be obtained, for example if strain 19 vaccine has been used recently, or where mucus is collected by means likely to cause irritation of the genital tract, such as tampons, or is mixed with blood as might occur immediately after an abortion. False-negative reactions are likely to occur if the animal is not infected in the genital tract.

Within these limitations the use of the test is indicated in the examination of 'normal' calvings in infected herds and in cases of abortion. However, in the latter case cultural examination of vaginal mucus is preferred.

Tests on Semen Agglutination tests may be performed on the seminal plasma obtained after addition of sodium azide to a semen sample followed by centrifugation to remove the spermatozoa. The test is useful in testing bulls which give persistent reactions to the serum agglutination test in excess of 30 i.u. and whose serum is anticomplementary.

Tests for Cell-mediated Immunity

Lymphocyte Stimulation Tests These consist of incubating whole blood, leukocyte or lymphocyte suspensions in tissue culture medium in the presence of antigen. Antigenic stimulation initiates lymphoblast formation which is accompanied by increased DNA, RNA and protein synthesis. Usually the process is monitored by measuring incorporation of tritiated thymidine into the lymphocyte DNA. Appropriate controls must be set up in parallel with the test system and usually include a plant mitogen to check the capacity of the lymphocytes to respond to stimulation, and antigen-free negative controls. The stimulation index is expressed as the ratio of the uptake of thymidine per unit in the presence of antigen:the uptake of thymidine per unit in the absence of antigen.

Most studies with brucella antigens have used impure or ill-defined preparations, making interpretation of the results difficult. A few studies have used purified antigens, including S-LPS and outer membrane proteins. These have shown that antigen preparations containing S-LPS are subject to interference by non-specific lymphocyte stimulation and crossreacting antigens. Tests using outer membrane proteins as antigens have not demonstrated adequate sensitivity for detecting all infected animals.

As this type of test requires freshly collected blood, radioisotope handling facilities and is difficult to standardize, it is not recommended as a routine diagnostic procedure for brucellosis.

Other Tests for Cell-mediated Immunity In vitro methods have included macrophage migration inhibition and leukocyte lysis or aggregation procedures. These are difficult to standardize and reproducible results are unlikely to be achieved when dealing with field samples. None of these procedures shows diagnostic potential at present.

Intradermal Test for Delayed Hypersensitivity This is the only type of test for detecting cell-mediated immune responses to brucella which has any diagnostic application at present. Several different types of antigen preparation have been used, all collectively described as 'brucellins'. These range from crude preparations of whole cells or culture supernatants to refined protein fractions such as 'brucellin-INRA' or acid extracts such as 'brucellin fraction F'. The purified preparations are reported not to provoke antibody responses which interfere with serological tests.

'Brucellin fraction F' is used in sheep, goats and swine but 'brucellin-INRA' is also used in cattle as well as the other species. It is administered as a dose of 100 μg contained in 0.1 ml injected into the skin of the neck. Reactions indicated by local swelling and induration are read at 24, 48 and 72 h. It is reported that the intradermal test becomes positive before serological tests in recently infected animals. However, the overall detection reaction is unlikely to exceed 70% of infected individuals and for this reason the test is best used on a herd basis. It has recently been evaluated for surveillance of beef herds in France, New Zealand and some parts of the United States, with encouraging results.

Prevention and Control

The only really effective means of eradicating bovine brucellosis is by operation of a test and slaughter policy. This has to be carried out in conjunction with effective measures for controlling the movement of animals. This is in turn dependent upon a reliable system for identifying individual cattle and for recording their movements.

Where the disease is prevalent, test and slaughter may not be a viable option for controlling the disease in the first instance. Under these circumstances intensive vaccination may be necessary to reduce the spread of infection and eventually lower the prevalence of the disease. When the latter has declined sufficiently a test and slaughter policy, operated on an area basis if necessary, can then be introduced. The factors to be considered when deciding on a vaccination and control strategy have been discussed in some detail in the section on vaccines.

Many developed countries have now eradicated bovine brucellosis or reduced its prevalence to a low level by operating such a strategy. In Britain, eradication was begun in the 1930s but was interrupted by the Second World War. The Brucellosis (Accredited Herds) Scheme was introduced in 1967 following a prolonged vaccination campaign with strain 19 vaccine introduced in 1944. This scheme was preceded by a National Survey of Brucellosis conducted between 1960 and 1962. It was succeeded by the Brucellosis Incentives Scheme in 1970 which was also voluntary but which differed in the method of compensation and in the introduction of the Rose Bengal plate test as a screening procedure. Compulsory eradication was introduced on an area basis in 1971. By the end of 1980 all parts of the country had been covered by the eradication scheme. The United Kingdom was declared 'brucellosis attested' on November 1 1981 and 'officially brucellosis-free' on October 1 1985. Currently surveillance is carried out by an annual blood test on all cattle over 12 months old except for lactating animals in which monitoring is performed by not less than four milk ring tests per year on herd milk.

Under European Economic Community regulations, the term 'officially brucellosis-free' means that brucella vaccines must not have been used in the herd within the past 3 years and all nonlactating animals over 12 months of age must have an annual blood test and give a negative result to the Rose Bengal plate test or a reaction to the serum agglutination test of less than 30 i.u. Animals giving a reaction to the serum agglutination test of up to 60 i.u. can be retained in the herd but are not acceptable for intracommunity trade. Lactating animals can be monitored by the milk ring test performed on bulk tank samples and must give a negative reaction to four tests performed not less than 2 months apart in any one year.

Detailed recommendations for designing strategies for the control of bovine and other forms of brucellosis have been made by the joint FAO/WHO Expert Committee on Brucellosis.

SHEEP AND GOATS

Brucellosis in sheep and goats is usually caused by biovars of *B. melitensis*. Occasionally, *B. abortus* infection occurs in individuals of these species but does not undergo lateral spread within the herd or flock nor is it readily transmitted between herds or flocks. *B. melitensis* infection is prevalent in the Iberian peninsula, in countries around the Mediterranean littoral, the Arabian peninsula, Iran, the Indian subcontinent, China, Mongolia, the Asian republics of the USSR and many countries in Latin America. It is also present in many African countries but the full extent is unknown. Of all the *Brucella* nomen species it is the most important in zoonotic terms, accounting for a high proportion of the more severe cases of human brucellosis.

The epidemiology, pathogenesis and pathology of *B. melitensis* infection in sheep and goats is similar to that of *B. abortus* infection in cattle. The main source of infection is infected genital discharges but excretion from the udder can be prolific for several months after parturition or abortion, and may continue intermittently for years. Sexual transmission probably occurs more frequently than in bovine brucellosis.

Most goat breeds are very susceptible to infection but there is considerable variation in the susceptibility of different breeds of sheep with some showing considerable natural resistance. Some sheep and goats can recover from infection spontaneously but

many others remain chronic carriers and reservoirs of infection for life.

In sheep flocks the abortion rates are often low, commonly between 5 and 15% although higher rates may occur. Factors that contribute to a higher incidence of infection are bad and overcrowded housing, lambing occurring over a long period of time, lack of sanitary measures and mixing of sheep and goats.

Diagnosis

The diagnosis of the disease is best based on the recovery of the causal organism from fetuses, placenta, vaginal discharge or milk. The cultural and biological methods used are those employed for bovine brucellosis. Diagnosis is often hindered by the difficulty of obtaining suitable material for examination; here the examination of vaginal swabs may be of assistance. The microscopical procedures used for demonstration of the organism in bovine abortion material can also be used for sheep and goats. Of the serological tests available, the complement fixation test is the most effective for diagnosing the disease in individual animals. The procedure used is similar to that for bovine brucellosis but the sera are usually inactivated at 62 °C for 30 min. The Rose Bengal plate test can be used as a screening test but it may be necessary to reduce the cell concentration of the antigen to achieve optimum sensitivity.

The serum agglutination test using 5% NaCl as diluent can be used on sheep and goat sera but has low sensitivity and specificity. The antiglobulin test is more effective but still may only detect 70% of infected animals.

The milk ring test has been used on sheep and goats but interpretation of results can be difficult as the milk of positive animals tends to give an agglutinate at either the top or bottom of the tube rather than a distinct ring at the top.

The intradermal test for delayed hypersensitivity is much more effective as a flock screening test. Either 'brucellin-INRA' or 'brucellin fraction F' may be used. In the former case, doses of 50 µg in 0.1 ml volumes are injected into the lower eyelid of sheep or the skin of the neck of goats. The local reactions are read after 48 h.

Animals may develop reactions as a result of active infection, exposure to infection or to vaccination, though not all infected animals give a reaction.

For these reasons, the allergic test is recommended as a flock or herd test and is of most value in nonvaccinated populations. Animals in flocks or herds with no history of exposure and with no serological reactions are usually negative to the allergic test whereas in known infected flocks a proportion of the animals will react to it. In such situations serological tests should also be done to identify the individual infected animals.

For control purposes, the removal of individual reactors from flocks or herds may not be sufficient to eradicate the disease because of the inefficiency of the diagnostic procedures in identifying all infected individuals. A further constraint is imposed by economic factors; the cost of elaborate tests can easily exceed the value of the animals, especially in less affluent countries.

Prevention and Control

Ultimately the only effective means of eradicating ovine and caprine brucellosis is by operation of a test and slaughter policy. In practice this is only operable in a situation where the disease is of low prevalence, the necessary technical resources are available and adequate funds exist for the payment of compensation for slaughtered animals. Unfortunately few of these conditions exist in most of the countries in which the disease is prevalent. The only practicable means of control in these circumstances is by vaccination.

Although various vaccines have been tried, there is general agreement that the most effective of those currently available is the *B. melitensis* Rev 1 live vaccine. This can be used at full dose level to vaccinate young animals or in reduced dose, to vaccinate sheep and goats of any age. Usually antibody titers decline within a few months but a small proportion of animals can retain the vaccine strain and develop persisting serological reactions.

With adequate application of the vaccine to the animal population at risk, the economic and zoonotic impact of the disease can be drastically reduced. Following a sustained vaccination program, a test and slaughter policy can then be applied when the prevalence of the disease has been reduced to a very low level.

In China, *B. suis* strain 2 vaccine given by the oral route has been effective in reducing the prevalence of ovine and caprine brucellosis.

A large proportion of the infections occurring in man could be prevented if adequate heat treatment was applied to sheep and goats milk used for human consumption.

Brucella ovis *Infection in Sheep*

Brucella ovis causes an infection which is of great economic importance in most of the sheep raising countries of the world. It has never been found in Britain,

however. The most serious impact of the disease is on the ram; ewes are relatively resistant and play a subsidiary role in the transmission and maintenance of the infection.

Infection is transmitted directly from ram to ram by sexual contact or indirectly via ewes contaminated with infected semen and in whom the disease may or may not become established. The disease has also been transmitted by shearing with contaminated shears. The incubation period can vary from 6 to 17 weeks before the lesions develop. For the first 1 or 2 weeks the infection remains localized to the site of entry and regional lymph nodes but later bacteremia develops and the infection spreads to distant lymph nodes, the spleen, kidneys, and throughout the genital tract.

Persistent nephritis with urinary excretion of *B. ovis* can develop in some rams but usually the most serious consequence of infection is invasion of the seminal vesicles, ampullae, testes and epididymines. The testicular lesions result in reduction in semen quality and lowered fertility.

In the ewe, the course of the disease is different. Organisms disappear from the site of entry soon after exposure, a prolonged bacteremia develops and infection appears in the genital tract at about the third month of gestation. Abortion will occur if the cumulative placental damage reaches the stage at which fetal survival cannot be maintained. However, many ewes proceed to lamb at term, in spite of heavily infected placentas. Direct ewe-to-ewe transmission of the disease following abortion is rare and the ewes play little role in maintaining *B. ovis* in the flock.

In flocks where abortion occurs, lamb yields can be reduced from 100 to 25% with further mortality of up to 16% of the lambs born alive within 6 weeks of birth.

Diagnosis

Clinical examination is of limited value as only a minority of infected rams develop the classical lesion of palpable thickening of the tail of the epididymis. Semen can be examined microscopically by immunospecific staining with labelled antibody to *B. ovis*, or by tinctorial staining with the modified Ziehl–Neelsen method.

Culture is best done on a medium containing 5–10% sheep blood or serum and the antibiotics vancomycin, colistimethate, nystatin and furadantin as selective agents. Incubation must be at 37 °C in 10% CO_2. Abortion material, milk, semen and tissues removed postmortem can all be cultured. Semen is best diluted and filtered through a 0.8 μm filter before culturing. Serological tests have to be performed with antigens prepared from *B. ovis*. The Coombs antiglobulin test and enzyme immunoassay are the most sensitive procedures, followed by the complement fixation and immunodiffusion tests. The serum agglutination test with *B. ovis* antigen, which must be stabilized at alkaline pH, is only positive during the first few weeks of infection.

Prevention and Control

B. abortus strain 19, *B. abortus* 45/20 and *B. melitensis* Rev 1 vaccines all give protection against *B. ovis* infection. The Rev 1 vaccine is probably the most effective but there is a reluctance to use it in countries in which *B. melitensis* infection is not present. Vaccines prepared from killed *B. ovis* cells have also been employed with some success.

The most effective way of eliminating the disease has been by test and slaughter of infected rams. Diagnosis on clinical examination alone is inadequate for this purpose and best results have been achieved when the *B. ovis* complement fixation test has been used. Possibly the more sensitive tests now available would improve on these results. The segregation of immature rams from the main flock and restricting the mating period to 2 months also helps to limit the spread of the disease.

PIGS

Porcine brucellosis is nearly always caused by *B. suis* biovars 1, 2 and 3 although strains of *B. abortus* and *B. melitensis* can infect pigs. Infections caused by *B. suis* biovar 1 are the most widespread and occur in the United States, parts of Central and South America, the Pacific Islands, southern China and among feral swine in Australia. Infections caused by *B. suis* biovar 2 are largely confined to Europe and tend to be maintained in wild hare (*Lepus europaeus*) populations. *B. suis* biovar 3 also has a fairly limited distribution and has been reported mainly from North America and southern China. *B. suis* has never been isolated from pigs in Britain and the disease is now rare in western European countries.

With the exception of some differences shown by biovar 2, the epidemiology, pathogenesis and pathology of the disease is similar for all biovars of *B. suis* causing porcine infection. Infection is usually acquired by ingestion of contaminated materials, including abortion products, or by sexual transmission. Hares act as a wildlife reservoir of *B. suis* biovar 2 and cause sporadic outbreaks in pig herds. Pigs of all ages, breeds and either sex are susceptible to infection. In young animals the organisms may produce an eventually self-limiting infection confined to lymph nodes, but a substantial proportion will develop bacteremia with localization in various organs including the genital tract. Bacteremia is more frequent in older pigs and localization commonly occurs in the male and female genital tract, mammary glands, bones, joints and the organs of the reticuloendothelial system.

Abscess formation is typical of *B. suis* infection but biovar 2 can also produce miliary lesions, consisting of discrete whitish-yellow nodules up to 10 mm in diameter in the testis, seminal vesicles and endometrium. Adjacent nodules may fuse producing extensive destructive lesions.

B. suis infection may produce no overt clinical signs and some animals recover spontaneously. In others abortion, orchitis, male and female infertility and sometimes posterior paralysis and lameness are the sequel to infection.

The first indication that the disease exists in a herd is often abortion, usually between the 4th and 12th weeks of gestation. Because of the individual placentation not all fetuses in a litter are necessarily aborted; pregnancy may go to term with the birth of stillborn, weak or normal piglets.

In sexually mature female pigs, the consequences of infection depend on the stage of gestation when exposure occurred. For example, when infection follows service by an infected boar there is no interference with fertilization or early attachment, but abortion occurs relatively early in pregnancy at around the 3rd week. Such early abortions are not always accompanied by vaginal discharges and may be overlooked. When exposure occurs after pregnancy has started but before the 3rd month, abortion can again occur at about 33 days after infection. If exposure occurs late in pregnancy, normal full-term litters may be born or the litters may contain mummified fetuses or stillborn or weak piglets. Late abortions are accompanied by copious bloody or purulent infected vaginal discharges and the placenta may be retained. Aborted placentas are usually edematous, covered with a yellow or brownish exudate and may show diffuse or focal hemorrhages.

When infected females are rebred, fertilization may fail to occur or the fetuses may die very early because of the unsuitable uterine environment. Many female pigs recover after a period of sexual rest and then conceive normally but in some the disease may persist indefinitely, providing a reservoir of infection.

Infected boars can develop an orchitis with very enlarged testicles, which is often followed by atrophy with infection in the epididymines, seminal vesicles, prostate and accessory glands. Fertility is usually reduced and the boar may become impotent. Bone involvement frequently occurs in both sexes, occasionally associated with lameness. In small self-contained herds the disease is often self-limiting but in larger herds it becomes endemic and persists in a mild form for long periods.

Diagnosis

Culture of abortion material, discharges, tissues collected postmortem, milk and semen can be done using media suitable for the isolation of *B. abortus*. Direct microscopical examination is also useful if suitable material is available.

Serological diagnosis presents difficulties in individual pigs as no single test can be relied upon to detect infected animals. The serum agglutination test has been widely used but is insensitive and also susceptible to interference by nonspecific agglutinins and crossreacting antibodies which can occur frequently in porcine sera. Buffered brucella antigen tests such as the Rose Bengal plate test are more effective and probably the most practicable method for examining large numbers of sera.

The complement fixation test has not proved as reliable for the diagnosis of brucellosis in pigs as it has been in other species. Enzyme immunoassay and the Coombs antiglobulin test have shown greater sensitivity in experimental studies but still did not detect all infected animals.

The intradermal test for delayed hypersensitivity has given good results and may be the best test for both individual and herd diagnosis.

Prevention and Control

Until recently no effective vaccine was available. The *B. suis* strain 2 vaccine developed in China is reported to protect pigs against infection by most routes but not natural service. The efficacy of this vaccine in controlling infection under field conditions remains to be established.

Porcine brucellosis can only be effectively controlled by a test and slaughter policy. This has been successful in drastically reducing the prevalence of the disease in the United States and in eradicating it from some countries, such as Denmark, Czechoslovakia. Several strategies can be used, including:

1. Slaughter of the entire herd, the most effective method.
2. Slaughter of adult swine and retention of weaning pigs as breeding stock; this requires an elaborate system of testing and isolation and because of the limitations of diagnostic tests, is very liable to failure. Embryo transfer is a much safer method of preserving valuable blood lines.
3. Repeated serological testing of the herd, with removal of reactors. This is only likely to be successful when the prevalence of infection is low.

Within the herd, the spread of infection can be limited by hygienic methods, including the segregation of sows in separate farrowing pens and the careful disposal of cyetic products. Any animals with reproductive disease should be slaughtered without delay. New stock should not be imported from herds of unknown testing status and boars should not be shared between farms.

As *B. suis*, particularly biovars 1 and 3, is readily transmissible to man and can cause a severe, often insidious disease great care needs to be observed in the handling and slaughter of infected pigs.

DOGS

Dogs and wild Canidae, including foxes and wolves, are susceptible to infection with *B. abortus*, *B. melitensis* and *B. suis*. This can produce a variety of clinical manifestations including abortion, orchitis, epididymitis, lymphadenopathy and arthritis. The organisms may also be excreted in the urine, and in the vaginal discharges of infected bitches. In such circumstances, infected animals can transmit the disease to other species including man although such incidents are uncommon. Both wild and domesticated Canidae can also play a mechanical role in transmission by carrying aborted fetuses or placentas from one farm to another.

In 1966, an organism subsequently designated *B. canis* was isolated from cases of abortion in beagles in the United States. This infection shows a strong host-specificity for the dog which has been attributed to the presence of a specific factor in canine serum; infection does not occur in other species with the exception of occasional transmission to man. It is now known to be very widespread and has been found in many European countries, North and South America and some Asian countries including China, India, Japan and the Philippines. Culturally confirmed cases have not been recorded in Britain, Australia or New Zealand. There is no breed specificity although all of the earlier cases were identified in beagles.

The disease is usually manifested as abortion or infertility in bitches and as epididymitis with scrotal dermatitis in male dogs but inapparent infections are common. Abortion usually occurs between 45 and 55 days of gestation but may be earlier. There is prolific shedding of brucella organisms in the placenta and the vaginal discharge and the latter may remain culturally positive for weeks. Other clinical manifestations are variable. A local or generalized lymphadenopathy may be present, and complications involving various organ systems including the eyes, limb joints and vertebrae have been described. A persistent, often afebrile, bacteremia occurs during the first 2 years of infection but tends to become intermittent later.

Infection occurs by ingestion or mucosal contamination by infected discharges following an abortion and by the venereal route. Infected males excrete the organism in the semen but this tends to be intermittent more than 1 or 2 months after initial infection. The semen is usually grossly abnormal and contains leukocytes and aggregated spermatozoa. Antispermatozoal autoantibodies have been implicated in the pathogenesis of infertility in the male.

Dogs may recover spontaneously from the infection after one or more years or may remain infected indefinitely.

Diagnosis

The clinical picture is not usually sufficiently distinctive to permit diagnosis on the basis of this alone. The most definitive method is by isolation of the organism. This will grow on good quality peptone-based media or on blood or serum agar. Isolations can usually be made from placenta, aborted fetal tissues or vaginal discharge. Blood culture is also often successful during the first 2 years of infection. Isolation from semen is less reliable once the acute stage of infection has passed. Microscopical examination can also be used to detect the organism in smears of placenta or discharges.

Various serological tests are available for *B. canis* infection. Unlike infections caused by *B. abortus*, *B. melitensis* or *B. suis*, serological tests for antibodies to *B. canis* must employ antigens prepared from this organism or *B. ovis*. The latter is sometimes used for the preparation of agglutinating antigens as it is easier to prepare stable suspensions of *B. ovis* than of *B. canis*.

A slide agglutination test using Rose Bengal-stained *B. canis* or *B. ovis* cells buffered at pH 7 or higher is useful for screening. A high proportion of false-positive reactions are encountered to this test, however, but many of these can be eliminated by raising the pH of the suspending buffer to 8.9 or by adding 2-mercaptoethanol to the sera before test.

Various modifications of the tube agglutination test are available. Currently, there is no agreement on the standardization of these, although an international standard for antiserum to *B. canis* has been proposed and should help to reduce discrepancies between different laboratories. In Britain, the tube agglutination test antigen is buffered at pH 8.9 to reduce the effect of nonspecific agglutinins and problems with hemolyzed serum samples. In the United States, a modified 2-mercaptoethanol agglutination test is used and is reported to give much more specific results than the unmodified agglutination test. Other tests have also been developed, including complement fixation, immunodiffusion, antiglobulin and immunoassay, but are not in general use.

Prevention and Control

Many attempts have been made to develop a vaccine, including the selection of attenuated mucoid-reduced variants of *B. canis*. None of these has proved effective. Various attempts have also been made to develop treatment regimens, with limited success. The most successful of these used minocycline at a dosage of 27.5 mg/kg plus streptomycin at 22 mg/kg twice daily for 2 weeks but even this did not produce bacteriological cure of all the animals tested.

Control is best achieved by testing females which abort or fail to conceive and males with genital disease. Any giving positive cultures should be destroyed. It is also advisable to eliminate reactors to serological tests when there are clinical grounds for suspecting the presence of the disease.

In kennels, it is advisable to continue testing until at least 3 monthly tests on all dogs have given negative results. New animals should not be admitted to kennels until they have given negative results to two tests 30 days apart.

Some countries now require a negative serological test result for *B. canis* as a condition of importation for dogs.

HORSES

B. abortus and less frequently *B. melitensis* and *B. suis* can cause infection in horses. In many animals the only indication of this is seroconversion but in some chronic complications may develop. These include arthritis, bursitis which may develop into the 'fistulous withers' or 'poll evil' syndromes, osteomyelitis and tenosynovitis. Abortion and infertility have also been reported as occasional consequences of equine brucellosis.

In an experimental study conducted at the Central Veterinary Laboratory, Weybridge, the only clinical manifestation of infection with *B. abortus* was a mild pyrexia during the early stages, accompanied by an intermittent bacteremia. Focal granulomata were detected in the lungs, liver, testes and synovial membranes of some of the horses but clinically apparent lesions did not develop. Infected mares given natural service became pregnant and produced normal foals at full term. Brucella organisms were not recovered from the excreta or cyetic products of any of the infected horses and pregnant cattle kept in contact with them did not become infected.

Diagnosis is by isolation of the organism from local lesions or by the use of serological procedures. The serum agglutination test, Rose Bengal plate test, immunodiffission test, complement fixation and antiglobulin methods can be used on horse sera. The antiglobulin test is evidently the most sensitive and specific for detecting chronic infection. Agglutination procedures detect antibodies produced during the early stages of infection but are less reliable later on. Furthermore, nonspecific agglutinins for *B. abortus* are common in equine sera.

The current indications are that horses are relatively resistant to brucella infection and present a minimal hazard to other species. The sources of infection for horses are invariably infected animals of other species, usually cattle. Thus the control of equine brucellosis is dependent upon the elimination of the disease from the normal host species. Treatment is sometimes required for the late complications of equine brucellosis. Vaccine therapy, using killed suspensions of *B. abortus*, has been used in the past. Subjective reports have indicated success with this treatment but objective evaluation has been lacking. The vaccine is no longer available in the United Kingdom and the current approach is to use antibiotic therapy in conjunction with surgical procedure, if required.

Complementary References

Alton, G. G. & Elberg, S. S. (1967) Rev 1 *Brucella melitensis* vaccine: a review of ten years of study. *Vet. Bull.*, **37**, 793–800.

Alton, G. G., Jones, L. M. & Pietz, D. E. (1975) *Laboratory Techniques in Brucellosis*, 2nd edn. Geneva: World Health Organization.

Brinley Morgan, W. J. (1982) *Brucella abortus*. In *Handbuch der bakteriellen Infektionen bei Tieren*, Vol. IV, eds H. Blobel & T. Schliesser, pp. 53–213. Jena: VEB Gustav Fischer Verlag.

Carmichael, L. E. & Kenney, R. M. (1968) Canine abortion caused by *Brucella canis*. *J. Amer. Vet. Med. Assoc.*, **152**, 605–616.

Corbel, M. J., Braceweell, C. D., Thomas, E. L. & Gill, K. P. W. (1971) Techniques in the identification and classification of *Brucella* species. In *Identification Methods for Microbiologists*, 2nd edn, eds F. A. Skinner and D. W. Lovelock. *Soc. Appl. Bacteriol. Tech. Ser. No. 14*, pp. 71–122. London: Academic Press.

Corbel, M. J. & Brinley Morgan, W. J. (1984) Genus *Brucella* Meyer and Shaw 1920, 173. In *Bergey's Manual of Systematic Bacteriology*, Vol. 1, eds N. R. Krieg & J. G. Holt, pp. 377–388. Baltimore: Williams & Wilkins.

Corbel, M. J., Gill, K. P. W. & Redwood, D. W. (1979) *Diagnostic Procedures for Non-smooth Brucella Strains*. London: Ministry of Agriculture, Fisheries & Food.

Crawford, R. P. & Hidalgo, R. J. (eds) (1977) *Bovine Brucellosis: International Symposium*. Texas: A & M University.

Elberg, S. S. (1981) Rev 1. *Brucella melitensis* vaccine. Part II. 1968–1980. *Vet. Bull.*, **51**, 67–73.

Hellmann, E. (1982) *Brucella melitensis*. In *Handbuch der bakteriellen Infektionen bei Tieren*, Vol. IV, eds H. Blobel & T. Schliesser, pp. 261–292. Jena: VEB Gustav Fischer Verlag.

Howe, C. W. S., Morisset, R. & Spink, W. W. (1973) In *Non-specific Factors Influencing Host Resistance*, pp. 358–370. Basel: S. Karger.

Joint FAO/WHO Expert Committee on Brucellosis (1986) Sixth Report. *Technical Report Series No. 740*. Geneva: World Health Organization.

Hendry, D. M. F. D., Corbel, M. J., Bell, R. A. & Stack, J. A. (1985) *Brucella Antigen Production and Standardization*. London: Ministry of Agriculture, Fisheries & Food.

Leech, F. B., Vesey, M. P., MacRae W. D., Lawson, J. R., MacKinnon, D. J. & Morgan, W. J. B. (1964) *Animal Disease Survey Report, MAFF, No. 4*. London: HMSO.

MacMillan, A. P., Baskerville, A., Hambleton, P. & Corbel, M. J. (1982) Experimental *Brucella abortus* infection in the horse: observations during the three months following inoculation. *Res. Vet. Sci.*, **33**, 351–359.

MacMillan, A. P. & Cockrem, D. S. (1986) Observation on the long-term effects of *Brucella abortus* in the horse, including effects during pregnancy and lactation. *Equine Vet. J.*, **18**, 388–390.

Madden, E. (1983) *Brucellosis. A History of the Disease and its Eradication from Cattle in Great Britain*. London: Ministry of Agriculture, Fisheries & Food.

Meyer, M. E. (1982) *Brucella ovis*. In *Handbuch der bakteriellen Infektionen bei Tieren*, eds H. Blobel & T. Schliesser, Vol. IV, pp. 309–328. Jena: VEB Gustav Fischer Verlag.

Ministry of Agriculture, Fisheries & Food (1972) *Guidelines for the Control and Eradication of Brucellosis in Infected Herds*. London: Ministry of Agriculture, Fisheries & Food and Department of Agriculture and Fisheries for Scotland.

Nielsen, K. & Wright, P. F. (1984) *Enzyme Immunoassay and its Application to the Detection of Bovine Antibody to Brucella abortus*. Ottawa: Agriculture Canada.

Regamey, R. H., de Barbieri, A., Hennessen, W., Ikić, D. & Perkins, F. T. (eds) (1970) International Symposium on Brucellosis Standardization and Control of Vaccines and Reagents. Tunis, December 6–8, 1968. *Symposia Series in Immunobiological Standardization 12*, Basel: S. Karger.

Regamey, R. H., Hulse, E. C. & Valette, L. (eds) (1976) International Symposium on Brucellosis (11). Rabat, Morocco, June 2–4 1975. *Developments in Biological Standardization 31*. Basel: S. Karger.

Thimm, B. M. (1982) *Brucellosis: Distribution in Man, Domestic and Wild Animals*, Berlin: Springer-Verlag.

Valette, L. & Hennessen, W. (1984) IIIrd International Symposium on Brucellosis, Algiers, April 18–20 1983. *Developments in Biological Standardization 56*. Basel: S. Karger.

Verger, J. M. and Plommet, M. (1985) *Brucella melitensis*. Dordrecht: Martinus Nijhoff, Publishers for the Commission of the European Communities.

Weber, A. (1982) *Brucella canis*. In *Handbuch der bakteriellen Infektionen bei Tieren*, eds H. Blobel & T. Schliesser, Vol. IV, pp. 329–369. Jena: VEB Gustav Fischer Verlag.

Wundt, W. (1982) *Brucellose des Menschen*. In *Handbuch der bakteriellen Infektionen bei Tieren*, eds H. Blobel & T. Schliesser, Vol. IV, pp. 408–465. Jena: VEB Gustav Fischer Verlag.

Xie, X. (1986) Orally administrable brucellosis vaccine: *Brucella suis* strain 2 vaccine. *Vaccine*, **4**, 212–216.

APPENDIX I: RECOMMENDED MEDIA FOR THE SELECTIVE ISOLATION OF *BRUCELLA*

Basal Medium

'Oxoid' blood agar base No. 2 40 g.
Distilled water to 1 l.
Stand for 10 min, gently heat to dissolve.
Autoclave at 121 °C for 15 min.
Cool to 56 °C in a water bath.
Add
50 ml sterile equine serum inactivated at 56 °C for 30 min.
40 ml of a 25% (w/v) solution of dextrose that has been sterilized at 105 °C for 15 min.

Serum Dextrose and Antibiotic Medium (Modified After Morgan)

To the serum dextrose agar medium add:

12.5 ml bacitracin solution containing 2000 i.u./ml
1.2 ml polymyxin B solution containing 5000 i.u./ml
10.0 ml cycloheximide solution containing 10 000 μg/ml.

Mix well and pour plates.

Farrell's Medium

To the serum dextrose basal medium add:

12.5 ml 2000 i.u./ml bacitracin solution
5.0 ml 5000 i.u./ml polymyxin B solution
5.0 ml 10 000 μg/ml cycloheximide solution
0.4 ml 50 000 μg/ml vancomycin solution
1.0 ml 5000 μg/ml nalidixic acid solution in 0.5 N NaOH
2.0 ml 50 000 i.u./ml nystatin solution.

Thoroughly mix. Pour plates.

Vancomycin–Colistimethate–Nystatin–Furadantin (VCNF) Medium

This is prepared from serum dextrose agar basal medium with the serum content increased to 10% v/v. The medium is made selective by adding the reconstituted contents of one ampoule of VCN inhibitor (Baltimore Biological Laboratories) containing vancomycin 3 mg, colistimethate sodium 7.5 mg and nystatin 12 500 units to 1 l of molten basal medium at 56 °C. This is followed by 1 ml of 1% w/v Furadantin in 0.1 N NaOH. Thoroughly mix. Pour plates.

Modified Brodie and Sinton's Liquid Medium

'Oxoid' tryptone soya broth	30 g
Distilled water	1000 ml
Sterile equine serum inactivated at 56 °C for 30 min	50 ml
Amphotericin B	1 mg
Bacitracin	25 mg
Cycloheximide	100 mg
D-Cycloserine	100 mg
Nalidixic acid	5 mg
Polymyxin B sulphate	6 mg
Vancomycin	20 mg

The basal medium is prepared by dissolving the tryptone soya broth powder in distilled water and autoclaving at 121 °C for 15 min. When cool, the sterile horse serum is added aseptically, followed by the antibiotics. The medium is dispensed in 5 or 10 ml volumes. Between 0.5 ml and 2 ml of sample is added to each bottle of medium which is then incubated in air plus 10% v/v CO_2 at 37 °C. Subcultures are made onto solid selective medium every few days.

Serum dextrose agar is suitable for the isolation of *Brucella* from uncontaminated materials. For potentially contaminated material one of the selective media is to be preferred. Farrell's medium is the most selective and is generally suitable for *B. abortus*, *B. melitensis* and *B. suis*, but may be too inhibitory for *B. canis* and *B. ovis* and fastidious strains of the other species. It may be combined with modified Brodie and Sinton's liquid medium in a two-phase Castañeda system or the liquid medium can be used for enrichment before plating on to Farrell's medium. VCNF medium is suitable for isolation of *B. ovis* and either this or serum dextrose and antibiotic medium can be used for *B. canis*.

13

Campylobacters

K. P. LANDER

Campylobacters have been recognized as causes of reproductive loss in sheep since 1909, and in cattle since 1913. The bacteria were originally included in the genus *Vibrio* but in 1963 the microaerophilic 'animal vibrios' were given their own generic name of *Campylobacter*. The recent discovery of the importance of some campylobacters as causes of human enteritis has stimulated a revival in interest in the whole genus resulting in, among other things, greatly improved diagnostic techniques and a welcome clarification of their taxonomy.

MORPHOLOGY AND ETIOLOGY

Campylobacters are slender, gram-negative, spirally curved rods, 0.2–0.8 µm in diameter and 0.5–8.0 µm in length. Rods may have one or more spirals or may appear s-shaped or as 'gull-wings' (Fig. 13.1). In older cultures the *C. fetus* group tends to form long filaments while the *C. jejuni* group may become predominantly coccoid. Campylobacters have a rapid, darting motility. The organisms are microaerophilic requiring an oxygen concentration

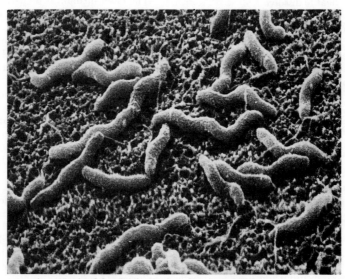

Fig. 13.1 Scanning electronmicrograph of *Campylobacter fetus fetus* (× 16 000).

Table 13.1 *Campylobacter* biotyping tests

	C. fetus fetus	C. fetus venerealis	C. fetus venerealis biotype intermedius	C. jejuni	C. cryaerophila	C. sputorum bubulus
Catalase production	+	+	+	+	+	−
Growth in air	−	−	−	−	+	−
Growth at 25 °C	+	+	+	−	+	d
Growth at 43 °C	−	−	−	+	−	−
Sensitivity to nalidixic acid	R	R	R	S	S	NK
Sensitivity to cephalothin	S	S	S	R	S	NK
Sensitivity to 1% glycine	R	S	S	R	d	R
H₂S production	+	−	+	+	−	+

d = Variable reaction.
R = Resistant.
S = Sensitive.
NK = Not known.

of 4–10%, and growth is improved by the addition of 10% carbon dioxide to the atmosphere. They also prefer media enriched with blood or serum, particularly for primary isolation. They are comparatively slow-growing; at 37 °C *C. fetus* takes 3 days, and *C. jejuni* 2 days, to form easily visible colonies on solid media. If the plates are damp the colonies may spread in a thin film across the plate. Various selective, enrichment and transport media have been developed for the isolation of campylobacters.

Campylobacters are remarkably unreactive in biochemical tests *in vitro*. The species are identified mainly on the basis of their ability to multiply in different growth conditions and in the presence of various inhibitory substances. Table 13.1 lists a range of such tests and shows the reactions of the six species/subspecies most likely to be found in the reproductive tracts of domestic animals.

The normal habitat of most campylobacters is the alimentary tract of animals, including birds and man; however, some are found only in the reproductive tract (for example, *C. fetus venerealis* in cattle, and *C. sputorum bubulus* in cattle and sheep). Of the organisms shown in Table 13.1, *C. sputorum bubulus* is nonpathogenic, and *C. cryaerophila*, although it has been recovered from aborted fetuses of cattle, sheep, pigs and horses and from the reproductive tracts of bulls, boars and sows, is not known to be pathogenic.

CATTLE

Two distinct syndromes of reproductive disease in cattle are associated with campylobacters—sporadic abortion, and infertility and abortion ('bovine venereal campylobacteriosis').

The former may be caused either by *C. fetus fetus* or, less commonly, by *C. jejuni*. Infection reaches the gravid uterus by hematogenous spread from the intestine. The condition is not common and rarely occurs in outbreaks.

Of much greater economic importance is the syndrome of venereal campylobacteriosis, caused by *C. fetus venerealis* or *C. fetus venerealis* biotype *intermedius*. The disease is characterized by temporary infertility in susceptible females, and occasional abortions. Transmission of infection is almost exclusively by the venereal route with bulls acting as healthy carriers; however, it is possible for infection to be spread indirectly between bulls via contaminated bedding, equipment or teaser animals. There is no doubt that, before the introduction of strict control measures including the antibiotic treatment of semen, artificial insemination (AI) using semen from infected bulls was responsible for much spread of campylobacteriosis. Nowadays, in contrast, AI using semen from a 'clean' bull is one of the most widely used methods for prevention and control of the disease.

Infection in the cow leads initially to mild inflammation of the cervix, endometrium and, sometimes, the oviducts. This may result in failure of implantation or early embryonic death; consequently there may be either regular or irregular returns to service. If the embryo survives, the placenta may become infected resulting in abortion, which occurs most frequently at 4–6 months of gestation but can be at any stage of pregnancy. Only rarely is infection in the nonpregnant female accompanied by overt vulval discharge.

Infection is cleared progressively from the oviducts, uterus, cervix and vagina, usually over a period of about 6–9 months. This spontaneous self-cure results in a return to normal fertility although some healthy cows may remain vaginal carriers for 2 years or more. A few cows develop chronic salpingitis causing permanent sterility. Recovered cows are usually resistant to reinfection but this immunity may wear off after several years.

The site of infection in bulls is the mucosa of the prepuce and penis, with the greatest concentration of organisms occurring at the fornix. There is little or no inflammatory reaction and neither the quality of the semen nor the libido is affected. Infection in untreated bulls, particularly those over 5 years of age, is usually lifelong.

Diagnosis

A herd history of poor fertility in susceptible females, with regular and irregular returns to service, should suggest the possibility of venereal campylobacteriosis. In newly infected herds the susceptible stock includes all breeding females, but in herds with long-established infection only the replacement stock will be fully susceptible. In analyzing the breeding history of a herd, accurate records are of great importance, but even with good records a confusing picture may be presented, especially if the herd has several bulls not all of which are infected, or, as commonly occurs, the herd management uses a combination of AI and natural service.

While a herd history may be suggestive of campylobacteriosis a definite diagnosis can be obtained only by laboratory tests. Although indirect tests are available the only unequivocal method at present is to isolate and identify the causal organism. Accurate identification of the organism is necessary because, as already stated, other species and subspecies of *Campylobacter* may be found in the reproductive tract and in aborted fetuses. The one most likely to be confused with *C. fetus venerealis* is the intestinal subspecies, *C. fetus fetus*, which can cause sporadic abortions and can colonize the bovine prepuce or vagina for periods of several months but is said not to cause infertility. Therefore the identity of an isolate will have considerable bearing on the choice of control measures.

Laboratory diagnosis can be made from samples taken from aborted fetuses, cows or bulls.

The Fetus

Routine examination of aborted fetuses should include gram-stained smears of stomach content and cotyledons, wet smears of stomach content (for detecting the characteristic motility of campylobacters) and bacteriological culture, using selective media and a microaerobic atmosphere, of cotyledons, stomach content, lung, liver and spleen. If the fetus is disembowelled or autolyzed the brain can be used for culture.

The Cow

Cervicovaginal mucus is examined for the presence of *C. fetus* or of specific antibodies to it. Mucus samples can be collected by suction, by tampons or, more effectively, by lavage of the vagina.

In recently infected and recently aborted cows *C. fetus* is usually present in mucus in sufficient numbers to allow for detection by direct culture. As the number of organisms declines it may be necessary to use an enrichment technique. As more laboratories become familiar with the techniques of *Campylobacter* isolation it is likely that the value of culture of vaginal mucus, as a method of diagnosis of this infection, will increasingly be recognized.

An alternative method of diagnosis is to demonstrate specific antibodies to *C. fetus* in the vaginal mucus. For many years the vaginal mucus agglutination test (VMAT) has been used. Although very useful as a herd test it is not sufficiently reliable for individual animals because of the variable response to infection in different cows: some produce no detectable agglutinins while in others the onset and duration of production can vary widely; furthermore, samples taken at estrus often give false-negative results. It is said that the VMAT is positive in only 50% of infected cows. Consequently in herd investigations it is important to take adequate numbers of samples, for example, 10% of the herd or a minimum of ten cows. A recently developed enzyme linked immunosorbent assay (ELISA) promises to be more effective, partly because it is more sensitive and partly because it detects a wider range of antibody types than the agglutination test.

Tests for serum antibodies, in bulls as well as cows, are of limited value in the diagnosis of venereal campylobacteriosis because of the large proportion of false-negative and false-positive results.

The Bull

Diagnosis in the bull is made by demonstrating infection in the prepuce or the semen.

The most accurate method is the test-mating of the suspect bull with virgin heifers, followed by examination of the heifers for evidence of infection. The heifers can be mated by natural service or by insemination with a mixture of freshly collected undiluted semen and preputial washings; infection may then be demonstrated either by isolation of the organisms from samples of cervicovaginal mucus or cervical biopsy, or by detecting antibodies in mucus. For the former method only one heifer is needed but for the latter at least four heifers should be used.

The test-mating procedure is expensive and time-consuming. Consequently a more common practice is to conduct laboratory tests on preputial samples collected from the suspect bulls. For these the quality of the preputial samples is of crucial importance. The most widely used method for collecting preputial samples is lavage. About 30–60 ml of sterile buffered saline is infused into the preputial cavity and the prepuce is massaged vigorously for 2 min before the fluid is withdrawn. The massage should be concentrated near the area of the fornix (25–50 cm behind the preputial orifice) and must be vigorous enough to dislodge the campylobacters which are buried deep in the folds of mucosa of the prepuce and penis.

The preputial sample is then examined by a fluorescent antibody test (FAT) or by culture or, preferably, by both methods. For the FAT the sample is centrifuged at high speed (6000g) and a smear made of the deposit. The smear is fixed, then stained with a *C. fetus* antiserum conjugated to a fluorescent dye. The stained preparation is examined, using an ultraviolet light microscope, for fluorescing particles with the morphology of *C. fetus*. The FAT is unaffected by the presence of contaminants and detects live and dead organisms; however, it requires experience to read the test, it is less sensitive than culture techniques and it does not distinguish between *C. fetus fetus* and *C. fetus venerealis*.

The cultural isolation of *C. fetus* from preputial samples is not easy because the samples invariably contain large numbers of microbial contaminants and campylobacters remain viable for only 6–8 h after collection of the samples. To control the growth of the contaminants, it is necessary to use selective techniques, the most effective being a combination of selective media and filtration of the sample through a 0.65 μm membrane filter which allows the passage of the slender, motile campylobacters while retaining most of the larger contaminants. The problem of poor viability can be overcome either by processing the preputial sample within a few hours of collection or by using transport media. Two such media, one Australian and one British, have been reported to give good results; both serve also as selective and enrichment media allowing the multiplication of *C. fetus* while inhibiting the contaminants.

Diagnostic tests in bulls are more reliable than those in cows, but only if particular care is taken at all stages—in collecting the preputial sample, delivering the sample to the laboratory and having the laboratory tests done by capable and experienced personnel. Even so, at least two samples, taken not less than 3 days apart, should be tested before a negative diagnosis can be made with any confidence.

Treatment and Control

If cows are treated with a suitable antibiotic such as streptomycin, by intramuscular injection or intra-uterine infusion, the period of infection and the time to clinical recovery are sometimes reduced. However, because of the lack of certainty and the fact that most cows make a spontaneous clinical recovery, treatment is not usually recommended.

Infected bulls can be treated successfully. The preferred method is to infuse the prepuce with 100 ml of an oil-based suspension of streptomycin (2 g) and penicillin (1 million iu) on 3 consecutive days, ensuring that the suspension is well distributed through the preputial sac. If antibiotics are given by systemic routes there is a risk of reduced spermatogenesis for several weeks after administration. The success of the treatment should be checked by a sensitive diagnostic method about 30 days later. Treated bulls are almost immediately susceptible to reinfection so should not be used for natural service with possibly infected females.

The control of venereal campylobacteriosis in cattle herds is based upon withholding the use of natural service except for animals known to be free of the disease. If there is any doubt, AI with clean semen should be used. In herds known to be infected it is possible, with exceptionally careful management, to run two herds—a clean herd, built up from a nucleus of virgin heifers and known clean bulls, where natural service may be used, and a 'dirty' herd consisting of all exposed cows, where AI must be used. The dirty herd can then be phased out over the course of a few years.

In countries where vaccines are available control, and even eradication, is greatly simplified. The vaccines have given very good results in both preventing and curing infection particularly in bulls. Thus vaccination, even of bulls alone, should result in a rapid decrease in the level of infection in a herd.

It is especially important that semen used for AI should be free of campylobacter infection. In most countries precautions against infection are taken at several stages in the production of semen. For example bulls and teaser animals are thoroughly tested before being allowed into AI centers; then they are tested or treated at regular intervals (for example, half-yearly) during their stay in the center; and finally, the semen itself is diluted in semen diluent to which antibiotics have been added.

SHEEP

Campylobacters are associated with abortion in sheep all over the world. In Britain they constitute the third most common cause, after *Chlamydia* and *Toxoplasma*.

Some aspects of the epidemiology of *Campylobacter* abortion are not well understood. The outbreaks nearly always occur in flocks which have not had the disease before and which, apart sometimes from a very low rate of abortions in the following year, do not experience a similar occurrence for many more years afterwards. Venereal transmission apparently plays no part in the spread of disease; infection of the gravid uterus probably occurs by hematogenous spread from the gut. The two species of *Campylobacter* involved—*C. fetus fetus* and *C. jejuni*—are both common inhabitants of the intestines of healthy sheep. It is possible that these normal inhabitants, in certain circumstances, become virulent; it is more likely, however, that abortions follow when new strains gain entry to the flock, for example by the introduction of new sheep or by wild birds. In some outbreaks the initial abortion is followed 2–4 weeks later by an abortion storm, the index case providing a reservoir of an abortifacient strain for the rest of the flock. Experimentally, abortion can be induced fairly readily by the intravenous inoculation of pathogenic strains of *Campylobacter* into pregnant ewes but only if they are more than 90 days into gestation. So far, no laboratory tests have been devised which distinguish abortion strains from normal intestinal strains. Such differentiation would be a major step towards a better understanding of the disease and its control.

Diagnosis

The disease is characterized by abortions in the late stages of pregnancy, stillbirths and births of weakly lambs. Although losses are usually about 15–20% of the ewe flock they may reach as high as 70%.

The aborted fetuses sometimes show characteristic pale necrotic focal lesions, up to 4 cm in diameter, on the surface of the liver (Fig. 13.2). There is frequently bloodstained fluid in the abdominal and thoracic cavities. There have been occasional reports of necrotic peritonitis, pleurisy and peri-

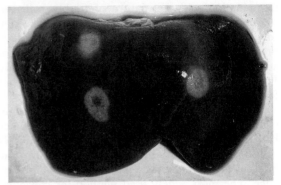

Fig. 13.2 *C. Fetus* infection. Ovine fetal liver with necrotic lesions.

carditis in the aborted fetus. The placental cotyledons may be pale and necrotic and there may be intercotyledonary foci of edema and necrosis.

Campylobacters are usually present in large numbers in the fetal stomach contents and often throughout the rest of the fetus. Laboratory examination of the fetus is similar to that recommended for the bovine fetus. If campylobacters are recovered from the placenta only, the possibility of fecal contamination being their source should be borne in mind. It should also be remembered that more than one infectious agent may be involved in an outbreak of abortions and even in the same fetus. Therefore it is wise to examine as much material as possible from each abortion outbreak.

Treatment and Control

Aborting ewes usually recover uneventfully after expelling the conceptus. Occasionally, however, they may require treatment with one of several antibiotics to which campylobacters are susceptible.

To prevent spread of infection ewes which have aborted should be isolated until all the discharges have ceased. The fetuses and membranes should be removed and, preferably, sent for laboratory diagnosis. The area in which the abortion occurred should be disinfected or fenced off.

Where an early diagnosis has been made further losses can be prevented by treating the remaining pregnant ewes either with antibiotics or by vaccination. However, although such treatments have given promising results in experimental work, the results in field outbreaks have been equivocal. If antibiotics are to be used a longacting formulation is more likely to be effective.

There is considerable evidence to suggest that ewes can acquire immunity either by natural exposure or vaccination. Commercial vaccines, where they are available, should be multivalent so as to protect against both *C. fetus fetus* and *C. jejuni*. However, because outbreaks of *Campylobacter* abortion occur so sporadically, the use of vaccines as a routine prophylactic measure may be uneconomic.

OTHER ANIMALS

There have been reports of campylobacters causing abortions in goats, pigs, dogs, mink and even humans. Because of the ubiquity of the organisms it would not be surprising if they were found as causes of sporadic abortions in yet more animals, but they are unlikely to be a cause of major economic losses. One possible exception, which merits further study, is the recently reported association between the aerotolerant *C. cryaerophila* and reproductive disorders in pigs.

Complementary References

Clark, B. L. (1971) Review of bovine vibriosis. *Aust. Vet. J.*, **47**, 103–107.

Clark, B. L. & Dufty, J. H. (1978) Isolation of *Campylobacter fetus* from bulls. *Aust. Vet. J.*, **54**, 262–263.

Garcia, M. M., Eaglesome, M. D. & Rigby, C. (1983) Campylobacters important in veterinary medicine. *Vet. Bull.*, **53**, 793–818.

Hewson, P. I., Lander, K. P. & Gill, K. P. W. (1985) Enzyme-linked immunosorbent assay for antibodies to *Campylobacter fetus* in bovine vaginal mucus. *Res. Vet. Sci.*, **38**, 41–45.

Lander, K. P. (1983) New technique for collection of vaginal mucus from cattle. *Vet. Rec.*, **112**, 570.

Lander, K. P. & Gill, K. P. W. (1985) Campylobacters. In *Isolation and Identification of Micro-organisms of Medical and Veterinary Importance*, eds C. H. Collins & J. M. Grange, pp. 123–142. Society for Applied Bacteriology Technical Series No 21. London: Academic Press.

Smibert, R. M. (1984) Campylobacter. In *Bergey's Manual of Determinative Bacteriology*, 9th edn, ed. J. G. Holt, pp. 111–118. Baltimore: Williams & Wilkins.

14

Fungal Infectious Agents

M. J. CORBEL

Fungi can produce reproductive failure in animals either as a direct result of establishing infection in the genital tract or by producing toxic metabolites (mycotoxins) *in vitro* which are subsequently ingested and absorbed.

Mycotic abortion is the most important consequence of fungal infection of the genital tract although fungi have been implicated occasionally in other syndromes such as vulvovaginitis or endometritis. Mycotoxicoses are occasionally implicated in abortion incidents, usually in association with signs of acute systemic intoxication but may also play a more subtle role in male and female infertility.

MYCOTIC ABORTION

This results from invasion of the placenta and fetal tissues by fungi, most of which are usually present in the environment or, in the case of yeasts, reside as commensals in the genital tract. Cattle are the most commonly affected species, but the disease also occurs in horses and has been reported infrequently in sheep and pigs. Mycotic abortion occurs worldwide but is most prevalent in countries of the cold temperate zone. In Britain, during a 6 year period it accounted for between 13.4% and 24.9% of diagnoses made on abortion material received at the Central Veterinary Laboratory. In the United States, between 0 and 16.4% of abortions were diagnosed as mycotic over a 25 year period; in two more recent studies the proportion ranged from 4.8 to 5.3%. In a Canadian survey 15.7% of abortions in a limited sample of dairy cows were attributed to fungal infection.

A similar prevalence has been reported in other surveys but it should be noted that wide variations occur within a country. The disease is most common in areas of high rainfall, and in Britain most of the diagnoses are made on material from the west of the country.

Causative Agents and Sources

At least 50 species of filamentous fungi and yeasts have been implicated in bovine mycotic abortion but *Aspergillus* species and several genera of mucoraceous fungi account for the majority of cases. In Britain, *Aspergillus fumigatus* accounts for about 65% of isolates, *A. nidulans*, *A. niger* and *A. terreus* for a further 10% and the mucoraceous species *Absidia corymbifera* (syn. *A. ramosa*), *Mortierella wolfii*, *Mucor pusillus* and *Rhizopus* spp., for approximately 15%. *Petriellidium boydii* (syn. *Allescheria boydii*) stat. conid. *Scedosporium apiospermum* (syn. *Monosporium apiospermum*) and miscellaneous filamentous fungi account for about half of the remaining isolates, with species of *Candida*, *Torulopsis*, *Geotrichum*, *Cryptococcus* and other yeasts accounting for about 3% of the total.

In New Zealand, *Mortierella* species, especially *M. wolfii*, account for the majority of cases diagnosed. There are indications that *Mortierella* species are more frequently implicated in other countries than the isolation reports would indicate. In New

Zealand, *M. wolfii* is frequently associated with the mycotic abortion–pneumonia syndrome.

Equine mycotic abortion has most frequently been associated with *Aspergillus* spp., especially *A. fumigatus*, and *Mucor* species but *P. boydii*, *Candida albicans*, *C. tropicalis* and *Cryptococcus laurentii* have also been implicated. The rare reports of mycotic abortion in sheep have identified *A. fumigatus* and unspecified mucoraceous fungi as the principal agents. *A. fumigatus* has also been implicated in porcine mycotic abortion, as also *Exophiala jeanselmei*, *Gliomastix* sp. and *P. boydii*.

The principal sources of infection are moldy feed, especially hay, and bedding. The fungal spore content of good quality hay is about 10^6 spores/g whereas grossly moldy material can contain $>10^{10}$ spores/g. A statistical correlation has been reported between the rainfall during the previous haymaking season and the percentage of abortions yielding aspergilli or mucoraceous fungi in the following year. *Aspergillus* infection was favored by high rainfall during June, whereas mucoraceous infection was favored by relatively low September rainfall. A more recent study conducted in Wales did not confirm this observation, however.

Mortierella spp. and *P. boydii* have been found in rotting hay and silage and abortions caused by these fungi have been associated with feeding this material.

Pathogenesis

It has not been established how the fungi responsible for mycotic abortion establish infection in the pregnant uterus. In cattle and sheep, the disease has been reproduced repeatedly by intravascular inoculation of spores and it is generally agreed that in natural infection the fungus reaches the genital tract by the hematogenous route. However, opinion is divided on the portal of entry of spores into the blood. Circumstantial evidence implicates both the respiratory and alimentary tracts but neither route has been confirmed experimentally.

There is little evidence that bovine mycotic abortion produced by the filamentous fungi results from infection ascending from the lower genital tract. However, abortions and early embryonic death associated with infection by the yeasts *Candida tropicalis* and *Acremonium kiliense* have been attributed to contaminated semen. In the mare, it has been suggested that fungal infection enters the uterus through the cervical canal during the estrus at which fertilization occurs.

Bovine placental cotyledons contain water-soluble material of low molecular weight which stimulates the growth of various fungi implicated in mycotic abortion. It is possible that this material promotes the development of these fungi *in vivo*. However, other factors are probably also involved, including the modification of local immune responses by the placenta.

Little is known about the immune mechanisms operating in mycotic abortion, although both antibody and cell-mediated responses to *A. fumigatus* antigens have been demonstrated in experimental infections in sheep and cattle. Further studies are indicated to determine whether protective immunity develops to subsequent fungal challenge, and if so the mechanisms responsible.

It is not known how fungal infection results in abortion. A toxic protein produced *in vitro* by *M. wolfii* has been characterized and toxic activity has been reported in various preparations from *A. fumigatus* but their role, if any, in mycotic abortion remains unclear.

Clinical Features

Mycotic abortion is sporadic, with usually only single animals affected at any one time. In cattle, the disease can occur at any time between the third month of gestation and full term but is most frequent in the last trimester. Similarly, in the mare, mycotic abortion usually occurs in the last 2–3 months of pregnancy. The incubation period of the natural disease is unknown; experimental studies have indicated an interval of 1–2 months between inoculation and abortion depending upon the stage of pregnancy, the size of the inoculum and the nature of the agent used.

No distinctive clinical signs precede abortion, but once this has occurred the appearance of the placenta and sometimes the fetus give an indication of the probable cause.

In the affected bovine placenta, the majority of placentomes are usually reddish-brown, swollen and necrotic with the maternal caruncles firmly adherent to the cotyledons. Central collapse is a distinctive feature, giving the placentomes a shallow cup shape. The intercotyledonary membranes are usually thickened, leathery, discolored red, brown or grayish and much less translucent than normal (Fig. 14.1). The amniotic and allantoic fluids are usually reddish-brown but not fetid.

The fetus may appear normal externally but in a minority of cases shows characteristic cutaneous lesions consisting of coin-shaped or irregular, raised plaques up to 2 cm in diameter. These may be grayish-white or erythematous and sometimes re-

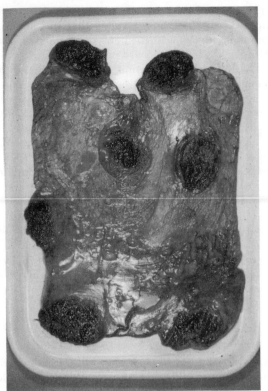

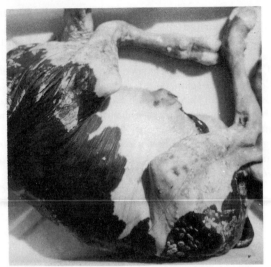

Fig. 14.2　Fetus expelled by a Friesian cow which developed mycotic placentitis caused by *Aspergillus fumigatus*. Characteristic skin lesions are present on the back and on the upper and outer surfaces of both forelimbs and hindlimbs.

Fig. 14.1　Placenta from a case of bovine mycotic abortion caused by *Aspergillus fumigatus*. Many placentomes are necrotic and show a central depression and the intercotyledonary membrane is thickened and leathery in places.

semble ringworm. They are most common on the back and sides and around the eyelids (Fig. 14.2).

In equine mycotic abortion, the chorion is frequently grossly thickened, pale grayish-yellow and fissured, especially around the cervical pole. Gross lesions in the fetus are uncommon, but small white nodules up to 5 mm in diameter are occasionally present in the lungs.

Mycotic abortion is inevitably accompanied by some degree of endometritis. This usually resolves spontaneously but secondary bacterial infection may develop, especially if part of the placenta is retained.

In the mycotic abortion–pneumonia syndrome, usually but not exclusively associated with *Mortierella* infection in cattle, the dam develops acute pneumonia accompanied by pyrexia and increasing signs of prostration 1–4 days after abortion. Death usually occurs within a few days of onset.

Laboratory Diagnosis

The most definitive diagnosis is achieved by histo-

logical examination of sections of placentome or fetal tissue fixed in neutral buffered formalin and stained by the periodic acid Schiff (PAS) light green, Gridley or Gomori–Grocott methenamine silver staining procedures. The branched septate hyphae of *Aspergillus* species, the nonseptate hyphae of mucoraceous fungi or the pseudomycelium and oval or round budding cells of yeasts are usually abundant in the exudate between caruncles and cotyledons and are readily stained by these methods. The delicate hyphae of *Mortierella* species may be difficult to identify in sections and staining with the periodic acid Schiff celestine blue method is recommended.

Fungal hyphae are usually abundant in the skin lesions of affected fetuses, particularly in infected hair follicles.

Histopathological examination is slow and not always feasible. Portions of placenta or fetal tissue can also be examined as wet mounts in 20% aqueous potassium hydroxide containing Ink Blue PP. Fungal mycelium is released from the digested tissue and the hyphae are stained blue by the dye (Fig. 14.3). A similar procedure can be used for examining the abomasal contents of aborted fetuses. The examination must be performed on freshly collected or formalin-preserved material to exclude postmortem growth of contaminating fungi.

Placenta is unlikely to give meaningful results on culture unless collected from the uterus. Culture of fetal skin lesions, lung, liver and abomasal contents

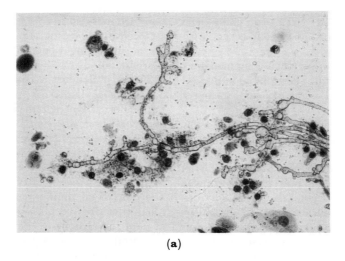

(a)

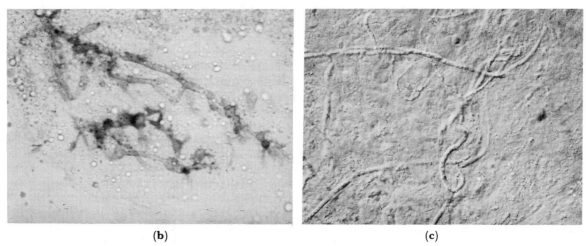

(b)   **(c)**

Fig. 14.3 (a) Fetal stomach contents from a case of bovine mycotic abortion, showing the typical branched septate hyphae of *Aspergillus fumigatus*. (20% KOH—Ink Blue PP × 1000.) (b) Alkaline digest of placental cotyledon from a case of bovine mycotic abortion caused by *Absidia corymbifera*, showing the nonseptate hyphae with terminal swellings. (20% KOH—Ink Blue PP × 1000.) (c) Fetal stomach contents from a case of bovine mycotic abortion showing the weakly stained narrow, unbranched nonseptate hyphae of *Mortierella wolfii*. (20% KOH—Ink Blue PP × 100.)

is to be preferred but must be done on fresh material. If placenta is cultured, the sample must be taken from the interior of placentomes after decontamination of the external surface. Cultures are made on malt extract agar containing 20 µg of benzyl penicillin and 40 µg of streptomycin per ml of medium. Cultures on appropriate bacteriological media incubated under aerobic and microaerophilic conditions should be set up in parallel as the gross appearance of mycotic abortion material can be indistinguishable from that resulting from some bacterial infections, including brucellosis.

Diagnostic significance should not be attached to the isolation of a fungus unless structures of similar morphology are disclosed by microscopic examination of the tissues.

Serological tests have received limited assessment in the diagnosis of mycotic abortion. Precipitins for *A. fumigatus* mycelial antigens have been detected in the sera of natural cases of mycotic abortion and in those of sheep and cattle in which mycotic placentitis was produced experimentally by intravascular injection of conidia. However, similar precipitins have also been detected in a variable proportion of nonpregnant and nonaborting pregnant cattle exposed to moldy hay. Antibodies to mycelial antigens of *P. boydii* and *M. wolfii* have also been detected in animals aborting from infection with these fungi.

Serology may be of some value as a confirmatory test in some types of mycotic abortion but at present cannot be recommended as the principal means of diagnosis.

Treatment and Control

As the disease cannot be diagnosed before abortion occurs treatment is limited to prevention of sequelae by removing retained placental tissue and administering antibiotics to eradicate persistent fungal or secondary bacterial infection. Nystatin irrigations have been used for removal of persistent fungal infections from the uterus of the mare. The newer imidazole antifungal agents may be potentially useful for systemic treatment but require clinical evaluation.

Ideally, the disease can be prevented by minimizing exposure of pregnant animals to fungal spores. In practice, this may be difficult to achieve but obviously moldy hay or silage should not be fed to pregnant animals nor should they be housed under conditions which favor exposure to high concentrations of airborne spores. In the mare, on the assumption that fungal infection of the uterus enters via the cervix, vaginal examinations should be carried out with full aseptic precautions, using the smallest speculum practicable.

MYCOTOXICOSES

Mycotoxins are produced when toxigenic fungi, usually of the genera *Aspergillus*, *Fusarium* and *Penicillium*, grow in a suitable substrate under appropriate conditions. For production in stored seeds, cereal grains and other feedstuffs a temperature between 12 and 25 °C, a relative humidity >85% and a residual moisture content exceeding 16% provide optimum conditions. These are most likely to occur in the uppermost and central portions of storage bins and the toxins may be quite localized within a batch of feed.

Abortions in cattle have followed ingestion of feed contaminated with aflatoxin B_1. In these cases, the cows have developed signs of acute intoxication resulting in death in a few days after abortion.

Aflatoxin B_1, aflatoxicol, ochratoxin and trichothecenes have also been suspected of causing reproductive failure in cattle, sheep and pigs when ingested at doses below the level required to produce acute intoxication. Aflatoxicol and zearale-

none are reported to compete with estradiol 17β for estrogen but not progestin receptors in the bovine uterus, indicating a potential for a specific effect on reproduction.

The ingestion of mycotoxin-contaminated feed has also been blamed for producing deterioration in the quality of bovine semen and reduction of spermatozoal viability *in vitro*.

Zearalenone (F-2 toxin of *Fusarium roseum* syn. *Gibberella zea*) has been consistently implicated in reproductive failure in pigs. Ingestion of feed contaminated by *F. roseum* toxins has been associated with abortions, fetal mummification, stillbirths, diminished litter size and birth of weak piglets. Ingestion of pure zearalenone at the rate of 100 ppm of diet has produced pseudopregnancy characterized by retention of corpora lutea. Dietary concentrations at half this level resulted in smaller litter sizes and low birth weights, whereas zearalenone at concentrations between 2 and 4 ppm of diet had no apparent effect on pregnancy.

Other trichothecene toxins such as deoxynivalenol and T-2 toxin may produce early embryonic loss and infertility in sows when present in the feed.

Ingestion of zearalenone by prepubertal gilts can produce signs of hyperestrogenism indicated by vulval tumescence and edema and precocious mammary development. Tenesmus is common and rectal and vaginal prolapses may occur and can result in death if not corrected. Boars exposed to zearalenone may develop preputial enlargement but effects on reproductive performance are usually minimal.

Cereal grains or meadow grass containing the sclerotia of ergot-producing fungi can produce ergotism in cattle, sheep and pigs, and reproductive failure has been attributed to this cause, although the evidence is inconclusive.

Diagnosis

Mycotoxicosis may be suspected on the basis of acute signs, for example hyperestrogenism in prepubertal gilts. The diagnosis can sometimes be confirmed by demonstration of the toxin in serum samples from the affected animals. The toxin may also be demonstrated in feed samples and toxigenic fungi may be isolated from these. However, the distribution of mycotoxin in feed samples tends to be irregular. Samples collected for mycotoxin analysis should be kept frozen if possible. The toxins are detected and identified by thin layer chromatography, gas liquid chromatography–mass spectrometry, high performance liquid chromatography, bioassay or immunoassay.

Treatment and Prevention

Treatment is by removal of the source of intoxication and by supportive measures.

Prevention is best achieved by storage of feed under conditions of low moisture content with adequate ventilation.

Complementary References

Ainsworth, G. C. & Austwick, P. K. C. (1973) *Fungal Diseases of Animals*, 2nd edn, pp. 74–80. Slough: Commonwealth Bureau of Animal Health, Farnham Royal.

Blaney, B. J., Bloomfield, R. C. & Moore, C. J. (1984) Zearalenone intoxication of pigs. *Aust. Vet. J.*, **61 (1)**, 24–27.

Blakenship, L. T., Dickey, J. F. & Bodine, A. B. (1982) *In vitro* mycotoxin binding to bovine uterine steroid hormone receptors. *Theriogenology*, **17 (3)**, 325–331.

Carter, M. E., Cordes, D. O., Di Menna, M. E. & Hunter, R. (1973). Fungi isolated from bovine mycotic abortion and pneumonia with special reference to *Mortierella wolfii*. *Res. Vet. Sci.*, **14**, 201–206.

Corbel, M. J., Day, C. A. & Cole, D. J. W. (1980) Examination of the relationship between pathological changes, immunological response and serum protein concentrations in pregnant sheep inoculated with *Aspergillus fumigatus*. *Mycopathologia*, **71**, 53–64.

Dion, W. M. & Dukes, T. W. (1979) Bovine mycotic abortion caused by *Acremonium kiliense* Grutz. *Sabouraudia*, **17**, 355–361.

Eades, S. M. & Corbel, M. J. (1973) The effect of soluble bovine placental extracts on the *in vitro* growth of fungi implicated in bovine mycotic abortion. *Proc. Soc. Gen. Microbiol.*, **1 (1)**, 27.

Eustis, S. L., Kirkbride, C. A., Gates, C. & Haley, C. D. (1981) Porcine abortions associated with fungi, actinomycetes and *Rhodococcus* sp. *Vet. Pathol.*, **18**, 608–613.

Gedek, B. (1984) Mykotoxineinflüsse auf die Trächtigkeit und Laktation der Sau. *Tierärztl. Umschau*, **39**, 461–464.

Haase, H., Lamner, P. & Feyerherd, L. (1983) Untersuchungen zur einer Spermaleistungsminderung bei Jungbullen. *Monats. Vet. Med.*, **38 (7)**, 265–268.

Knudtson, W. U., Kirkbride, C. A. & Thurston, J. R. (1975) Bovine mycotic abortion. *Proc. Amer. Assoc. Vet. Lab. Diagnost.*, October.

Long, G. G., Diekman, M. A., Tuite, J. F., Shannon, G. M. & Vesonder, R. F. (1983) Effect of *Fusarium roseum* (*Gibberella zea*) on pregnancy and the estrous cycle in gilts fed molded corn on days 7–17 post-estrus. *Vet. Res. Comm.*, **6 (3)**, 199–204.

MacDonald, S. M. & Corbel, M. J. (1981) *Mortierella wolfii* infection in cattle in Britain. *Vet. Rec.*, **109**, 419–421.

Mahaffey, L. W. & Adam, N. M. (1964) Abortions associated with mycotic lesions of the placenta in mares. *J. Amer. Vet. Assoc.*, **144**, 24–32.

Ministry of Agriculture, Fisheries & Food (1984) *Manual of Veterinary Investigation Laboratory Techniques*, 3rd edn. MAFF/ADAS Reference Book 389, vol. 1, p. 136. London: Her Majesty's Stationery Office.

Monga, D. P., Tiwari, S. C. & Prasad, S. (1983) Mycotic abortions in equines. *Mykosen*, **26 (12)**, 612–614.

Pepin, G. A. (1983) Bovine mycotic abortion. *The Veterinary Annual*, 23rd issue, 79–88.

Ray, A. C., Abbitt, B., Cotter, S. R., Murphy, M. J., Reagor, J. C., Robinson, R. M., West, J. E. & Whitford, H. W. (1986) Bovine abortion and death associated with aflatoxin-contaminated peanuts. *J. Amer. Vet. Med. Assoc.*, **118**, 1187–1188.

Ruhr, L. P., Osweiler, G. D. & Foley, C. W. (1983) Effect of the estrogenic mycotoxin zearalenone on reproductive potential in the boar. *Amer. J. Vet. Res.*, **44 (3)**, 483–485.

Shreeve, B. J., Patterson, D. S. P., Roberts, B. A. & Wrathall, A. E. (1978) Effect of mouldy feed containing zearalenone on pregnant sows. *Brit. Vet. J.*, **134**, 421–427.

Williams, B. M., Shreeve, B. J., Herbert, C. N. & Swire P. W. (1977) Bovine mycotic abortion: some epidemiological aspects. *Vet. Rec.*, **100**, 382–385.

15

Chlamydia

M. DAWSON

MORPHOLOGY AND ETIOLOGY

Chlamydiae are obligate intracellular bacteria with a unique biphasic replication cycle. The infectious form, the elementary body (EB), is spherical with a rigid cell wall and a diameter of 250–300 nm. Following entry into the parasitized host cell by an endocytosis-like mechanism, a structural, morphological and biochemical transformation of the EB occurs; its cell wall rigidity is lost and particle diameter increases fourfold. This stage, the reticulate or initial body, is metabolically active and replicates by binary fission within a membrane-bound cytoplasmic vesicle, and competes with the host cell for high energy nucleotides. Daughter cells ultimately condense into the EB phase and a new generation of infective particles are released when the vesicle ruptures.

The order Chlamydiales consists of a single family, Chlamydiaceae, with a single genus *Chlamydia*, and two species *C. trachomatis* and *C. psittaci*. The host range of *C. trachomatis* is almost entirely retricted to man whereas *C. psittaci* is probably the most ubiquitous potential pathogen in the animal kingdom and has been causally associated with a variety of diseases in many host species, including diseases of the reproductive system of domestic livestock. Attempts so far to serotype *C. psittaci* have been limited, although it has been possible to identify two serological groups of ovine isolates, using a plaque reduction neutralization assay, one consisting of abortion and enteric strains and the other of polyarthritis and conjunctivitis strains. A similar grouping has been recorded for isolates of bovine origin. Greater resolution of antigenic types is needed and should be forthcoming with the increasing application of monoclonal antibody technology.

CHLAMYDIAL REPRODUCTIVE DISEASES

Chlamydia psittaci has been isolated from genital tract disease in cattle, sheep, goats and pigs, being mainly associated with abortion in the female and seminal vesiculitis in the male.

Abortion

Sheep

The disease, known as ovine enzootic abortion (OEA) or enzootic abortion of ewes (EAE), occurs in many sheep rearing areas of the world and is particularly associated with intensive flock management practices.

Infection of susceptible ewes results not only in abortion, usually later than 100 days of gestation and typically in the last 3 weeks, but stillborn, weak or apparently normal lambs may be delivered. In flocks experiencing the disease for the first time, as many as 30% of lambings may be affected. In subsequent years the incidence falls to 10% with disease occurring mainly in the younger ewes. Evidence of a localized or extensive necrotic placentitis is usually evident on the expelled fetal membranes. Affected cotyledons are necrotic and usually covered with plugs or flakes of 'cheesey' exudate. The intercotyledonary membrane is inflamed, being opaque and edematous in the acute stages and progressing to a leathery corrugated appearance in chronically affected areas.

The contaminated lambing environment is the major source of infection for previously unexposed ewes and lambs. Infection is presumed to occur via the mucous membranes of the upper respiratory tract, eyes and orpharynx. Following experimental parenteral challenge of pregnant or nonpregnant ewes there is a brief chlamydemia during which the organism is distributed around the body, probably to the gut, and possibly to gut and uterine-associated lymphoid tissue. Other than possible fecal shedding, infection remains inapparent until late gestation, at which time chlamydiae can be recovered from uterine and placental tissue. The majority of cases of abortion occur in the lambing season after that in which infection was acquired. Ewe lambs which acquire infection in their own perinatal period may abort in their first pregnancy.

A naturally acquired immunity develops following infection. In some sheep, possibly the majority, it becomes effective shortly after exposure and is sufficient to prevent the establishment of uterine infection, or uterine replication is restricted to the extent that disease is not apparent. In more susceptible ewes, the protective immune state is not achieved until after the first affected lambing; thereafter, subsequent breeding is unaffected. Effector mechanisms contributing to immunity in chlamydial abortion are not well characterized, but probably include delayed-type hypersensitivity and neutralizing antibody.

Measures to control the disease in an affected flock should include the prompt disposal of placentas and the isolation of aborted ewes until uterine discharges have ceased, thus limiting further spread of infection. Susceptible ewes including those purchased as replacement breeding stock should be vaccinated before tupping. Where a serious problem is anticipated, for instance if there have been a few confirmed early cases, strategically timed injections of longacting oxytetracycline given to the whole flock should reduce clinical losses. Such an option is most likely to be effective in flocks where tupping was synchronized and a concentrated lambing period is expected. Injections repeated at 10–14 day intervals after 100 days of gestation have proved effective in controlling disease, but not in eliminating infection.

For previously unaffected flocks, care should be taken in the selection of female stock intended as breeding replacements. Ideally they should be purchased directly from disease-free sources, otherwise there is a significant risk of obtaining latently infected ewes destined to abort. The role of wildlife as local vectors of disease cannot be excluded and foxes or crows have been suspected of carrying infection across farm boundaries.

In Britain, an inactivated egg-derived vaccine has been available since the mid-1950s and after its introduction the disease ceased to be a significant problem for several years. However, the incidence of the disease has risen steadily in the last 10 years, and it is now the most frequently diagnosed infectious ovine fetopathy, accounting for approximately 20% of all abortion incidents investigated.

Breakdowns have occurred in vaccinated flocks. Experimental studies in sheep and mice have demonstrated that variation exists amongst recent field isolates, possibly influencing their antigenicity or virulence. One such isolate has been incorporated into the vaccine in an attempt to improve its efficacy.

That more effective control, and particularly a better vaccine, is desirable has been emphasized by the several recent well-documented cases of human fetopathy which have been attributed to ovine abortion isolates of *C. psittaci*, and have involved women attending affected sheep flocks.

Goats

As with sheep, chlamydial-induced fetopathy in goats is manifest clinically as late abortions, stillbirths or delivery of weak kids. However, there are significant differences in pathogenesis and epidemiology. The incubation period from challenge to abortion may be as short as 2 weeks, compared to at least 6 weeks in sheep. Goats which are destined to abort discharge chlamydiae in vaginal secretions for several days beforehand; sheep rarely, if ever, do so. The combined effects of a shorter incubation and early vaginal excretion contribute to a more rapid spread of infection and consequently, relative to sheep flocks, a higher proportion of the herd may be affected in an initial outbreak. Abortion rates of 25–90% have been described, and subsequently aborted goats may succumb to metritis or respiratory disease, and some may die.

Human health risks associated with caprine chlamydial abortion should also be considered, not only due to the handling of affected stock, but also through the consumption of unpasteurized milk.

Cattle

Bovine chlamydial abortions tend to be sporadic, occurring generally in the last third of pregnancy, and only occasionally as early as the last month. Retention of fetal membranes and metritis are not uncommon. The disease has been studied most extensively in the United States where epizootics have been described in hill beef herds, particularly in California. A tick vector may be involved. The placental pathology is similar to that in the ovine disease.

Pigs

Reports of chlamydial abortion in pigs are few and originate mainly from eastern Europe. Abortions tend to be late and a proportion of the litter are mummified, but some weak pigs may be born which can survive.

Diseases of the Male Genital Tract

Genital tract disease in the male, associated with chlamydial infection, is uncommon but has been described in rams and bulls, occurring mainly as seminal vesiculitis and/or epididymitis. The semen of affected bulls has a low count of poorly motile spermatozoa and cows inseminated with chlamydia-infected semen tend to return to service. Chlamydiae do not have a direct effect on the embryo because they are unable to penetrate the zona pellucida. It seems more likely that the uterine environment associated with endometrial infection is unable to support the early developing embryo.

LABORATORY DIAGNOSIS OF CHLAMYDIAL DISEASES

Progress in gaining a better understanding of the role of chlamydiae in livestock diseases has been impeded by the inadequacy of diagnostic methods.

Direct Examination of Tissue Smears

The original identification of chlamydiae as the etiological agent of ovine enzootic abortion (OEA) followed the demonstration of elementary bodies in fixed impression smears of aborted placentas which were stained by the modified Ziehl–Neelsen tech-

nique. The method is still widely applied in diagnostic laboratories, and the experienced observer can usually differentiate chlamydiae from *Coxiella burnetii*. To achieve greater specificity, increasing use is being made of immune labelling techniques, including fluorescent monoclonal antibody.

Culture Techniques

More efficient and sensitive cell culture isolation techniques are now routinely employed, whereby the inoculation is centrifuged onto tube coverslip cultures, usually of McCoy or L929 cells. A metabolic inhibitor, such as cycloheximide, is incorporated into the culture medium which blocks host cell protein synthesis, thus diverting available amino acid pools to support chlamydia replication. Coverslips are fixed at 48–72 h and examined for cytoplasmic inclusions after modified Ziehl–Neelsen, Giemsa, methylene blue or fluorescent antibody staining.

Serology

The cell wall of both chlamydial species contains a heat-stable, genus-specific, lipopolysaccharide (LPS) antigen, which is the basis of the standard complement fixation test (CFT). Aborted sheep and goats generally have high titers of complement-fixing IgG_1, and the CFT has proved to be a useful diagnostic aid when used on a group, rather than individual basis. The test has proved less satisfactory for cattle, and recent immunoblotting studies indicate that this is because the predominant antibody subclass responding to the genus specific LPS is noncomplement-fixing IgG_2. The limitations of the CFT in diagnostic chlamydial serology are becoming more evident and it is gradually being superceded by simpler and more discriminatory enzyme immunoassay techniques.

Complementary References

Aitken, I. (1986) Chlamydial abortion in sheep. *In Pract.*, **8 (6)**, 236–237.
Appleyard, W. T. (1986) Chlamydial abortion in goats. *Goat Vet. J.*, **7 (2)**, 45–47.
Perez-Martinez, J. A. & Storz, J. (1985) Chlamydial infection in cattle—part 2. *Mod. Vet. Pract.*, **66**, 603–608.
Plagemann, O. (1981) Chlamydia as a cause of abortion in sows and differential diagnosis from the SMEDI complex. *Tierarztl. Umschau*, **36 (12)**, 842–846.

16

Other Infectious Agents

T. W. A. LITTLE

LEPTOSPIROSIS

With the virtual eradication of brucellosis in many parts of the world, the role of other abortifacient agents has in some cases become clearer. This applies particularly to the leptospira which are now recognized as important causes of abortion and possibly infertility in cattle and pigs.

The leptospira are widely distributed in nature: one species, *Leptospira biflexa* occurs as a saprophyte in both fresh and sea water, and damp soil; the other major group, *L. interrogans*, is parasitic and has been isolated from a large range of both freeliving and domestic animals throughout the world. An isolate from a bull, described as *L. illini*, has been suggested to be a possible third species.

Currently, the leptospira are further classified by serological means; over 200 serovars of *L. interrogans* have been described and for convenience these have been placed in 20 antigenically related serogroups. Similarly many *L. biflexa* serovars have been identified forming over 40 serogroups.

Bacteriology

Leptospiral cells are flexible, helical rods which have 18 or more coils. They are 0.1 μm in diameter and 6 to over 12 μm in length. The unstained leptospira are not visible under bright field microscopy but are visible by dark field illumination and phase contrast microscopy. They are highly motile and the characteristic movements appear as alternating rotation along the long axis. Under the electron-microscope the leptospira have the same basic morphology as other spirochetes with two periplasmic flagella, often referred to as axial fibrils. With the exception of *L. illini* the basic bodies of the periplasmic flagella are similar to the flagella of gram-negative bacteria. In liquid media, either one or both ends of the cell are often typically hooked.

Leptospira stain very weakly with aniline dyes and only faintly with Giemsa stains. They are best stained either by a silver impregnation technique such as Warthin Starry, or by a fluorescent antibody stain or immunoperoxidase methods.

Leptospira were originally grown in simple media containing rabbit serum such as Korthof's medium, Stuart's medium or Fletcher's semisolid medium. However, many of the more fastidious serovars important in veterinary medicine such as *L. hardjo* will only grow in more complex media containing Tween 80, bovine serum albumin and various other growth promoters. The increased understanding of the nutrition of leptospira has enabled the isolation of many new serovars. Leptospira are usually grown in either liquid or semisolid media; they will, however, form discrete or sometimes diffuse subsurface colonies in media containing 1% agar.

Leptospires can pass through membrane filters of average pore size 0.22 μm. The guanine and cytosine content of their DNA is 35–41 mol%.

The initial part of the identification of a leptospiral isolate is to place it in its correct species. *L. interrogans* is usually pathogenic, and growth is usually inhibited by 8-azaguanine and does not occur at 13 °C. *L. biflexa* will grow at 13 °C and in the presence of 8-azaguanine and is not pathogenic. *L. illini* is the only leptospira able to grow in trypticase soy broth and has a GC ratio of 53 mol%.

Leptospira are further identified to the serogroup level by carrying out agglutination tests against a battery of sera selected to be representative of each of the 20 serogroups. The agglutination tests are read using a microscope with dark field illumination and the test is called the microscopic agglutination test (MAT).

Having placed a leptospira in its specific serogroup it can be further identified to the serovar level by comparison with reference cultures using the cross agglutination absorption test (CAAT), usually only performed in a reference laboratory. The test determines the antigenic structure of a leptospira by its ability to absorb antibodies from sera prepared against reference strains and similarly the ability of reference strains to absorb antibodies from sera prepared from the strain under test.

A quicker method of identification, referred to as factor analysis, is to use specifically absorbed antisera to identify specific antigens on the leptospira. However, these sera are not available commercially.

More recently, serovars have been reexamined using the restriction endonuclease analysis method. Serovars have been shown not to be homologous and the subtypes or genotypes may have important epidemiological and pathological differences. Thus two genotypes of *hardjo* have been described; the original type culture is now described as *hardjo prajitno* but its presence in Britain is rare, most strains being classed as *hardjo bovis*.

Leptospira are considered to be very fragile; while it is true they cannot tolerate desiccation or excessive sunlight, under optimum conditions of moisture, warmth and a pH near neutrality, some strains of *L. interrogans* may survive for several months; the natural habitat of *L. biflexa* is damp soil and fresh water but halophilic strains have now been isolated from sea water.

It has become increasingly obvious that most of the serovars of *L. interrogans* have a preferred or maintenance host which ensures the perpetuation of a particular serovar without the intervention of other accidental or incidental hosts; it is as important to recognize the different classes of hosts as the different serovars of leptospira in the study of the epidemiology of the infection and that these relationships may vary in different parts of the world.

The characteristics of a maintenance host in terms of leptospiral infection have been defined as follows:

1. High susceptibility of the host to the specific infection (i.e. low infective dose).
2. Relatively low pathogenicity of the organism for the host.
3. Longterm kidney infection relative to the systemic phase of infection.
4. Natural transmission within the host species.

In contrast, accidental (incidental) hosts are characterized by:
1. Low susceptibility to infection.
2. If the infection becomes established, the pathogenic effect may be severe.
3. A short renal phase.
4. Inefficient intraspecies transmission.

This has real implications for both the epidemiology and the pathogenesis of infection and is best exemplified by *L. interrogans* serovar *pomona*.

The pig provides a maintenance population for *pomona* in many parts of the world and demonstrates all the characteristics of a maintenance host. The pig can be readily infected with small numbers of leptospira and large numbers may be present in the kidney without provoking any marked cellular response. Clinical signs are minimal unless the pig is pregnant (when abortion may follow), excretion is prolonged and transmission readily takes place from one generation to the next to produce a maintenance population.

Cattle and sheep infected with *pomona* demonstrate most of the features of accidental hosts. Infection in cattle and sheep is sporadic even in situations where *pomona* infection is widespread in pigs. However, when infection occurs, a serious and sometimes fatal disease ensues. Excretion of the organism in survivors only lasts a few weeks and transmission to other cattle and sheep appears to be rare; the infection does not persist in these populations.

Pathogenesis

Although the most important natural route of infection has not been determined, it has been demonstrated that infection may occur via the mucous membranes of the eye, mouth or nose or through abraded or damaged skin. Venereal spread has been demonstrated in cattle and pigs and this route may be more important than previously realized. Infection may also occur by ingestion of infected prey by predators. Following an incubation period of 4–10 days there is a period of leptospiremia which may or may not be accompanied by clinical signs. This period usually lasts for up to a week and is terminated by a sharp rise in antibodies. An acute hemolytic anemia may occur at the time of leptospiremia which may be seen as bloodstained urine or jaundice in some animals.

Following the period of leptospiremia, the organism localizes in the renal tubules. Leptospiruria is usually detected approximately 2 weeks after infection and its intensity is highest during the first months of shedding, and more than a million leptospires may be present in each ml of urine. A period of more intermittent, low intensity leptospiremia ensues which may in some hosts be lifelong.

Infection may also cross the placenta in infected animals leading in some cases to fetal death. This may occur rapidly in some hosts or be more prolonged leading to the birth of stillborn or weak but infected offspring. Infection has also been demonstrated in the Fallopian tubes of nonpregnant cattle and in the testes and accessory sex glands of boars.

Diagnosis

The clinical signs of leptospirosis are variable and vague and there may only be an occasional abortion or a general lowering of fertility. This is particularly true in the maintenance host situation. The more acute and serious forms seen in accidental hosts may be manifested as either acute hemolytic anemia leading to death in some cases or jaundice. Occasionally there is evidence of meningitis.

In most cases laboratory diagnosis is either by the use of serological tests or isolation of the leptospira by culture or of antigen detection by immunological means such as fluorescent antibody tests or ELISA tests.

Of the serological tests the most widely used is the microscopic agglutination test (MAT) using live antigens, and this is the reference test for evaluating other tests. The MAT shows considerable serogroup specificity and is capable of detecting low levels of circulating antibodies. The test will detect both IgM and IgG and titers will remain for long periods after initial infection. Thus the test is of value in both restrospective diagnosis of acute cases and for serological surveys. It is performed with batteries of antigens which should represent at least all serogroups known to exist in a particular country and preferably representative antigens for all known serogroups. For screening purposes, antigens can be pooled. The main difficulties in carrying out this test are the maintenance and standardization of a supply of live antigens. Formalin-killed antigens have been used but are less sensitive and show much greater serogroup crossreactivity.

Complement fixation tests have been widely used and by using polyvalent antigens can be a useful test.

The ELISA test is currently being widely investigated using a variety of antigen preparations, enzymes, substrates and methodology. It potentially offers many advantages over the MAT in using antigens possibly of greater specificity, and in detecting different immunoglobulins. However, there is a need for a standardized approach if results from different laboratories are to be comparable.

Isolation of Leptospira

During the acute phase of infection, leptospira can be isolated from blood, milk, cerebrospinal fluid and various tissues. In the chronic phase, they can usually be isolated from the kidneys and urine and possibly from the female genital tract. In the fetus, the kidneys or lungs are tissues which may contain leptospira.

Apart from the fastidious nature of some leptospira, two other problems need to be overcome—the presence of contaminating microorganisms and the presence of inhibitory substances in tissues. These can both be alleviated by making serial dilutions of the inoculum in the growth media up to at least 1000–5000-fold. As purines but not pyrimidines are incorporated by leptospira from culture medium, leptospira are resistant to the pyrimidine analog 5-fluorouracil (5-Fu) which inhibits the growth of most other bacteria. This compound at the rate of up to 200 μg/ml is often used to assist the isolation of leptospira. The incubation of cultures may need to be continued for up to 16 weeks before leptospira are detectable thus considerably reducing the usefulness of culture as a means of diagnosis.

Microscopy

The use of dark ground microscopy has been advocated as a means of demonstrating leptospira in body fluids. However, it is generally accepted that the numbers are too low to be detected and cell debris artifacts frequently bear a striking resemblance to dead leptospira; therefore this method is rarely used today.

Silver staining of tissues using modifications of the Warthin Starry method is recommended where the numbers of leptospira in tissue are sufficient to be seen. The silver is selectively coated on to the leptospira but frequently tissue membranes may take up the stain producing artifacts which are difficult to distinguish from leptospira.

The most successful technique for visualizing leptospira in tissue is undoubtedly the fluorescent antibody technique (FAT). It can demonstrate leptospira in fetal tissues even when the organisms are nonviable. It does, however, require high quality conjugates which are not available commercially, and relatively expensive high quality incident light fluorescent microscope. It is probably the best currently available technique for investigating the products of abortion and the results have been shown to be comparable with isolation methods.

Immunoperoxidase staining techniques have been described and are currently being further investigated. They have the advantage that they can be read with a normal light microscope.

Leptospirosis in Cattle

Hardjo *Infection*

Hardjo is an obligate parasite of cattle. There does not appear to be a wildlife reservoir and cattle are regarded as the maintenance host. Infection is occasionally recorded in other farm species and there is some evidence that the serovar may be adapting to sheep.

Cattle appear to act as the maintenance host of *L. interrogans* serovar *hardjo* in many parts of the world. It is a widespread infection in Britain, Australia, New Zealand and North America. In many endemically infected herds, clinical signs of infection are minimal and often overlooked. The clinical signs of leptospirosis in cattle fall into two types: the acute form which is seen as agalactia or milk drop syndrome; and a more chronic form seen as either abortion, stillbirth and birth of premature or weak calves or infertility.

The acute form has been increasingly recognized in recent years particularly when it occurs as an outbreak when infection first enters a herd or a large group of susceptible cattle. It should not, however, be forgotten that individual cases of agalactia may occur in endemically infected herds.

The milk drop syndrome occurs shortly after infection during the bacteremic phase; it is characterized by a sudden drop in milk yield and a flaccid udder with all four quarters involved. Any milk produced is very thick, like colostrum, and may be slightly blood-tinged. Cell counts are very high. The affected animals are mildly pyrexic (up to 41 °C) and may show mild anorexia or depression. Milk production returns to previous levels within 5–14 days. The severity of infection varies considerably, some herds only showing some loss in milk yield and increased cell counts with no obvious clinical signs. These outbreaks occur typically in spring-calving and summer-calving herds often from May to September when the herd is in peak production.

Laboratory studies and in depth epidemiological studies clearly show that *hardjo* is an important primary abortifacient agent. Earlier confusion of the role of *hardjo* was primarily due to diagnostic difficulties using only serological tests before the introduction of the fluorescent antibody techniques and their evaluation by advanced cultural techniques. The high prevalence of antibodies in cattle makes the use of serological tests in diagnosis in individual animals of doubtful value, although they can be valuable when larger numbers of cattle are sampled.

Abortion, stillbirth, premature calving and the production of full-term weak calves are all recognized sequels to *hardjo* infection. Although leptospiral abortion was traditionally considered to occur in the last 3 months of pregnancy, *hardjo* has been demonstrated in fetuses aborted from the 4th month of gestation until term. The increase in return to service which often follows a milk drop outbreak also suggests that fetal death may occur even earlier. The majority of abortions occur between October and January and factors which may influence this seasonal distribution are the high level of moisture in the environment at this time, winter housing of cattle and an increase in urine drinking by housed cattle.

Diagnosis may be confirmed by immunofluorescence backed up by cultural examination. Fetal serology is also useful at times since a proportion of infected fetuses has detectable levels of circulating antibodies.

The role of *hardjo* in infertility is gradually becoming more apparent. Epidemiological studies have associated higher levels of infertility in naturally infected herds with an apparent improvement following vaccination; recent studies have placed this association on a much firmer base. *Hardjo* has been isolated from the genital tract of nonpregnant cattle in Northern Ireland, particularly from the oviduct and the uterus, and also in some cases from the ovaries and vagina. The similar prevalence of infection found in heifers and older cattle suggests that *hardjo* may persist in the genital tract for as long as it does in the kidney.

Although transmission is still considered to be primarily due to exposure to infected urine, the possibility of venereal transmission should now be considered. Experimental studies with serovar *pomona* have demonstrated this possibility with both natural service and artificial insemination.

Control of hardjo *Infection* Various strategies for the control of leptospirosis in cattle have been proposed including early exposure to allow the development of natural immunity, the use of dihydrostreptomycin and vaccination.

Deliberate exposure of young cattle to infected cattle is unreliable because of the uncertainty of transmission which may be delayed for several months. It also assumes that a lifelong immunity follows natural infection. The method has often failed to achieve its objective and provides a continuous source of infection for uninfected cattle and farm workers. Manipulating herd management to facilitate infection of young stock may not always be convenient and herds free from infection will remain at risk. The method has little to recommend it.

Dihydrostreptomycin at the rate of 25 mg/kg body weight is very effective in reducing the number of leptospira excreted in the urine and has been the basis of various control programs. Trials have shown that the method is not completely effective under field conditions where both environmental persistence of the organism and residual kidney infection may prevent a successful outcome.

Vaccination is currently the method of choice for control and commercial vaccines are now widely available.

Vaccinal strains of *hardjo* are grown in protein-free media, killed by formalin and the vaccines are rigorously standardized using hamster protection tests. Their use can form the basis for the elimination of *hardjo* from infected herds over a period of years. Whole herd vaccination will provide a high level of control but vaccination during an outbreak will not stop all subsequent abortions. In some herds a policy of vaccinating only heifers has been advocated but in an endemically infected herd such animals may abort in subsequent years.

Infection of Cattle with Other Serovars

Cattle may on occasion become accidentally infected with other serovars. In Britain a member of the *pomona* serogroup *mozdok* has been found on rare occasions to cause death of young calves and abortion and hematuria in older stock. The infection is maintained in small rodents. Cattle in Britain also occasionally become infected with other serogroup strains such as *L. icterohaemorrhagiae, canicola* and *australis*. In other countries, *L. grippotyphosa* and *tarassovi* may cause severe problems.

Cattle-related Infections in Man

In Britain, leptospirosis is becoming increasingly recognized as an occupational disease of farm workers, particularly dairymen. *Hardjo* infection in man is usually seen as a flu-like illness with fever, severe headache and often accompanying mental confusion. In untreated cases recovery may be pro-

longed with depression and lethargy as common features; some cases develop a lymphocytic meningitis. Human cases of abortion have also been recorded.

Leptospirosis in Pigs

L. interrogans serovar *pomona* although absent from pigs in Britain is by far the most commonly isolated leptospira from pigs occurring widely in southern Europe, North and South America, Asia, Australia and New Zealand. Because of its economic importance it has received more attention than any other leptospiral serovar in domestic animals.

As with other domestic species, infection occurs via the mucous membrane of the eye, nose or mouth and venereal infection must now also be considered, since as few as 100 organisms can establish infection via the vaginal route.

Very few cases of leptospirosis are diagnosed during the acute phase when the only clinical signs are of pyrexia, anorexia and listlessness; these coincide with the period of leptospiremia occurring 2–10 days after infection and lasting for about 7 days. The acute hemolytic anemia seen with *pomona* infection in cattle and sheep is not observed in pigs. Following the period of leptospiremia the leptospira localize in the kidney tubules and leptospiruria is usually detectable approximately 2 weeks after infection. The intensity is very high during the first months of shedding and over a million organisms may be present in each ml of urine. Leptospiruria may continue for up to 16 months after infection. There is a rapid serological response to infection and agglutinins appear 1 week after infection and reach a peak level at approximately 3 weeks. Peak titers are very variable but are often in the range of 1/100 000 and then slowly decline. Low level titers are usually detectable for several years.

The major importance of *pomona* in pigs is as a cause of reproductive disease. Pregnant sows in the last third of pregnancy often abort about 4 weeks after infection. Abortion typically occurs in the last 3 weeks of pregnancy and whole litters of dead piglets are expelled. Sometimes a few weak and jaundiced piglets are born alive but they usually die within 48 h. Following abortion sows appear to be solidly immune.

The pathogenesis of reproductive disease due to *pomona* is poorly understood but it is now generally believed that transplacental infection during the period of leptospiremia is the sole cause; this is followed by septicemia with large numbers of leptospira present in all fetal tissues.

In adult pigs the only lesions seen at postmortem

examination are small grayish-white foci on the surface of the kidneys. In the fetus the only consistent finding is the appearance of small grayish-white foci in the liver.

Infection with *pomona* enters a herd with the introduction of infected stock or by exposure to a contaminated environment. Once introduced into a pig herd a high prevalence of infection is rapidly established and the typical endemic cycle seen with a maintenance host is established. Young piglets are protected via the colostrum for the first 4 months of life, and then either become infected by contact with older stock or from a urine-contaminated environment.

Control is best achieved by introduction of a vaccination program. Control is not absolute as some infected pigs will become leptospiruric after exposure to infections. However, by avoiding the introduction of infected breeding stock and continued application of a vaccination policy the infection can be eradicated from most herds.

In England a small number of self-limiting outbreaks of abortion in pig herds has been observed and titers to *pomona* serogroup antigens observed. These outbreaks were recognized to be different because the infection never became endemic in infected herds. The causal strain has been isolated and identified as *mozdok*, a serovar maintained by small rodents such as field voles.

Principally in Eastern Europe—Bulgaria, Hungary, Czechoslovakia and Russia—the serovar *tarassovi* of the *tarassovi* serogroup is maintained in pig populations and presents a similar but somewhat milder syndrome to that observed with *pomona*.

Australis *Serogroup Infection*

Extensive surveys have failed to demonstrate the presence of *pomona* or *tarassovi* in pigs in the United Kingdom and leptospirosis of pigs was until quite recently considered not to be a problem. However, it is now evident that *australis* serogroup infection is widespread in pigs and may be an important cause of abortion. The infection was not detected until recently because the internationally recognized antigen for this serogroup—serovar *australis*—does not detect infection in pigs with serovars *muenchen* and *bratislava* which are present in pigs; these antigens were not used in diagnostic laboratories until 1977. In a recent survey approximately 20% of sera were seropositive to these *australis* serogroup antigens. The analysis of serological results revealed an association between seropositive pigs and poor reproductive performance.

Extensive studies in Northern Ireland have pro-duced evidence that leptospira of the *australis* serogroup are of real importance in reproductive disease of pigs; in one study leptospira of the *australis* serogroup were isolated from over 60% of aborted or stillborn fetuses. The strains isolated were either serovar *bratislava* or serovar *muenchen*. In a further study *australis* serogroup strains were recovered from the genital tract of 20 sows which had previously aborted, in one case 140 days after the abortion. The leptospira were isolated principally from the oviduct and uterus and this may explain their implication in infertility. A boar from an infected farm was also examined, and leptospira of this serogroup were isolated from the testes, seminal vesicles, the urethral and prostate glands. These findings suggest that the genital tract is a site where leptospira can survive equally well as in the kidneys producing further confirmation that venereal transmission is a feature of this disease.

Infection with the *australis* serogroup strains does not appear to stimulate the high titers as seen, for example, in *pomona* infection and many infected pigs are seronegative. This situation often occurs in the maintenance host of a particular serovar and is further evidence of the high degree of adaptation of these serovars to pigs. The maintenance host of *bratislava* is traditionally described as being the hedgehog which maintains the strain in nature and field voles in the case of *muenchen*. However, the high serological and bacteriological prevalences of these serovars in pigs suggest that the strains may have adapted to pigs and are being maintained in pig populations.

As vaccines are not yet available, control can only be attempted by the use of dihydrostreptomycin and separation of healthy animals from either infected pigs or wildlife.

Other Domestic Species

There is little evidence that leptospira are a serious cause of reproductive disease in sheep, goats and horses. However, these species may occasionally become accidentally infected with serovars such as *pomona* or *hardjo* leading to sporadic abortion.

LISTERIOSIS

Listeria monocytogenes causes a sporadic infection in a wide range of mammals and birds and it may often be subclinical and manifests itself in a variety of different ways. Thus infection of the uterus leads to abortion, while septicemia of the young unweaned animal leads to production of widespread miliary lesions and is frequently fatal. The third form is an encephalitis affecting animals of all ages.

History

The organism was first isolated in an epidemic in laboratory rabbits and guinea-pigs. Experimental reproduction of the infection in rabbits showed that it produced a very marked monocytosis, hence the name 'monocytogenes'. This feature is fairly diagnostic in laboratory animals but not in domestic ruminants.

Listeriosis was first described as a disease of domestic animals in New Zealand where the causal agent was found in sheep suffering from 'circling disease'. It has subsequently been found in most parts of the world in birds and mammals including man as well as in their environment.

Etiology

Listeria monocytogenes is a pleomorphic, gram-positive rod, some 1–2 μm in length resembling in many ways *Erysipelothrix*. It is actively motile at 25 °C but much less so at 37 °C and will grow under aerobic and microaerophilic conditions.

On blood agar plates it produces small transparent colonies some 1–2 mm in size which show varying amount of hemolysis.

There are five major serotypes which are divided into a number of subtypes.

Listeria monocytogenes can be readily isolated from uncontaminated material such as fresh fetuses on 5% sheep blood agar when it can be seen to produce slight to quite pronounced hemolysis.

From contaminated material such as placenta it is best isolated on selective media such as blood agar plates containing nalidixic acid (0.004%) and thallium acetate. To isolate from soil or silage, media containing nalidixic acid and potassium thiocyanate are used.

It is often difficult to isolate *Listeria* from brain material using the above methods but the 'cold enrichment' technique may be useful. This consists of placing a suspension of brain material in trypticase phosphate broth and holding at 4 °C for periods up to several months and periodically plating out onto selective medium. This method may also be useful for isolating from contaminated material. On plates the *Listeria* colonies can be easily recognized in either reflected or transmitted light (Henri's technique) by their characteristic lilac to blue-green coloration.

The isolates can be identified by their cellular morphology, colonial appearance, characteristic tumbling motility at 25 °C, positive catalase reaction, and their ability to hydrolyze esculin. The identity can be confirmed by slide agglutination tests using polyvalent *Listeria* antiserum.

Epidemiology

Listeria monocytogenes is present in most countries throughout the world and many species of animal including man excrete the organism in their feces without showing any symptoms.

The organism is extremely resistant to desiccation, sunlight and freezing. It is thus widely distributed in the environment and can readily be isolated from soil, sewage of both human and animal origin and some animal feedstuffs including silage.

The peak incidence of listeriosis in sheep in Great Britain is in February to April and in the past has been associated with severe cold weather. The winter housing of sheep does not appear to have influenced this increase.

The number of outbreaks of listeriosis in sheep has apparently risen recently in a number of countries and appears to be due to the increased use of silage as a source of winter roughage for sheep. If silage is cut too late in the year it does not develop a sufficiently acid pH and is more prone to spoilage. In the outer layer of silage where there is aerobic spoilage, *Listeria* appears to multiply to produce counts of over 12 000 organisms/g. Listeriosis appears to be more common in Scotland and the North of England possibly because the climate leads to the production of lower quality silage. The bulk of silage is usually free from *Listeria*, but small areas of spoilage may have very high counts which may explain the sporadic nature of many outbreaks.

Clinical Signs

Usually only one form of listeriosis occurs on a farm and it is unusual for both abortion and the encephalitic form to occur together. In animals which abort there are usually no observed clinical signs preceding the abortion, although in experimental infection it can be shown that there is a period of fever, anorexia and dullness before the abortion, which usually occurs in the last 4 weeks of pregnancy in sheep and during the last quarter of the pregnancy in cattle. In both species *L. monocytogenes* is present in the vaginal discharge for several days or longer if the placenta is retained and metritis occurs. Young lambs with the septicemic form are often found dead without any previous warning signs.

Often the first sign in the encephalic form is

drooping of one ear. The head may be on one side with the neck held stiffly and the animal may walk round in circles in one direction; sometimes an eyelid is allowed to droop and conjunctivitis may be present. Eventually the animal becomes incoordinated then recumbent prior to death.

Pathogenesis

The route of transmission may determine the type of disease which follows infection. In experimental infection either by the oral route or by intravenous injection, the result is usually either abortion or a septicemia with no central nervous system involvement.

However, infection by the conjunctiva and possibly the upper respiratory tract may lead to encephalitis. It is also thought that this form of the disease may occur from infected tooth sockets when the deciduous teeth are lost. The infection may pass to the brain via the trigeminal or one of the facial nerves.

The lesions in the placenta in cases of abortion consist of tiny yellow necrotic foci occurring in the tips of the cotyledonary villi. Similarly in the fetus, miliary necrotic foci may be found in the liver and spleen.

Diagnosis

Diagnosis of abortion is based on the isolation and identification of *L. monocytogenes* from fetal stomach contents, liver or placental membranes.

Histological examination is useful in the diagnosis of the cephalic form. Serological examination is of very limited value because of the ubiquitous nature of the infection. However, by using a trypsinized antigen and mercaptoethanol-treated sera, the demonstration of a rising titer in paired samples taken after an abortion may be of some value.

Treatment and Control

Tetracyclines and longacting penicillins may be used to prevent further abortions in infected flocks but the results are not convincing as to their value.

As the role of silage becomes clearer in the etiology of *Listeria* abortion, the need for care in the preparation and storage of silage is obvious. Silage should be cut early when the grass is in full leaf. Spoiled silage from the edge of a clamp or from the surface of torn big bales should not be fed to pregnant animals.

As the specific immunological protection against listeriosis is based primarily on the cell-mediated immune system, live vaccines should perform better and a live attenuated vaccine containing two serovars of *L. monocytogenes* has been developed and used extensively in Bulgaria. A recent trial of this vaccine in Norway also demonstrated some protective effect. At present there are no vaccines licenced for use in Great Britain.

Killed vaccines have been of little value.

MYCOBACTERIAL INFECTION OF THE GENITAL TRACT OF CATTLE

The eradication of tuberculosis in most developed countries has progressed to the point where the disease can no longer be regarded as an important cause of infertility. The disease tends to be more prevalent in the absence of control measures, where cattle are housed, and varying incidences of disease are found. The infection is almost exclusively caused by *Mycobacterium bovis* and although both *M. tuberculosis* and *M. avium* are occasionally isolated from cattle, they very rarely result in a generalized infection affecting the reproductive tract.

Mycobacterium bovis infection

In surveys carried out in the earlier part of the century it was found that about 20% of cattle with generalized tuberculosis had lesions of the endometrium representing about 4% of all tuberculous cattle. The frequency of the infection of bulls is unknown but there are reports of primary tuberculosis of the penis and its associated lymph nodes and of hematogenous spread to the testes and epididymis.

It has been estimated that over 90% of cattle become infected by the aerogenous route, although some can become infected by ingestion of contaminated food. However, tuberculous endometritis is a dangerous type of open lesion which may result in a bull developing lesions on the penis leading to venereal spread. Infection via contaminated instruments such as intrauterine catheters is also recorded.

Cows with tuberculous endometritis are particularly dangerous to other animals and attendants because the affected animal excretes the organism for life.

In cattle the primary focus of infection is usually in the lung and may remain quiescent for a long period before the animal develops progressive disease.

Lymphohematogenous dissemination of *M. bovis* leads to secondary foci of infection in many organs of the body including the uterus or testes. However,

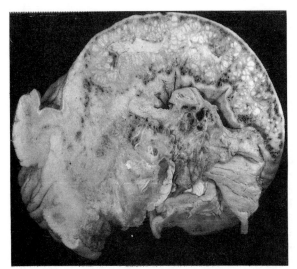

Fig. 16.1 Longitudinal section through the right uterine horn of a cow showing tubercules in the uterine wall.

as mentioned above, infection is occasionally spread venereally or via contaminated instruments.

The lesions found in the genital organs are similar to those in other sites, their character and extent varying with the age of the lesion. They may occur in the ovaries and Fallopian tubes as well as in the uterus. Lesions may extend into the cotyledons leading to infection of the fetus, resulting in abortion and the expulsion of a tuberculous fetus and placenta.

The primary symptom observed in the cow is usually infertility associated with a chronic vaginal discharge. Sometimes there may be a history of irregular or absent estrous periods.

The discharge is usually fairly copious and may be seen adhering to the ventral surface of the tail. It may be clear with flecks of whitish pus or wholly purulent and yellowish in color. Vaginal examination shows the discharge in the vagina originating from the cervix. The gross enlargement of the vulva, which sometimes occurs, is readily recognizable and nodules may be palpated in the vulva.

Rectal examination may reveal the presence of extensive adhesions in the region of the ovaries and perhaps also uterine enlargement with thickening of the wall of the uterus (Fig. 16.1). When there is extensive calcification of the uterine lesions their granular character may be palpated. However, these lesions are by no means a constant feature of tuberculosis of the female genital tract. Abortion is a not infrequent sequel, usually occurring in late pregnancy.

In the bull, painless nodular swelling of the testicles or ulceration of the penile mucosa may be observed with palpable enlargement of the associated lymph nodes. The bull may be impotent with reduced number and quality of spermatozoa.

As lesions are not usually restricted to the genital tract, the animal may have other signs of generalized tuberculosis, such as persistent cough, anorexia and loss of condition together with enlargement of palpable lymph nodes and induration of the udder.

Tuberculosis may be suspected on clinical grounds but must be confirmed by isolation of *M. bovis*. Large numbers of acid-fast bacilli may be found in the uterine discharge in smears stained by the Ziehl–Neelsen method. However, in many cases they can only be detected with difficulty, or not at all, depending on whether endometrial lesions have ulcerated or not. Acid-fast bacilli may also be detected in the fetal placenta following abortion but may be difficult to demonstrate in the fetus.

In the case of the bull, the clinical findings are again only suspicious and must be confirmed by isolation of *M. bovis*. Semen, puncture samples from testicles and material from penile ulcers should be examined. The animal could be subjected to a tuberculin test using a mammalian purified protein derivative (PPD). However, cattle with advanced generalized tuberculosis may be anergic and fail to react.

Material should be sent to a specialized laboratory for the isolation and identification of the causal organism. This involves decontamination of the material followed by cultural and/or biological tests.

Mycobacterium paratuberculosis infection

It should also be recognized that in the final stages of Johne's disease, caused by *Mycobacterium paratuberculosis*, the infection becomes generalized and may lead to abortion. In one series of investigations, Doyle examined 24 fetuses from such cases and isolated *M. paratuberculosis* from the cotyledons of 13 fetal placentas and from the spleen of eight and the liver of five fetuses. Such organisms would not be isolated using the techniques used for *M. bovis* as *M. paratuberculosis* does not infect guinea-pigs and requires medium containing mycobactin for growth.

Mycobacterium avium infection

Although *M. avium* infection is not uncommon in cattle it very rarely produces a generalized infection. It has been reported, however, that *M. avium* produces a rare mild endometritis which does not progress, but infected animals may abort.

MYCOPLASMOSIS

Three different genera of the Mycoplasmataceae, namely the *Acholeplasma*, the *Mycoplasma* and the *Ureaplasma* are found in the urogenital tract of animals.

Mycoplasmas are similar to bacteria which have lost their rigid cell walls, and are instead surrounded by a cell envelope which resembles the cytoplasmic membrane of mammalian cells. The organisms are extremely pleomorphic and may appear as small elementary bodies or as filaments, globules or ring forms. The smallest form which will pass through some filters are 0.1–0.15 μm in size. They stain poorly with most stains but can be stained with Giemsa. They are identified on the basis of their biological and serological characteristics.

Mycoplasmas are the pathogenic or, more properly, the parasitic types which require a complex medium for their growth containing in particular cholesterol, serum, yeast extract and other proteins.

Acholeplasmas are the saprophytic types found in sewage, soil, compost and manure. They are less exacting in their growth requirements and do not require cholesterol for growth.

Both mycoplasmas and acholeplasmas produce small colonies on solid agar which grow to about 1.0 mm in diameter after 3–4 days of incubation. As the center of the colony grows onto the agar, the colonies are often said to have a typical fried egg appearance.

The third genus of Mycoplasmataceae, originally called the T strains because of the tiny colonies they produce, are now classified as *Ureaplasma* because of their ability to split urea. They are strictly parasitic.

Cattle

All three genera of mycoplasmas have been isolated from the lower genital tract of both cows and bulls.

Acholeplasma laidlawii was one of the earliest to be isolated, and although now generally regarded as a nonpathogenic saprophyte, it has been isolated from the oviducts of infertile cows with evidence of salpingitis and bursal adhesions and also from aborted fetuses. As these organisms are so common in the environment all such reports should be interpreted with great caution.

Mycoplasma bovigenitalium was isolated in early studies from the bovine urogenital tract and has since attracted much attention and study. It has also been identified as a cause of bovine mastitis. It is frequently isolated from cervicovaginal mucus from both healthy and infertile cows. It also has been,

rarely, isolated from aborted fetuses. But again its role, if any, is not clear. *M. bovigenitalium* has also been associated with bovine granular vulvovaginitis and has been frequently isolated from such cases but the disease can only be reproduced if the vulval epithelium is scarified prior to inoculation. This condition is considered in more detail under ureaplasmas (see below).

The role of *M. bovigenitalium* in the bull is also controversial. Although this mycoplasma has been isolated from natural cases of seminal vesiculitis and the disease has been experimentally reproduced, cultures from the prepuce and semen of healthy bulls have shown a high level of isolation with no evidence of reduced fertility. Although venereal spread of *M. bovigenitalium* takes place there is little evidence that infection lowers either male or female fertility.

Experimental studies have also indicated that *M. bovis* can produce endometritis and salpingitis following the use of contaminated semen, but the organism has rarely been recovered from infertile cows. Similarly *M. bovirhinis*, *M. canadense*, *M. organini* and several others have been isolated from aborted fetuses but their role is not considered to be important.

Recently attention has focussed on the ureaplasmas, the species present in cattle being called *Ureaplasma diversum*. This species is now considered to be the cause of bovine granular vulvovaginitis. The condition appears 3–6 days after breeding but direct transmission from cow to cow also occurs. The main sign of infection is the presence of a sticky purulent vulval discharge on the hair of the tail or vulva. This is followed in a few days by the appearance of buff-colored granular lesions 1–4 mm in diameter in the vulvovaginal epithelium especially near the clitoris. The acute form persists for up to 10 days but may recur, and the granular nodules sometimes persist for several months.

Studies in Canada have associated the condition with a marked drop in fertility, the conception rate at first service dropping by up to 50% and then slowly improving. It has been suggested that infection is transferred from the vagina to the uterus at artificial insemination but will also occur following natural service. Control has been achieved by infusing 1 g of Terramycin into the uterus 24 h after insemination and this has been claimed to lead to an improvement in fertility.

Bulls are widely infected with ureaplasmas, but infection usually remains restricted to the prepuce and is the main source of semen contamination with ureaplasmas. The antibiotics used in semen extenders are more effective against mycoplasma than ureaplasmas. Wide variations are reported in the pathogenicity of ureaplasmas and this is an area requiring further elucidation.

Ureaplasmas can be isolated from most cases in the acute stage using suitable media containing penicillin and thallium acetate to control bacterial contamination.

Sheep

Ureaplasmas are widely present in ewes and infection levels rise after first mating. In a study in the United States, ewes served by an infected ram showed poorer fertility and the birth of smaller and weaker lambs than the control group. Vulvitis in sheep has also been associated with ureaplasmas.

Pigs

Workers in Czechoslovakia have isolated ureaplasmas from boars' semen and have also reported lower fertility levels in sows inseminated with semen contaminated with ureaplasmas.

Q FEVER

Q fever is a zoonotic disease of man which is becoming increasingly diagnosed in populations at risk. The source of this infection is often cattle, sheep and goats in which no clinical signs are usually observed.

The first outbreak was described by Derrick in 1935 in abattoir workers in Australia. He described a fever which occurred without a rash and gave it the name Q (for 'query') fever. Derrick could not isolate the causal organism but succeeded in passaging the infection in guinea-pigs using both blood and urine from infected patients. Burnet identified typical rickettsia organism in smears from a sample of liver from an infected guinea-pig and in further studies concluded that the agent of Q fever was similar to the agents causing other rickettsial fevers.

In 1938 Cox isolated a filter-passing infectious agent from specimens of *Dermacentor andersonii* from Nine Mile Creek in Montana in the United States. A laboratory worker subsequently became infected and the disease produced was recognized by Dyer as being very similar to the disease described in Australia. This new agent showed some marked differences from other rickettsias and was eventually called *Coxiella burnetii* in recognition of its two discoverers.

Typically the disease in man is a flu-like illness lasting 1–2 weeks with fever, malaise, muscular pain and usually a very severe headache. There may be pneumonia and bronchitis with a dry cough and both hepatomegaly and splenomegaly are recorded. Most cases recover uneventfully but about 10% of cases become chronic developing endocarditis and occasionally pericarditis. Q fever is currently responsible for about 3% of all cases of endocarditis. Cases occur typically in people occupationally exposed to livestock such as farmers, abattoir workers and veterinary surgeons. Approximately 100 cases a year are diagnosed in Great Britain. Veterinary surgeons in large animal practices are particularly at risk. One serological survey in the northwest of England found antibodies in 28% and in another in Northern Ireland in 24% of veterinary surgeons.

Thus the main importance of Q fever in domestic animals is as a source of infection for man.

The Causal Organism

Coxiella burnetii is a typical member of the Rickettsiales, a group of organisms with properties intermediate between those of bacteria and viruses. Although generally smaller than bacteria, they can readily be seen under the light microscope. They do not stain readily but Giemsa stain is satisfactory. They are between 0.2 and 0.6 μm in diameter and are either spherical or rod-shaped. Their cell wall is rigid and structurally similar to those of the gram-negative bacteria and contains muramic acid; they reproduce by binary fusion, contain both DNA and RNA and are susceptible to broad-spectrum antibiotics such as tetracyclines, all of which supports the belief in a phylogenic link with bacteria. However, they will only grow in cells, the best site still being the yolk sac of the developing chick embryo although they will also grow in some tissue cultures.

Coxiella does, however, differ from rickettsia in several important respects justifying its classification as a separate genus. The genome size of both rickettsia and coxiella is very similar at 1.04×10^9 daltons but the guanine plus cytosine content differs, the rickettsia falling between 29.0% and 33%, while *C. burnetii* is 42%.

Coxiella are smaller than rickettsia, and will pass through a Seitz EK filter, and unlike rickettsia, do not cause a rash to develop in man or the development of Weil–Felix agglutinins. In cells coxiella proliferate within lysosomal vacuoles while rickettsia develop in the cytoplasm.

However, the main difference is in their mode of transmission. Rickettsia are arthropod-borne infections, while coxiella, because of its exceptional resistance to chemical and physical agents, survives desiccation and can maintain itself in nature without an arthropod vector, and airborne transmission is normal in some situations.

Tick Cycles

The rickettsia provide one of the best examples of insect or arthropod-borne infection and *C. burnetii* is no exception. The rickettsia multiply in the lumen and epithelial lining of the alimentary canal and salivary gland of ticks, lice, fleas and mites, and become infected from the blood of infected hosts. A new vertebrate host becomes infected either from an insect bite or when a crushed insect or its feces gains access through an abrasion of the skin caused by scratching.

Coxiella burnetii has been isolated from over 40 species of tick throughout the world and tick tissue and tick feces are the richest known source of the organism. In its original host *Dermacentor andersonii*, tissue from the tick was found to be infectious to guinea-pigs at a dilution of $10^{11.7}$ and from the feces at 10^{10}.

In the species of tick found in America, *Dermacentor andersonii*, *Rhipicephalus sanguineus* and *Ornithodorus moubota*, *C. burnetii* is transmitted transovariomally from one generation of tick to another. However, unlike some rickettsia which appear to exist synergistically in ticks, *C. burnetii* does not appear to be maintained through several generations of ticks without passing through another host.

In Britain, *C. burnettii* has only been isolated from ticks (*Haemophysalis punctata*) infecting sheep in the Romney Marsh. Although *C. burnetii* is present in *Ixodes ricinus* in continental Europe, it has not been demonstrated in the Ixodid tick in Britain.

In some habitats, *C. burnetii* has a sylvatic cycle and exists independently of domestic animals. One such cycle is well documented on Morten Island of the coast of Australia where there are no domestic livestock. This involves a mammalian host, the Australian bandicoot, *Isoodon torasus* and its tick *Haemophysalis humerosa*. When cattle enter such a habitat—as in mainland Australia—*C. burnetii* demonstrates its versatility by adapting to survival without an arthropod host.

Cattle

In cattle and other domestic ruminants, *C. burnetii* is able to localize and multiply in the genital tract and the udder without apparent harm to the host. Early workers in both Australia and California quickly associated human infection with infection in cattle. The agent was discovered to be excreted in enormous numbers in birth fluids and placenta of cattle

that have produced normal live calves and from the milk. The placenta was found to contain up to 10^8 guinea-pig infection doses/g.

There was no evidence of reduced milk yield nor of any detrimental effect on the fetus resulting in abortion. Postmortem examination of infected cows failed to reveal lesions, although *C. burnetti* was isolated from both mammary tissue and the associated lymph nodes. Experimental infection by a number of different routes produces infection but no clinical disease.

It is assumed that cattle and people working with cattle become infected by inhaling dust from either dried fetal fluids or perhaps tick feces.

Infection was first demonstrated in cattle in Britain in 1944 by Slavin who reported a serological prevalence of 2.1%. However, by examining bulk milk samples he found a herd prevalence of 6.9% in England, 2% in Wales and 0.8% in Scotland. In the mid 1970s a survey of cattle in the Midlands showed a serological prevalence of 4.5% among cattle which had aborted and 3.1% among normal calving cattle.

In individual herds up to 10% of cattle have been found to be excreting coxiella at any one time and cows may go on excreting for over 2 years.

The prevalence of infection appears to be greater in warmer climates where dust is a problem, and appears to be increasing, for example, in California.

Sheep

Studies in England in the 1950s suggested an epidemiological association between infection in man and contact with sheep, and an increase in human cases was noted at lambing time.

Studies in California showed that naturally infected sheep excreted *C. burnetii* in the placenta, birth fluids, feces and milk at, and following, lambing. The placenta may contain 10^9 infection doses/g of tissue and can lead to a heavily infected environment. *C. burnetii* has been isolated from the air in lambing pens and from soil and water. Artificially infected sheep do not excrete significant numbers of coxiella until lambing has occurred. Sheep are usually infected via the respiratory tract and the infection lies dormant until the ewe becomes pregnant when multiplication takes place in the placenta and excretion only occurs at parturition.

Unlike cattle, in sheep there are some cases where abortion is attributed to *C. burnetii*. Such cases are rare and *C. burnetii* has been demonstrated in the liver and brain of the fetus in addition to the placenta.

Although a serological prevalence of about 3%

has been described in sheep in Britain, it is possible that up to 30% of flocks are infected.

Goats

Infection with coxiella is widespread in goats in the Mediterranean and in other parts of the world, and abortion storms have been reported. Coxiella has been shown to be excreted in the milk of goats for up to 3 years and people have become infected when attending goats while kidding. Goats were thought to be responsible for the extensive outbreaks of Q fever which occurred in troops in Greece at the end of World War II and more recently in Cyprus.

Diagnosis

In many cases an investigation in domestic animals is conducted for public health reasons to attempt to establish a source of infection. The demonstration of coxiella in the placenta is not sufficient to establish a cause of abortion as it is so frequently present in animals giving birth to normal offspring. The laboratory procedures used include the microscopic examination of smears, various serological tests and the isolation of the organism in embryonated hens' eggs, tissue culture or laboratory animals.

Smears of placental or fetal tissue may be stained with techniques used for *Brucella* such as modified Ziehl–Neelsen stain. The organisms are small red coccoid bodies which lie both intracellularly and extracellularly and in sheep may be confused with the agent of enzootic abortion. Other stains such as Giemsa and fluorescent antibody have been described.

Isolation of *C. burnetii* is often attempted from milk, blood samples, and tissue such as placenta and fetal liver. The material, as free from contamination as possible, is homogenized to a 10% solution in normal saline containing penicillin (1000 units/ml) and streptomycin (250 units/ml) and 1 ml of this material is injected either intramuscularly or intraperitoneally into either guinea-pigs or hamsters whose sera have previously been screened for *C. burnetii* antibodies. A febrile response may occur if *C. burnetii* is present, and the organism can be seen in stained impression smears from the spleen if the guinea-pig is killed at this stage. Usually the guinea-pigs are retained and bled 28 days after inoculation and the sera tested for seroconversion.

Embryonated eggs remain the best way of propagating *C. burnetii*. Material is injected into the yolk sac on the 5th to 7th day of incubation and the yolk sacs of eggs which die after the 3rd day are used to prepare smears which are stained for microscopic examination. The greatest number of *C. burnetii* are found about 11 days after inoculation. Isolates can be identified by inoculation into experimental animals or antigen extracted for serological identification by homogenization, differential centrifugation and passage through density gradients.

A number of serological tests has been described to detect coxiella antibodies, the most successful being the complement fixation test although this is now being replaced by the ELISA test.

However, before discussing these tests it is necessary to describe briefly the antigenic changes which occur when *C. burnetii* is passaged through eggs. The naturally occurring organism in milk, placenta, ticks or when passaged through laboratory animals is said to be in phase I. It remains in phase I during its first few passages in eggs then undergoes an antigenic shift (loss of some surface antigens), into phase II, a process which can be reversed by a single passage through a mammalian host. Whether this phase variation is of survival value to *C. burnetii* is uncertain but it is of great diagnostic importance. Antigens prepared from phase I antigens react with the sera of convalescent patients while phase II antigens react with acute sera, although antibodies to phase II antigens may be present for years. Most veterinary laboratories use phase II antigens which are commercially available.

Methods of Control

The main object of control is the prevention of human infection. The main human population at risk are those exposed to the birth fluids of animals, abattoir workers and people drinking raw milk. Heating milk at 71.7 °C (161 °F) for 15 s kills all coxiella so that pasteurized milk is safe. The organism has, however, also been isolated from goats' and ewes' milk, and from butter and cheese made from unpasteurized milk.

Human cases are usually treated with tetracyclines for long periods to attempt to prevent the development of chronic infection leading to endocarditis. Similar regimes have failed to stop the excretion of coxiella by domestic animals.

Vaccination has been successfully used in man and vaccines now available are prepared from phase I of *C. burnetii* which do not cause the severe reactions seen with earlier vaccine. The requirement is to stimulate a cell-mediated immunity and subjects should be tested prior to vaccination. Similar vaccines have shown promise in preventing both cattle and sheep excreting *C. burnetii* but the vaccines are not available commercially.

Several large islands such as New Zealand,

Japan, Iceland, the Philippines and most of Scandinavia are thought to be free from Q fever and quarantine and serological tests are used to prevent its introduction.

SALMONELLOSIS

Salmonellae are ubiquitous organisms distributed widely in nature. A very large number of serotypes has been described but in any particular habitat a small number of serotypes tend to predominate and some serotypes appear to be strongly host-adapted. Infection of animals often is symptomless and they may harbor the infection in a 'latent' or carrier form.

Some serotypes induce an acute infection characterized by fever followed by diarrhea and abortion; in the young animal, this form may occur as an acute septicemia with a high morbidity. Some serotypes often cause chronic infection in which no symptoms other than abortion are observed. Three host-adapted species, *Salmonella abortus ovis*, *S. abortus equii* and *S. dublin* tend to produce abortion.

Salmonella typhimurium on the other hand may infect a wide range of hosts, appears to be increasing in prevalence, and may produce severe acute disease in livestock.

Salmonellae have considerable public health importance but this account only covers their significance in relation to fertility.

Cattle

Over the last 20 years in England and Wales a large increase in the number of reported incidents of salmonella infection in cattle was seen reaching a peak in 1969 when over 4000 incidents were reported. Since then, the number of incidents has declined to around 1200 a year. This increase was largely due to *S. dublin* which between 1968 and 1974 was responsible for over 76% of the salmonella incidents in cattle, but by 1984, *S. dublin* was implicated in only 25% of incidents and *S. typhimurium* has become the dominant strain. Together *S. dublin* and *S. typhimurium* are currently responsible for nearly 90% of incidents in cattle. This cyclic behavior of salmonella serotypes may be observed in other countries. *S. dublin*, for example, has been quiescent for years in the United States but it now appears to be spreading quite rapidly.

About one-third of the recorded isolations of *S. dublin* are from cases of abortion, and in the past it has been the most important identified cause of abortion in cattle. The infection is most prevalent in the southwest of England and in Wales. Infection is usually acquired by the oral route. Although *S. dublin* may occur as an acute infection in adult cattle with fever and dysentery, in the majority of cases the only observed symptom is abortion; these occur about the 7th month of gestation and most cases occur in younger animals particularly in the autumn.

In adult cattle, after acute disease with dysentery, excretion of *S. dublin* in feces is persistent. In some cattle, the organism may invade the tissues and remain dormant without fecal excretion. Such 'latent' carriers may excrete *S. dublin* if stressed by disease or at parturition and may abort without any previous clinical signs. The 'latent' carrier is important in the spread of *S. dublin* infection. Although calves which recover from *S. dublin* infection cease to excrete organisms in the feces it has been suggested that in some of these the infection may lie dormant until activated by parturition leading to the birth of an infected offspring.

Salmonella dublin infection is often thought to be activated by liver fluke (*Fasciola hepatica*) infection. Low level fluke infection appears to predispose to clinical salmonellosis and persistent excretion of *S. dublin*. The lack of fluke challenge in recent years may be of significance in the decline of the number of *S. dublin* incidents. The extensive use of a live attenuated *S. dublin* vaccine in calves may also have reduced clinical disease, if not infection.

Salmonella typhimurium differs from *S. dublin* in several ways. It is the most ubiquitous organism, being isolated from a wide range of animals and is the commonest salmonella involved in human food poisoning, unlike *S. dublin* which appears to be especially adapted to cattle. *S. typhimurium* may cause acute disease in adult cattle characterized by fever, anorexia and reduced milk yield, quickly followed by acute diarrhoea. Pregnant animals commonly abort during the course of the illness. Cattle which survive excrete *S. typhimurium* for a limited period of a few weeks or months, unlike cattle infected with *S. dublin* which may excrete for years ('active carriers'). *S. typhimurium* infection is found throughout Britain and is usually sporadic, unlike *S. dublin* which is endemic in parts of Wales and the southwest of England.

Diagnosis

Diagnosis is normally based on the isolation of the organism from the fetus or placenta (Fig. 16.2). This can normally be achieved by direct overnight culture on MacConkey agar or deoxycholate citrate (DCA) agar. If the material is contaminated, prior

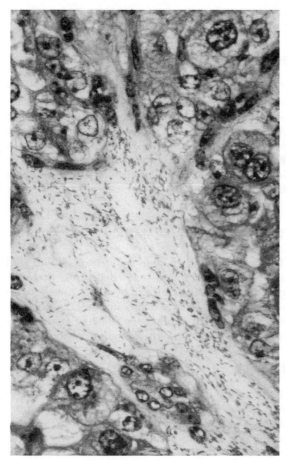

Fig. 16.2 Salmonellae in placental tissue.

incubation in a selective medium such as selenite broth may be necessary before the organism can be recovered on agar plates. The typical nonlactose fermenting colonies are further identified by biochemical tests and slide agglutination tests using polyvalent O and H agglutinating sera.

Serological tests are a useful adjunct to bacterial examination and both O (somatic) and H (flagella) antibody titers should be determined.

Control

The control of salmonellosis in cattle is currently based largely on the detection and elimination of carrier animals, hygienic measures to prevent the spread of infection in both calves and adult animals, control of liver fluke infection in relation to *S. dublin* and the vaccination of calves.

The detection of all carrier cattle is usually unsatisfactory with the exception of active carriers of *S. dublin*, but by definition it is impossible in 'latently' infected cattle. More emphasis must be placed on hygiene, particularly in relation to the rearing of calves.

A live attenuated *S. dublin* vaccine is licenced for use in calves, while formalin-killed vaccines containing both *S. typhimurium* and *S. dublin* are commercially available in the United Kingdom and are licenced for use in both calves and adult animals. Both have some value in the control of abortion.

Sheep

The serotypes of salmonella isolated from sheep in recent years in Britain and, in particular, those associated with abortion have undergone some very marked changes. *S. abortus ovis*, a serotype which appears to be host-adapted to sheep and a serious cause of abortion, used to be very prevalent in Britain. During the period 1958–67, 63% of incidents in sheep were caused by *S. abortus ovis* infection. However, during the period 1968–74, *S. dublin* became dominant, mirroring the situation in cattle, being responsible for 45% of incidents, whereas *S. abortus ovis* became second in importance being responsible for 36% of incidents. Since 1976, *S. abortus ovis* has virtually disappeared, only a single incident being recorded during 1984.

Currently the salmonella most frequently isolated from sheep is *S. typhimurium*, followed by *S. montevideo*, *S. arizona* and *S. dublin*.

Salmonella abortus ovis, a host specific serotype, causes little systemic illness in adult sheep, the only clinical sign being abortion which usually occurs in the last 6 weeks of pregnancy. Usually the rate of abortion is around 10% but may vary from a single abortion to over 60% of the flock. A few ewes may develop metritis which can be fatal. Occasionally lambs in contact with infected ewes may die suddenly from septicemia or develop diarrhea.

There are no characteristic lesions in the aborted fetus but occasionally the placenta may show chronic thickening similar to that seen with chlamydia abortion. Stained smears reveal large numbers of organisms in the fetal stomach contents and fetal membranes. Diagnosis is made by isolating the organism and typing it serologically. *S. abortus ovis* grows much more slowly than most other salmonellae, and colonies may take 48–72 h to reach a significant size on solid media.

Serological examination is of relatively little value in diagnosis as approximately 17% of apparently healthy sheep have high titers to the flagellar antigens of *S. abortus ovis*. Before the virtual disappearance of the latter it was largely confined to the southwest of England yet significant antibody levels are present in sheep in many parts of the country probably due to the presence of other organisms which share common antigens with *S. abortus ovis*.

Infection is normally introduced into susceptible flocks by the introduction of infected sheep although infection may persist on pastures for some time. Although a carrier state has been postulated, the virtual disappearance of *S. abortus ovis* in recent years suggests that it does not become endemic in infected flocks.

Salmonella typhimurium behaves in sheep in a similar manner to that in cattle. It usually produces fever (41 °C), and a profuse diarrhea; some ewes may die of septicemia and others from dehydration. Thus a range of clinical signs from sudden death to acute scour will occur along with abortions.

Salmonella dublin behaves in a similar manner to *S. typhimurium* in sheep producing fever, anorexia and diarrhea along with some abortions. The decline in the number of *S. dublin* incidents reported in Britain parallels the decline in cattle numbers.

Salmonella montevideo on the other hand behaves like *S. abortus ovis* and appears to be well adapted to sheep. Only abortion is observed in many flocks. The prevalence of infection has increased particularly in the southeast of Scotland. Wild birds, particularly gulls, are postulated to spread this serotype mechanically on their feet whilst scavenging on the products of abortion. *S. arizona* (serotype 61:K:1,5,7) is also regarded as being well-adapted to sheep and has recently become established in northern England. Although it has been isolated from aborting sheep in the majority of cases, other abortifacient agents such as chlamydia or toxoplasma were also present.

A large range of other salmonella serotypes has been isolated from aborting sheep, many of these 'exotic' serotypes possibly being introduced in feedstuffs.

Control and Treatment

The acute nature of salmonellosis in sheep with some serotypes, inevitably means that treatment with parenteral antibiotics is indicated, together with suitable supportive treatment to correct dehydration.

As a large number of other ewes may be at risk, treatment of the whole flock with furazolidone or other antibiotics in the food has been attempted but results are somewhat equivocal.

S. abortus ovis has apparently been successfully controlled with the use of killed vaccines but the results are difficult to assess particularly in view of the

evidence in Britain that the infection may be self-limiting.

Horses

Salmonella abortus equi is a serotype which was well-adapted to the horse causing few clinical symptoms other than abortion. In both Europe and North America it appears to have declined markedly in prevalence. It has not been reported recently in Britain where currently the most common serotype in horses is *S. typhimurium*, principally a cause of fever and diarrhea.

TICKBORNE FEVER (TBF)

Tickborne fever is a benign rickettsiosis of both wild and domestic ruminants caused by *Cytoectes phagocytophilia* and characterized by a prolonged parasitemia, high fever, drop in milk yield and depression of B lymphocytes allowing other infections to develop; pregnant animals may abort.

Etiology

The condition was first discovered in Scotland when it was accidentally transmitted to sheep from nymphs of *Ixodes ricinis* while investigating the cause of louping ill. It was also shown to infect cattle, goats and deer.

The rickettsia may be demonstrated in the neutrophils or monocytes of infected animals as round bodies 0.2–0.6 μm in size with up to five bodies in each cell. The rickettsias are readily stained with either Giemsa, Leishmann or Romanowsky stain.

The name *Rickettsia phagocytophilia* was proposed originally for this organism on the basis of its morphology, its size, its morphological similarity to other members of the group, its intracellular location and because it has an arthropod vector. It was suggested that it should be placed in the genus *Ehrlichia* which are rickettsia that usually parasitize mononuclear leukocytes; subsequently it was proposed that the tickborne fever agent should be placed with the vole rickettsia in the genus *Cytoectes* because they both parasitize polymorphonuclear leukocytes and its current name is *Cytoectes phagocytophilia*.

All European isolates share a number of common antigens which can be demonstrated either by complement fixation or immunofluorescent test. The organism divides by binary fission. The small bodies are phagocytosed by eosinophils and neutrophils and lie in an intracytoplasmic vacuole. Here the organisms enlarge and divide to fill the vacuole in a few hours; the organisms are then released to parasitize further cells.

Epidemiology

Tickborne fever has been recognized in the temperate parts of Europe, but not in the United States, and infects cattle, sheep, goats and deer. The principal arthropod vector is the sheep tick, *Ixodes ricinus*. Although transovarian infection has not been demonstrated in *I. ricinus*, infection acquired at one stage of its life cycle is retained as it passes from nymph to larva to adult and will survive in adults for up to 1 year. The greatest incidence of infection in sheep tends to occur at the time of the 'spring rise' in tick numbers.

Unlike louping ill which is somewhat restricted in its distribution, *C. phagocytophilia* occurs in *I. ricinus* almost everywhere it is found; and on infected pastures most ticks will harbor the infection. Tickborne fever can also be transmitted during blood sampling if a contaminated needle is used.

Symptoms

Infection occurs either soon after adult cattle or sheep are exposed to the tick bites for the first time and to lambs born on tick infected pastures.

The incubation period varies from 5 to 12 days and this is followed by sudden onset of a fever between 40 and 42°C. The virulence of strains varies and the fibrile reaction may fall rapidly or decline slowly over 10 days. Pregnant sheep abort 2–8 days after onset of fever; cows may also abort after a similar period. There is nothing characteristic in the appearance of either the fetus or the placenta.

In cattle a sudden and marked drop in milk yield is observed which may last for up to 20 days after the onset of fever. Death from tickborne fever is rare except in aborting ewes where retention of the placenta may lead to considerable mortality. However, the immunosuppressive effect of tickborne fever may lead to exacerbation of a number of other conditions, the principal one being tick pyemia in lambs, where *C. phagocytophilia* enhances the invasion and multiplication of *S. aureus*. A similar enhancement of listeriosis, pasteurellosis, chlamydial infection and louping ill has been demonstrated in sheep.

It has been suggested that the prolonged fever caused by *C. phagocytophilia* may impair spermatogenesis in the ram but this is disputed. Rickettsia may be observed in impression smears of liver and spleen and possibly lung where rickettsia have been demonstrated in alveolar macrophages. There are no characteristic lesions in aborted fetuses and rickettsia-like bodies are not observed in impression smears made from fetal or placental material.

Diagnosis

Diagnosis relies initially on the history of recent exposure of cattle or sheep to ticks for the first time. This is aided by knowledge of tick distribution in an area, the history of the farm, the season and the age of the stock. Fever and abortion are the principal signs in sheep while drop in milk yield is also important in cattle.

The provisional diagnosis must be confirmed by demonstrating the rickettsia-like organism in the neutrophils in blood films or in spleen or liver smears suitably stained by either Giemsa or Leishmann staining.

Carrier sheep can usually only be detected by inoculating blood into susceptible sheep and observing the development of the disease although complement fixation tests may be of value.

The changes in the total and differential leukocytic counts are of diagnostic importance in tickborne fever. Initially, with the onset of fever, there is little change in the total count, but the relative proportions change, with an increase in the number of neutrophils and a decrease in the number of lymphocytes. This is followed by a fall in total count due to a progressive neutropenia. The lymphocytopenia and neutropenia may persist for several weeks.

C. phagocytophilia is found most readily during the initial increase in neutrophils but rarely in the neutropenic phase. It persists in the body for several weeks after infection and sometimes longer. The lowered resistance to other microorganisms which accompanies *C. phagocytophilia* infection is related— the neutropenia, the functional impairment of the infected neutrophils and the lymphocytopenia arising from the depression of the B lymphocytes and consequent suppression of antibody response to other infecting agents.

There is little gross pathological change in lambs which die or in adult animals killed during the acute phase except an enlarged spleen in some cases; occasionally petechiation of the intestinal mucosa, hemorrhages into the colon and some serosal and endocardial hemorrhages are observed.

Histopathological examination may reveal the presence of rickettsia-like bodies in Kupffer cells in the liver and neutrophils in the spleen.

Treatment and Control

One of the best methods of control, long practiced by flockmasters, is to purchase the sheep with the land when farms change hands thus avoiding the introduction of susceptible sheep to tick-infested pastures. It is especially important to avoid the introduction of susceptible pregnant animals to tick-infested pastures.

Extensive pasture improvement, from the use of techniques such as bracken burning, liming and reseeding will alter the tick habitat sufficiently to reduce tick numbers drastically, but this means that care must be taken to avoid livestock being moved back even temporarily to unimproved pasture.

Dipping is relatively ineffective in reducing the tick burden of an area although it may give livestock some temporary relief. Very small numbers of ticks remaining in an improved pasture are sufficient to reinfect livestock.

Tetracyline is the drug most widely used to treat the disease. A single dose may cause the fever to abate and clear the parasitemia but allows a mild relapse which ensures resistance to reinfection.

Replacement rams may need to be housed or kept separately before use where the disease is a problem. Dipping before use offers only temporary protection.

TOXOPLASMOSIS

Toxoplasma gondii is an intestinal coccidium of the cat family with a very wide range of intermediate hosts. It is an important cause of abortion in sheep, which are an intermediate host of *T. gondii*.

Toxoplasma gondii was found originally in 1908 in rodents in Tunis, and in laboratory rabbits in Brazil. Its economic importance as a cause of loss to the sheep industry was recognized in the 1950s, but it was not until 1970 when it was discovered that *T. gondii* was a coccidian parasite of cats that its various life cycles became clear.

In man toxoplasmosis is recognized to be a fairly common but relatively mild infection except when acquired congenitally where it can cause occular disease, principally a retinochoroiditis, hydrocephalus and intracerebral calcification.

Life Cycles

Toxoplasma gondii occurs worldwide and has been recorded in a large range of mammals and birds. However, only the cat family acts as the definitive host in which the parasite multiplies sexually in the

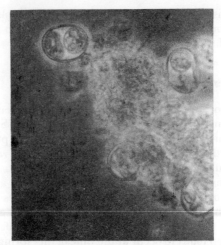

Fig. 16.3 *Toxoplasma gondii* in placental tissue.

intestinal epithelium leading to the production of oocytes. In Britain the only definitive host is the domestic cat, but in other countries it has been described in mountain lions, ocelots, bobcats and tigers.

A cat may become infected either by ingesting oocytes or by eating one of the intermediate hosts such as the small rodents whose tissues contain toxoplasma cysts. In the stomach and small intestine of the cat the tissue cyst wall is dissolved by proteolytic enzymes releasing the bradyzoites which penetrate the epithelial cells of the small intestine and pass through several stages of the life cycle before sexual reproduction begins in which microgametes develop which penetrate mature macrogametes. A thick wall forms round the resulting fertilized gamete which is shed into the lumen of the intestine and passes out in the feces. Sporulation takes from 1 to 5 days to complete, depending on the temperature and aeration. The final oocyte contains two ellipsoidal sporocysts each comprising four sporozoites. The oocytes are very resistant and survive on the ground for over a year.

Cats begin to shed oocytes 4–5 days after infection and continue to do so for 7–12 days; over 10^8 oocytes may be produced. Infection stimulates an effective immunity and reinfection seldom produces any significant amount of oocyte production.

An intermediate host may become infected either by ingesting oocytes or tissue cysts. Again the bradyzoites are released but penetrate the intestinal wall, invade the extraintestinal tissues and multiply rapidly in host cells as tachyzoites. These are crescent-shaped organisms 5 μm by 1.5–2 μm (Fig. 16.3) which gave toxoplasma its name from the Greek *toxon* meaning an arc. Infected host cells burst

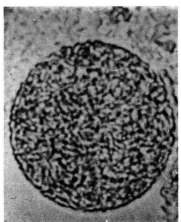

Fig. 16.4 Toxoplasma cyst in mouse brain emulsion.

and release more tachyzoites which are carried throughout the body by both the blood and lymph streams and continue to attack more cells; they may even cross the placenta to infect the fetus. This active phase of asexual multiplication is eventually suppressed by the host's immune response and some of the tachyzoites multiply more slowly without lysing the host cells which eventually become packed with bradyzoites and become the tissue cysts (Fig. 16.4). These cysts survive because the cyst wall is formed from the hosts' cell membrane and does not provoke an immunological response. This represents a latent form of infection which may be lifelong. An antibody response to the tachyzoites persists and leads to resistance to reinfection.

The important reservoirs of infection are oocytes on the ground which primarily infect herbivores, and the tissue cysts representing a second reservoir of infection in intermediate hosts which infect carnivores. The third method of infection is the congenital route which may occur in any host. Some fetuses survive infection and are born with toxoplasma tissue cysts.

There is neither evidence of direct transmission between sheep nor that venereal transmission can take place. All the evidence points to sheep as being intermediate hosts of *T. gondii* becoming infected by the ingestion of oocytes. The high prevalence of antibodies to *T. gondii* in sheep, around 33% in Britain, has led to the hypothesis that all infection in sheep relates to ingestion of oocytes from cats being questioned.

There is more infection in lowland than in hill sheep; most farms support a sizable population of cats and the farm environment supports the toxoplasma cycle in cats and small rodents. Infection in sheep flocks tends to be sporadic, often occurring in

a previously healthy flock; it is usually restricted to one lambing season, with an abortion rate of around 12%. These points suggest that chance contact between sheep and oocytes must occur, the appearance of outbreaks being the result of sudden exposure of susceptible flocks to infection at the most susceptible stage of their pregnancy. This suggests either movement into an infected environment or the presence of oocytes in the food.

Pathogenesis

Following infection of the ewe by the ingestion of oocytes, the period of parasitemia, when tachyzoites are present in the blood, lasts for a very short time. The tachyzoites tend to localize in the muscles, the central nervous system and the fetal cotyledons. Destruction of placental tissue allows the tachyzoites to enter the fetal circulation.

The stage of gestation at which infection occurs is of critical importance. During the first 2 months of pregnancy infection will lead to fetal resorption and the appearance of barren ewes. From 70 to 100 days, infection will lead to either abortion or fetal mummification, and from around 110 days on the fetus may survive leading to congenitally infected lambs.

Where abortion occurs, the most characteristic lesions are in the fetal membranes; the cotyledons are bright to dark red and speckled with white foci 1–2 mm across which may vary in number or be very numerous, and often have a gritty consistency because of calcification (Fig. 16.5). Microscopically the earliest lesions seen in fetal membranes consist of focal mononuclear cell infiltrations and hyperplastic trophoblastic epithelium. These are followed by coagulative necrosis and finally calcification. It is not easy to detect toxoplasma in sections but occasionally clumps are seen within intact trophoblastic epithelium.

Mummified fetuses appear as small brown miniatures of lambs with a small placenta. The fresh fetus has no characteristic macroscopic lesions. Sections of fetal brain, however, show a characteristic leukoencephalomalacia. There may also be mild perivascular cuffing and distinctive foci of glial cells.

Diagnosis

Toxoplasmosis has little effect on nonpregnant sheep except a mild fever followed by the production of antibodies 10–14 days after infection. In pregnant sheep, infection leads to abortion, fetal mummification, stillbirth and neonatal deaths

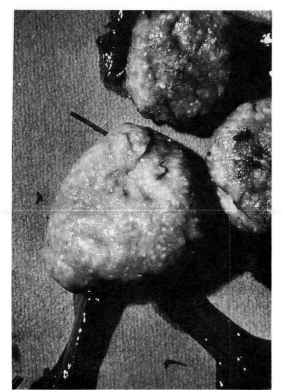

Fig. 16.5 Toxoplasma infected placenta showing necrotic foci in cotyledons.

specific antibody acts on the tachyzoites so that they no longer stain with methylene blue. Titers of $\geq 1/20$ are regarded as positive.

The indirect fluorescent antibody test gives similar titers to the dye test, but is safer in that killed tachyzoites are used. The test has been successfully used to detect antibodies in various fetal fluids. A wide battery of other tests has been used including the indirect hemagglutination test, the complement fixation test, radioimmunoassays and ELISA tests. The latter two lend themselves to automation and can detect either IgG or IgM antibody. Commercial kits are now available for some of these tests.

Control and Treatment

Although infection produces prolonged immunity, no successful vaccine against toxoplasmosis has yet been developed. Attempts to manage the disease by exposure of newly purchased ewes to infection may be effective in stimulating immunity, but the sporadic nature of infection makes this method of control difficult.

Treatment in the face of an outbreak of abortion is impracticable, but toxoplasma are susceptible to sulfonamides and particularly potentiated sulfonamides which may on occasion be used to treat individual animals.

usually starting about 3 weeks before lambing should commence.

Diagnosis of toxoplasmosis must be confirmed by laboratory examinations by either (a) isolation by mouse inoculation; (b) examination of fetal membranes and fetal tissues by conventional histological methods, or by immunofluorescent of immunoperoxidase methods; or (c) examination of sera from ewes or serum or body fluids from lambs for specific antibodies.

The isolation of *T. gondii* is both time-consuming and expensive, and involves the use of laboratory mice which are very much more sensitive than embryonated hens' eggs. Suspensions of fetal brain or placenta are inoculated intraperitoneally or subcutaneously into mice, and stained smears of ascitic fluid are searched for tachyzoites 7–14 days after infection, or tissue cysts sought in drops of brain suspension on slides stained with Giemsa. Antibodies can also be detected in mice 19 days after inoculation.

The most reliable serological test is still the Sabin and Feldman dye test. This requires the use of live virulent tachyzoites, a complement-like accessory factor and the test sera. The basis of the test is that

TRICHOMONIASIS

Trichomoniasis is a contagious venereal disease of cattle characterized by early embryonic death and occasionally abortion and pyometra. It is caused by a pear-shaped flagellated protozoan parasite, *Tritrichomonas fetus*.

The disease was first fully documented in Germany between 1928 and 1932. It is now found throughout the world and is a particular threat to large beef herds in Australia and the United States. The widespread use of artificial insemination in dairy cattle has considerably reduced the prevalence of infection in dairy herds. Trichomoniasis was last diagnosed in cattle in Britain in 1973.

The Causal Organism

The Trichomonadidae family is composed of three genera, the *Tritrichomonas* with three anterior flagella, the *Trichomonas* with four, and the *Pentatrichomonas* with five. Organisms are frequently found as part of the normal intestinal flora of most vertebrates and in the nasal cavity of some animals. *Tritri-*

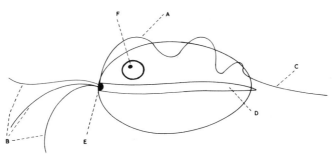

Fig. 16.6 *Tritrichomonas fetus*. A: undulating membrane; B: anterior flagella; C: posterior flagellum; D: axostyle; E: blepharoblast; F: nucleus.

chomonas fetus is found in the genital tract of both bulls and cows.

In unstained preparations examined at a magnification of about 100, *T. fetus* is a pear-shaped organism 10–15 μm long and 5–10 μm wide; motile protozoa can be recognized as *T. fetus* by the presence of the undulating membrane, the posteriorly projecting part of axostyle and the anterior flagella, whose number cannot be determined in living preparations (Fig. 16.6). The organisms remain freely motile at temperatures close to 37 °C. Stained preparations are necessary to demonstrate the three anterior flagella and the posterior flagellum which is a continuation of the outer edge of the undulating membrane.

T. fetus can be cultivated in laboratory medium such as peptone broth on an inspissated horse serum slope. A number of other liquid media have been devised—some containing penicillin, streptomycin and nystatin—to control contaminants. *T. fetus* is readily killed by drying, moderate heat and most disinfectants. However, a small number of organisms may survive the freezing processes used for storing semen.

Three serologically different types of *T. fetus* have been described in cattle, the Manley, Belfast and Brisbane strains.

Epidemiology

Trichomoniasis is transmitted only at coitus and an infected bull will pass the infection to over 90% of the females he serves. Most bulls remain permanently infected unless successfully treated but the majority of cows will recover spontaneously. As mentioned above, *T. fetus* may survive the freezing processes used for semen storage, but the diagnostic tests applied to bulls before their use for artificial breeding has considerably reduced the possibility of spread by artificial insemination and widespread use of artificial insemination has done much to re-

duce the prevalence of *T. fetus*. In herds where bulls are used, the disease is often confined to a group served by a single infected bull. The majority of cows and heifers are susceptible to infection and the disease is quickly established in the group. As many cows will return to service, a second bull may be used further spreading infection.

Both field and experimental evidence indicates that older bulls are more susceptible to infection while 1 or 2 year old bulls are not readily infected.

Infection may also be spread by insanitary or careless procedures used by personnel carrying out artificial insemination or while examining the genital tract.

Pathogenesis

In the bull, *T. fetus* colonizes the prepuce but often in only small numbers. While they are found throughout the prepuce and on the penis, the greatest numbers are found in the fornix and on the glans penis. The infection in no way interferes with spermatogenesis or the ability to copulate.

In recently infected cows or heifers, *T. fetus* is found in large numbers in the vagina 12–19 days after coitus. From then on the number and activity of the trichomonads vary in relation to the estrous cycle or stage of pregnancy.

After the initial exposure and the multiplication of *T. fetus* in the vagina, the organism invades the uterus; vaginal colonization remains until the first estrus after infection, and from then on *T. fetus* is only detectable in the vagina during the last few days before estrus. The trichomonads persist in the uterus between estrous periods and it is assumed that they prevent implantation of the fertilized ova causing lowering of fertility. There is no interference with the normal cyclical regression of the corpus luteum. Not all fertilized ova die, some become implanted and continue to develop. Others are aborted at times varying between 3 weeks and 7 months. In a small number of cases, the fetus dies in the uterus and becomes macerated leading to the development of pyometra.

During pregnancy the trichomonads are found in the uterus, in the amniotic and allantoic sacs and in the fetal alimentary tract.

Cows which fail to become pregnant free themselves of infection after a number of estrous cycles, and the rationale of resting such animals for 90 days is to allow them to do this. Cows which abort or which go on to term rapidly free themselves from infection usually by the time of the first estrous period postpartum.

It has been pointed out that the *T. fetus* is only able to colonize the genital tract when there is an active corpus luteum during the estrous cycle, or during pregnancy or pyometra. There may be some specific effect of estrogens which makes the uterine environment unfavorable for *T. fetus*.

Resistance to reinfection occurs. The mechanism of protection may be due to the local production of antibodies in the genital tract. Specific agglutinins to *T. fetus* are present in the vaginal mucus of animals which have recovered.

Clinical Signs

The principal symptom of trichomoniasis in cattle is infertility with a significant increase in the inter-calving intervals. This is due to early embryonic death in the first 50–100 days after conception. The owner will complain of animals with repeat breeding and irregular estrous cycles.

If the pregnancy continues, some result in early abortion. Most cows which carry their calves beyond the 4th month will go on to deliver a live calf. In less than 5% of cows, postcoital pyometra will develop, estrus does not occur and the condition will persist for months if no treatment is instituted.

On initial infection of a herd the main sign is repeat breeding with estrus cycles varying considerably in length. However, eventually most cows will conceive and have healthy calves.

After several months some cows will still return to service without any obvious evidence of abortion. At the 4th month and beyond, some abortions may be seen and in open cases of pyometra there will be some discharge of mucopurulent material. Some animals thought to be pregnant will be found to be cases of pyometra.

In subsequent breeding seasons, if infected bulls continue to be used, symptoms will usually be seen mostly in replacement heifers.

Diagnosis

While the herd history and clinical signs may be suggestive of trichomoniasis a definite diagnosis can only be made by demonstrating the presence of *T. fetus*. The organism can readily be demonstrated in the placental fluids and stomach contents of a freshly aborted fetus. If a fetus is not available, vaginal mucus from suspicious animals must be examined.

Those most likely to yield positive results are:

1. Cows or heifers during proestrus—that is, during the week before estrus when the cervix is beginning to relax.
2. Cows or heifers 7–21 days after their first exposure to infection.
3. Cows or heifers known to be discharging mucopurulent material from the vagina or those which have been found on rectal examination to have pyometra.
4. Cows which are between 3 and 5 months pregnant.

Mucus may be collected from the vagina using a speculum with a spoon, vulsellum forceps or by washing out with saline using a suitable aspiration tube.

If trichomonads are not found in the vaginal mucus, material from the prepuces of suspected bulls must be examined. The smegma may be collected with a pipette and suction bulb, or the prepuce and glans penis are washed with normal saline. Mucus and fluid washings must be examined as soon after collection as possible and must never be refrigerated. Preputial washings, smegma and vaginal fluid may be examined directly or centrifuged and the deposit examined for motile trichomonads. The material should also be cultured in suitable medium containing antibiotics and antifungal drugs to control contaminants.

The sensitivity of the cultural test on bulls is between 80 and 90%, but on vaginal mucus is less than 60%. This limits the value of any single examination and in cows four or five tests are needed to demonstrate freedom from infection.

Serological tests such as agglutination and complement fixation tests on sera have proved disappointing because of the presence of antibodies in normal cattle. However, the demonstration of agglutinins specific to *T. fetus* in vaginal mucus is of value. The best time to collect mucus for this test is 5–10 days after estrus.

Treatment and Control

Control is based on the assumption that transmission only takes place at coitus. In most herds the introduction of artificial insemination for a period of 2 years will lead to freedom from infection as most cows recover spontaneously.

Animals with pyometra may be cured by treatment to induce regression of the corpus luteum, but it is advisable to examine the reproductive tract to determine so far as possible if any damage has been caused which might interfere with conceptions. Where bulls are used, it may be possible to divide the herd into two groups, consisting of those known to be exposed and those unexposed. The unexposed group should be bred using a clean bull. The exposed group should not be served for 90 days and then may be bred from successfully provided their estrous cycle is normal.

The relative resistance to infection by young bulls may be exploited by removing all bulls over 4 years of age and using only young bulls.

Systemic treatment of bulls with either dimetridazole, ipronidazole or metronidazole has been described but there may be unpleasant side-effects. Local treatment of bulls with acriflavin ointments and solutions is time-consuming, tedious and expensive and the slaughter of infected bulls rather than treatment is usually recommended.

In countries where trichomoniasis is still a problem potential carriers of *T. fetus* must be isolated and tested. Bulls used for AI must be examined before use to insure that they are free from infection.

OTHER BACTERIAL INFECTIONS ASSOCIATED WITH INFERTILITY

Cattle

A very wide variety of bacteria have been recovered from bovine fetal material, but often their significance as a cause of abortion is debatable.

Actinomyces pyogenes (previously *Corynebacterium pyogenes*) is not infrequently found, and in one study in West Germany *A. pyogenes* was present in 17.3% of cases from which microorganisms were isolated.

Haemophilus somnus was originally recognized as a cause of thromboembolic meningoencephalitis in feedlot cattle in North America. However, *H. somnus* has increasingly been recognized as a cause of respiratory disease, polyarthritis and reproductive disease including endometritis and abortion. In several parts of the world including Australia, Canada and Switzerland, *H. somnus* has been isolated from the vagina of normal cattle and from the prepuce of bulls.

Yersinia pseudotuberculosis has been reported as a cause of sporadic abortion. The infection causes minute necrotic foci in the fetal liver and the organism is readily recoverable from both fetus and placenta. *Bacillus licheniformis*, *Serratia marcescens* and *Nocardia asteroides* are also organisms which are not infrequently isolated from aborted fetuses.

Sheep

In Australia, *A. pyogenes*, *Corynebacterium pseudotuberculosis*, and *Rhodococcus equi* (previously *C. equi*) and other unidentified coryneform species have been isolated from aborted ovine fetuses and various coryneform species have been isolated from similar material in Britain.

Similarly, *A. pyogenes* and other *Corynebacterium* species have been isolated from cases of orchitis and epididymitis in the ram. Such animals are usually infertile.

A relatively fastidious gram-negative coccobacillus referred to as *Histophilus ovis*, has also been isolated from cases of epididymitis in Australia and New Zealand and a case has recently been described in Britain. A similar organism, *Actinobacillus seminis* has been isolated from cases of ovine epididymitis.

A wide variety of other bacteria including *Bacillus* species, *Y. pseudotuberculosis* and *Nocardia* species have been isolated from cases of abortion.

Pigs

The examination of the products of abortion from sows yields a wide variety of bacteria including *Aerobacter* species, staphylococci, streptococci, *E. coli* and others. Their significance is doubtful. Occasionally *Erysipelothrix rhusiopathiae* is isolated from expelled fetuses, sometimes from small outbreaks of abortion.

Erysipelas mainly affects growing piglets where it may occur in an acute form with septicemia, high temperature and skin discoloration occurring as purple diamond-shaped lesions. The more chronic form is manifested as chronic arthritis and vegetative endocarditis. Mortality from the acute form may be high in young pigs. Older pigs may survive but pregnant sows often abort. Control by regular vaccination is advocated as *E. rhusiopathiae* is widespread in the environment as well as in carrier pigs.

Complementary References

Anon (1983) A common code of practice for the control of contagious equine metritis and other equine reproductive diseases for the 1984 covering season in France, Ireland and the United Kingdom. *Vet. Rec.*, **113**, 512–515.

Anon (1986) Trichomoniasis. In *Manual of Veterinary Parasitological Laboratory Techniques*. MAFF. 3rd edn, pp. 93–98. London: HMSO.

Baca, O. G. & Paretsky, D. (1983). Q fever and *Coxiella burnetii*: a model for host–parasitic interactions. *Microbiol. Rev.*, **47**, 127–149.

Ball, H. J., McCaughey, W. J. & Irwin, D. (1984) Persistence of unreaplasma genital infection in naturally infected ewes. *Brit. Vet. J.*, **140**, 347–353.

Bartlett, P. C., Kirk, J. H., Wilke, M. A., Kaneene, J. B. & Mather, E. C. (1986) Metritis complex in Michigan Holstein–Friesian cattle, incidence, description, epidemiology and estimated economic impact. *Prevent. Vet. Med.*, **4**, 235–248.

Blewett, D. A. (1985) The epidemiology of ovine toxoplasmosis. In *The Veterinary Annual*, 25th Issue, eds Hill, F. W. G. & Grunsell, C. S. G., pp. 120–24. Bristol: Scientechnica.

Blewett, D. A. & Watson, W. A. (1984) The epidemiology of ovine toxoplasmosis. III: Observations on outbreaks of clinical toxoplasmosis in relation to possible mechanisms of transmission. *Brit. Vet. J.*, **140**, 54–63.

Brewer, R. A. (1983) Contagious equine metritis: a review/summary. *Vet. Bull.*, **53**(**10**), 881–891.

Burn, K. J. (1976) Tuberculosis. In *Handbook on Animal Diseases in the Tropics*, ed. Robertson, A., pp. 158–162. London: British Veterinary Association.

Buxton, D. & Finlayson, J. (1986) Experimental infection of pregnant sheep with *Toxoplasma gondii*: pathological and immunological observations on the placenta and foetus. *J. Comp. Pathol.*, **96**, 319–333.

Dawson, F. L. M. (1983) Reproduction and infertility. In *The Veterinary Annual*, 23rd Issue, eds Hill, F. W. G. & Grunsell, C. S. G., pp. 1–19. Bristol: Scientechnica.

Doig, P. A., Ruhnke, H. L., MacKay, A. L. & Palmer, N. C. (1979) Bovine granular vulvitis associated with ureaplasma infection. *Can. Vet. J.*, **20**, 89–94.

Doig, P. A. (1981) Bovine genital mycoplasmosis. *Can. Vet. J.*, **22**, 339–343.

Doyle, T. M. (1959) Johne's disease. In *Infectious Diseases of Animals. Diseases Due to Bacteria*, eds Stableforth, A. W. & Galloway, I. A., pp. 319–345. London: Butterworths.

Cranwell, M. P. & Gibbons, J. A. (1986) Tick-borne fever in a dairy herd. *Vet. Rec.*, **119**, 531–532.

de Bois, C. H. W., Nitschelm, D., van der Holst, W. & Keller, H. (1986) Reproductive diseases in the mare and stallion. In *Equine Diseases*, ed. H.-J. Wintzer, pp. 162–212. Berlin and Hamburg: Verlag Paul Parey.

Dubey, J. P. & Towle, A. (1986) *Toxoplasmosis in Sheep: A Review and Annotated Bibliography*. Farnham Royal: Commonwealth Agricultural Bureau.

Ellis, W. A. & Little, T. W. A. (eds) (1986) *The Present State of Leptospirosis Diagnosis and Control*. Dordrecht: Martinus Nijhoff.

Ellis, W. A., Cassells, J. A. & Doyle, J. (1986) Genital leptospirosis in bulls. *Vet. Rec.*, **118**, 333.

Ellis, W. A., O'Brien, J. J., Bryson, D. G. & Mackie, D. P. (1985) Bovine leptospirosis: some clinical features of serovar *hardjo* infection. *Vet. Rec.*, **117**, 101–104.

Ellis, W. A., McParland, P. J., Bryson, D. G. & Cassells, J. A. (1986a) Prevalence of *Leptospira* infection in aborted pigs in Northern Ireland. *Vet. Rec.*, **118**, 63–65.

Ellis, W. A., McParland, P. J., Bryson, D. G. & Cassells, J. A. (1986b) Boars as carriers of leptospires of the *australis* serogroup on farms with an abortion problem. *Vet. Rec.* **118**, 563.

Gitter, M. (1985) Listeriosis in farm animals in Great Britain. In *Isolation and Identification of Microorganisms of Medical and Veterinary Importance*, eds Collins, C. H. & Grange, J. M., pp. 191–200. London: Academic Press. Society for Applied Bacteriology, Technical Series No. 12.

Gitter, M., Richardson, C. & Boughton, E. (1986) Experimental infection of pregnant ewes with *Listeria monocytogenes*. *Vet. Rec.*, **118**, 575–578.

Goodger, W. J. & Skirrow, S. Z. (1986) Epidemiological and economic analyses of an unusually long epizootic of trichomoniasis in a large California dairy herd. *J. Amer. Vet. Med. Assoc.*, **189**, 772–776.

Griffin, J. F. T., Hartigan, P. J. & Nunn, W. R. (1974) Non-specific uterine infection and bovine fertility. I: Infection patterns and endometritis during the first seven weeks post partum. *Theriogenology*, **1**, 91–105.

Hathaway, S. C. & Little, T. W. A. (1983) Epidemiological study of *Leptospira hardjo* infection in second calf dairy cows. *Vet. Rec.*, **112**, 215–218.

Hathaway, S. C., Little, T. W. A. & Pritchard, D. G. (1986) Problems associated with the serological diagnosis of *Leptospira interrogans* serovar *hardjo* infection in bovine populations. *Vet. Rec.*, **117**, 84–86.

Humphrey, J. D. & Stephens, L. R. (1983) *Haemophilus somnus*: a review. *Vet. Bull.*, **53**(**II**), 987–1004.

Linklater, K. A. (1983) Abortion in sheep associated with *S. montevideo* infection. *Vet. Rec.*, **112**, 372–374.

Little, T. W. A. (1983) Q fever, an enigma. *Brit. Vet. J.*, **139**, 277–283.

Little, T. W. A. & Hathaway, S. C. (1983) Leptospirosis in pigs. In *The Veterinary Annual*, 23rd Issue, eds Hill, F. W. G. & Grunsell, C. S. G., pp. 116–121. Bristol: Scientechnica.

Livingston, C. W. & Gauer, B. B. (1982) Effect of venereal transmission of ovine ureaplasma on reproductive efficiency of ewes. *Amer. J. Vet. Res.*, **43**, 1190–1193.

Low, J. C. & Graham, M. M. (1985) *Histophilus ovis* epididymitis in a ram in the UK. *Vet. Rec.*, **117**, 64–65.

Low, J. C. & Renton, C. P. (1985) Septicaemia, encephalitis and abortion in a housed flock of sheep caused by *Listeria monocytogenes* type 1/2. *Vet. Rec.*, **116**, 147–150.

Pepper, R. T. & Dobson, H. (1987) Preliminary results of treatment and endocrinology of chronic endometritis in the dairy cow. *Vet. Rec.*, **120**, 53–56.

Sandals, W. C. D., Curtis, R. A., Cote, J. F. & Martin, S. W. (1979) The effect of retained placenta and metritis complex on reproductive performance of dairy cattle—a case control study. *Can. Vet. J.*, **20**, 131–135.

Scott, G. R. (1984) Tick-borne fever in sheep. In *The Veterinary Annual*, 24th Issue, eds Hill, F. W. G. & Grunsell, C. S. G., pp. 100–106. Bristol: Scientechnica.

Sojka, W. J., Wray, C., Shreeve, J. E. & Bell, J. C. (1983) The incidence of *Salmonella* infection in sheep in

England and Wales 1975 to 1981. *Brit. Vet. J.*, **139**, 386–392.

Stipkovits, L., Rashwan, A., Takacs, J. & Lopis, K. (1978) Occurrence of ureaplasmas in swine semen. *Zentralbl. Vet. Med. B.*, **25**, 605–608.

Wilesmith, J. W. & Gitter, M. (1986) Epidemiology of ovine listeriosis in Great Britain. *Vet. Rec.*, **119**, 467–470.

Wray, C. (1985) Is salmonellosis still a serious problem in veterinary practice? *Vet. Rec.*, **116**, 485–489.

17

Infectious Causes of Reproductive Failure in Cats and Dogs

R. M. GASKELL and C. J. GASKELL

THE CAT

A number of infectious agents have been implicated in reproductive failure in the cat. Typically this is manifest by pregnancy failure, the birth of stillborn kittens, or neonatal losses, but occasionally systemic infections may result in temporary loss of libido. Fetal resorption, and to a lesser extent abortion, is thought to be relatively common in the cat, although it is difficult to quantify; a figure of 2.8% was considered by Scott to be an underestimate. Stillbirth rates generally appear to be of the order of 6–12%, with preweaning mortality figures of up to 30%. Although a significant proportion of this mortality, particularly in a colony situation, is likely to be due to various microbiological agents, even in a specific pathogen-free colony mortality rates may reach 15%. Thus other causes of reproductive failure, such as genetic, hormonal, nutritional or management problems, should also always be considered.

Feline Leukemia Virus Infection

Feline leukemia virus (FeLV) is probably the most important single cause of reproductive failure in the cat. Fetal resorption is the most common manifestation of FeLV infertility, but abortion, stillbirths and neonatal losses also occur. Typically, conceptual swellings are palpable at 3–4 weeks' gestation,

and other signs of pregnancy such as abdominal distension or increased appetite are also present. Then at 5–7 weeks' gestation, the uterine masses disappear, there is a sudden reduction in abdominal size, and possibly a slight vaginal discharge. The mechanism of resorption is not known, although it is postulated that it is due to damage to maternal–fetal attachments.

Not all queens with persistent FeLV infection will have reproductive problems, however, and indeed even an affected queen may have previously had one or two normal pregnancies. Clinical signs are not usually seen in queens at the time of FeLV-induced reproductive failure, although it should be noted that all cats with persistent infection have a very high risk of developing an FeLV-related disease at some time; such diseases include lymphosarcoma, leukemia, anemia, immunosuppression, bone marrow aplasia, and possibly glomerulonephritis.

All kittens born to infected queens will be persistently viremic, probably as a result of in utero passage of virus to the developing embryos. Such kittens will generally develop an FeLV-related disease within a short period. Thymic atrophy and accompanying immunosuppression makes the kittens susceptible to a variety of secondary bacterial and viral, respiratory and enteric infections.

Recently a latent carrier state for FeLV virus has been demonstrated in many apparently recovered cats. While no infectious virus is found in blood, latent virus may be found in bone marrow. Present evidence suggests that such animals are only very rarely infectious by contact with other cats. However, it appears that in the occasional latently infected queen, virus may be transmitted to the offspring via the milk.

Diagnosis of FeLV-associated infertility should be based on testing for infection using virus isolation, immunofluorescence, or an ELISA test, with the aim of eliminating FeLV-positive cats. The procedure for this has been described fully elsewhere, together with a discussion of the disposal of positive cats. In some countries vaccines are available to aid prophylaxis of the disease. Vaccination does not, however, control preexisting infection.

Feline Herpesvirus 1 Infection

Feline herpesvirus 1 (FHV1) is a major respiratory pathogen of cats, causing a generally severe upper respiratory syndrome characterized by pyrexia, depression, sneezing, marked ocular and nasal discharges, conjunctivitis, and sometimes dyspnea and coughing. The disease may be particularly severe in young kittens, where complications such as pneumonia, keratitis, and generalized disease may also occur and which may lead to high mortality.

Many herpesviruses of other species are known to induce not only respiratory disease, but also genital and reproductive problems. Since abortions and possibly genital infections have been seen occasionally in association with naturally occurring FHV1 infection, attempts have been made to determine the pathogenicity of FHV1 for the genital tract under experimental conditions. Transplacental infection and abortion has been demonstrated following intravenous inoculation of virus, but although abortions also occurred following the more natural intranasal route of inoculation, virus was not recovered from aborted material. Thus abortion was attributed to nonspecific effects of the severe debilitating upper respiratory infection and not to the effects of virus itself. Vaginitis and congenital infections have also been shown experimentally following intravaginal infection of pregnant queens. Kittens born to such queens in the later stages of gestation often had generalized disease with hepatic lesions.

However, although involvement of FHV1 with the genital tract may be shown experimentally, in the field it would seem to be a rare event. In utero transmission of virus does not seem to occur, and kittens born to FHV1 infected queens are generally infected when they lose their passive immunity. This

is often of short and variable duration (2–10 weeks, with mean levels falling below detectable levels at 6–9 weeks of age). The source of the infecting virus is generally a carrier cat within the colony, often the mother. At least 80% of cats recovered from FHV1 infection are latently infected with virus. Carrier cats may shed virus intermittently, but particularly following stress such as a change of housing, or during lactation. Thus they are ideally placed to transmit virus to the next generation, and although most infected kittens will show clinical signs, in some cases kittens may be subclinically infected and become latent carriers under cover of passive immunity.

Diagnosis of FHV1 infection is generally based on clinical signs and virus isolation; in some laboratories an immunofluorescent test has also been used. Prevention and control of the disease is best achieved through a combination of vaccination and management procedures (reviewed elsewhere). Both intranasal and systemic vaccines are available, and are reasonably effective in protecting previously unexposed cats against the disease. However, vaccination does not necessarily protect against subsequent infection and the development of a latent carrier state, nor does it 'cure' preexisting carriers. Treatment of FHV1 infection is supportive, although antiviral substances developed for use in other species may prove to be of use.

Feline Calicivirus Infection

Feline calicivirus is also a major respiratory pathogen of cats, although the disease seen is typically milder than that seen with FHV1, and often characterized by mouth ulceration. There are also a number of different strains of feline calicivirus of slightly varying pathogenicity. Although there is no recorded genital tropism for any of these strains, occasional cases of in utero transmission of virus to fetuses have been observed with virus isolated from aborted fetuses. This undoubtedly is a very rare event, and feline calicivirus generally only affects reproductive performance through occasional severe infection and mortality in neonatal kittens.

Feline Infectious Peritonitis

Feline infectious peritonitis (FIP) is a sporadic, fatally progressive disease of cats caused by a coronavirus, and characterized by the accumulation of fluid in peritoneal or other body cavities. An extraperitoneal or noneffusive form of the disease with granulomatous lesions also occurs, and in the male cat lesions may occasionally be found in the testes. A possible association of FIP virus with reproductive failure in queens and neonatal death in kittens has been suggested, based largely on circumstantial evidence. Others have suggested from epidemiological observations that transplacental transmission might perhaps occur, although there is no definitive evidence to support this.

Feline Panleukopenia

Feline panleukopenia is an acute febrile disease of cats characterized by a marked decrease in circulating white cells (hence panleukopenia) and severe enteritis. The disease is caused by a member of the parvovirus family, a group of viruses which has an affinity and requirement for actively dividing cells. It is this feature of the agent that determines its pathogenicity, since its primary target cells are the rapidly dividing cells of the lymphoid tissue and bone marrow leading to panleukopenia, and the crypt epithelium of the intestinal mucosa leading to enteritis.

However, in view of this predilection of feline panleukopenia virus for actively dividing cells, it is not surprising that transplacental infection may also occur. The virus infects and replicates in placental cells, and has the ability to cross the placenta to infect the fetus. Infection then occurs throughout the fetus, causing fetal resorption, abortion, stillbirth, or teratogenic effects. The precise changes that result will depend on the stage of gestation at the time of infection. Thus it has been postulated that infection early in pregnancy may lead to early fetal death and resorption, but later on (from the middle third of gestation to immediately postnatally) it has been shown that it will lead to cerebellar hypoplasia. Histologically, there is a marked reduction in the numbers of granular and Purkinje cells.

Although present at birth, clinical signs of cerebellar hypoplasia are not usually apparent until the kittens attempt to walk at 2–3 weeks of age, and not all the litter are necessarily affected. Affected kittens show a symmetrical ataxia and incoordination, which persists for life. Nevertheless, the kittens may learn to compensate and continue to thrive in other respects.

Diagnosis of feline panleukopenia is by characteristic clinical signs and histopathology; virus isolation may also be attempted. In general, the disease may be prevented very successfully by regular vaccination. Both modified live and inactivated vaccines are available and are both highly effective. Modified live vaccines should not be given in pregnancy, however, as they may also cross the placental barrier. Where a clinical case has occurred, the environment will be heavily contaminated. Since feline panleukopenia virus is remarkably stable and may persist in infected premises for up to a year, it is wise to thoroughly clean and disinfect the premises (with hypochlorite or formalin), in addition to instituting a vaccination program.

Feline *Chlamydia psittaci*

The feline strain of *Chlamydia psittaci* is predominantly a conjunctival pathogen of cats, although sometimes mild upper respiratory signs may also be seen. The conjuntivitis is characterized by marked ocular discharge, blepharospasm, hyperemia and chemosis, and signs may persist in a chronic or recurrent form for some time.

In some other species, *C. psittaci* has a genital tract tropism, and this has led to speculation that it may be involved in reproductive failure in the cat. However, although vaginitis has been induced under experimental conditions following direct inoculation of the organism into the reproductive tract, genital tract signs do not seem to occur following more natural routes of infection. Nevertheless vaginal shedding of the organism has been noted following both natural and experimental conjunctival infection, and it may be that this occasionally plays a role in reproductive failure or in neonatal infection in kittens.

Feline Mycoplasmas

The importance of feline mycoplasmas is difficult to assess, since they are found in a significant proportion of apparently normal cats. The most common isolates are *M. gatae*, *M. felis*, *M. argini* and *Acholesplasma laidlawii*, and they have mostly been isolated from upper respiratory and urogenital tracts. Abortion has been reproduced in cats experimentally with ureaplasmas, but the significance of this in the field is unknown.

Bacteria

In general, bacteria are uncommon causes of reproductive failure in cats, but sometimes they may be involved in fetal deaths or abortion, and acute and chronic endometritis. A number of species, including *E. coli*, *Staphylococcus* spp., and *Streptococcus* spp., may be involved, although such bacteria can also be found in the reproductive tract of cats with a normal reproductive history. As in other species, bacterial growth is enhanced when the uterus is under the influence of progesterone. *Salmonella choleraesius* has also been implicated in a case of feline abortion.

Toxoplasmosis

Toxoplasmosis is caused by a protozoan parasite, *Toxoplasma gondii*. The cat is the only definitive host for this parasite, although a variety of other species of animals, including man, can be infected as intermediate hosts. Infection in cats is relatively common, but mostly subclinical. As any body tissue is susceptible to invasion by the parasite, clinical signs, when they occur, are very variable; respiratory, gastrointestinal and hepatic signs may occur and, in the chronic form, ocular and CNS signs may be present. Pregnant cats may abort, and neonatal infection may occur. However, toxoplasmosis is not considered a common cause of reproductive failure in cats. The diagnosis and treatment and control of the disease has been discussed in detail elsewhere. Although serology is often used in diagnosis, its usefulness is limited.

Cystic Endometrial Hyperplasia; Pyometra

Pyometra is recognized less frequently in cats than in dogs, but is similar in that it follows hormonal 'priming' of the uterus and subsequent bacterial infection. The clinical signs of pyometra may be more or less conspicuous, with some queens showing little apart from a record of infertility. Others may show more classic depression, inappetance, vaginal discharge and polydypsia though these may not always be noticed by the owner. Similarly, abdominal distension is not often a major feature. When present, the vaginal discharge may vary from a pale to a dark red-brown colour and may be viscous in character. Diagnosis is based on the clinical signs, abdominal palpation and radiographic examination; hematological examination typically reveals a marked neutrophilia with a shift to the left.

Treatment is usually by ovariohysterectomy, with appropriate support before and following surgery for the systemic effects of the condition. Medical treatment has been attempted in breeding queens and the use of estrogens has been suggested to dilate the cervix and induce drainage, given in combination with antibacterial therapy. Prostaglandin treatment similar to that used in the bitch has also been suggested for the management of pyometra in cats.

Endometritis, without the accumulation of fluid within the uterus, is more difficult to diagnose and queens often show little apart from an apparent inability to conceive. The diagnosis may only be satisfactorily achieved at laparotomy, either on gross examination or on histology following uterine biopsy. Some animals may breed successfully following antibiotic therapy and rest for two or three cycles.

THE DOG

There are perhaps fewer specific infectious agents implicated in reproductive failure in the dog than in the cat. As with the cat, however, and indeed in other species, problems associated with infectious agents will generally be exacerbated in kennel situations where groups of dogs are housed closely together. Similarly, other factors such as management and nutrition, and selection of breeding stock should also be considered in any investigation of canine infertility even where the cause appears at first sight to be an infectious agent. Indeed in many cases the etiology will be multifactorial.

Canine Herpesvirus 1 Infection

Canine herpesvirus 1 (CHV1) causes a severe, frequently fatal, generalized disease of neonatal puppies. In older dogs, the disease is generally mild or inapparent and restricted to the respiratory or genital tract. Generalized disease only occurs in puppies less than 2–3 weeks of age, possibly to some extent because of the predilection of the virus for growth at the often lower, and poorly regulated, body temperature of the neonatal pup. Clinical signs in puppies may be minimal, or they may cry, show abdominal pain and difficulty in breathing, and cease feeding; most animals die rapidly or within a few days. Focal necrotizing and hemorrhagic lesions are present in many organs throughout the body; the distinctive hemorrhagic foci generally present on the surface of the kidney are of diagnostic significance.

In older dogs, mild rhinitis has been observed by some workers following experimental oronasal inoculation, and mild conjunctivitis after instillation of virus into the conjunctival sac. Naturally occurring, recurrent vaginal lesions associated with a clinical history of infertility, abortions and stillbirths have been observed in association with canine herpesvirus infection, and vaginitis and balanoposthitis have also been reproduced experimentally by intravaginal or intrapreputial inoculation of the virus.

The virus is transmitted mainly by contact between susceptible puppies and infective oronasal or vaginal secretions. These are usually from the bitch, but may also be through direct or indirect contact with other dogs or puppies on the premises. Recovered dogs probably remain as latent virus carriers, as with FHV1. Periodic episodes of virus shedding in the nasal secretions of recovered dogs have been recorded, and vaginal shedding has also been detected both in a case of recurrent vaginitis, and in a bitch 18 days after whelping a litter of puppies which died from infection with CHV1. Experimentally, intravaginal inoculation of pregnant bitches 1 or 2 weeks before whelping has been shown to lead to neonatal infection. Presumably where the virus is shed from the vagina, puppies may be infected either immediately postnatally or during passage through the birth canal.

Natural transplacental infection with in utero infection of puppies and fetal death has also been observed, but does not seem to occur very commonly. Experimentally, transplacental infection, and fetal death, mummification, abortion, or premature birth have been demonstrated following intravenous inoculation of the virus in the 2nd or 3rd trimesters of pregnancy.

Despite the probable latency of CHV1, it seems that bitches that have lost litters due to CHV1 do not necessarily produce subsequent litters with the disease. However, this has been recorded and thus it might be wise to segregate such bitches from others at whelping. Puppies with maternal antibody are apparently protected against disease but not infection, and thus the administration of hyperimmune serum to puppies at birth may help in obtaining healthy litters. However, this will be of no benefit to puppies infected prenatally.

Other Canine Virus Infections

Although there is some evidence to suggest that the other major canine viral diseases, namely canine distemper, canine parvovirus infection, and canine adenovirus infection may on occasion cross the placenta and induce neonatal infections, in general these diseases occur in older pups and young adults unprotected by vaccination or maternal antibody.

When canine parvovirus (CPV) infection first appeared in the dog population in 1978, all ages of dogs were susceptible. Since the pathogenesis of CPV infection is determined by its requirement for actively dividing cells, the disease seen reflects the mitotic rate of various target tissues and this in turn is determined by the age of the dog. Thus neonatal, and possibly on occasion, in utero infection results in the myocarditis syndrome, and occasionally, generalized disease. In older puppies and adult dogs, the major target cells are the intestinal epithelium, leading to enteritis, and the bone marrow and lymphatic system, leading to leukopenia. Since CPV infection became endemic in the dog population, however,

the pattern of disease has changed. Immune bitches now provide protection in utero and via colostrum in the first few weeks of life, and thus CPV is now rarely involved in neonatal infection and the myocarditis syndrome.

Canine Brucellosis

Infection in dogs due to *Brucella canis* is an important cause of canine abortion and infertility problems in some parts of the world, notably the United States (see also Chapter 12). Dogs are the only known natural host of this organism, although occasional human infections have been recorded (see Chapter 12).

Infection occurs predominantly in dogs in breeding kennels. In pregnant bitches, the most typical finding is abortion after the 30th day of gestation, usually between the 45th and 55th day. Occasionally puppies are stillborn or die soon after birth. Early embryonic death and fetal resorption may occur also. In male dogs epididymitis and orchitis, often followed by testicular atrophy, may occur, but sometimes infertility may be the only sign of the disease. Semen samples show the presence of abnormal sperm and inflammatory cells, and a reduction in sperm motility and concentration. In both sexes, there may be slight lymphadenopathy, but there is no fever, and in some cases infected animals may appear clinically normal.

Transmission occurs mainly through infected vaginal discharges following an abortion, or through seminal fluid from males during mating. Urinary excretion also occurs but is not thought to be important. Although dogs are most infectious during the initial stages of infection, organisms may be shed intermittently in semen for over a year. Prolonged bacteremia, which may after several months become intermittent, is also a feature of the disease. A number of treatment schedules have been suggested, but the organism is difficult to eliminate from infected animals. Control measures should include: the identification of carrier dogs by means of serum agglutination tests and blood cultures; the isolation and removal of infected animals; and the use of suitable hygiene and disinfection procedures.

Canine Mycoplasmas

A number of mycoplasma species has been isolated from dogs, both from apparently healthy animals and from those with a variety of clinical signs. The most commonly isolated species from both upper respiratory and genital tracts is *M. canis*, and experimentally an isolate of *M. canis* has been shown to induce chronic orchitis and epididymitis in the dog and endometritis in the bitch. Slightly higher isolation rates of mycoplasmas and ureaplasmas have also been found in infertile stud dogs and breeding bitches, compared to clinically normal animals, but these differences were significant only in the male.

In general, however, the role of mycoplasmas in canine reproductive problems is difficult to assess and needs to be clarified. Nevertheless where inflammatory discharges are present or infertility is a problem swabs for mycoplasma culture should be taken, and if grown in high numbers, appropriate chemotherapy instituted.

Other Bacteria

The role of bacteria in canine reproductive problems is difficult to assess for, as with mycoplasmas, they are generally present in both healthy dogs and in those with clinical signs. The most commonly isolated species from both clinically normal bitches and from those with vaginitis are *E. coli*, *Staphylococcus* and *Streptococcus* spp. There is some evidence to suggest, however, that higher numbers of bacteria may be found in those bitches with vaginal exudates compared to controls.

Cystic Endometrial Hyperplasia; Pyometra Complex

The precise etiology of pyometra in the bitch is obscure. The combined effects of estrogen and progesterone on the endometrium lead to cystic hyperplasia of the endometrial glands, and it is generally accepted that subsequent infection with bacteria may lead to an endometritis and the accumulation of infected fluid within the uterus. *E. coli* is the bacterium most frequently isolated, and it has been suggested that this may be due to the ability of this organism to adhere via the K-antigen to the progesterone-stimulated endometrium and myometrium. However care must be exercised in interpreting the results of vaginal swabs, as the organisms so cultured may not be representative of those found within the uterus.

Clinical Signs

The clinical signs of pyometra classically occur in the metestral stage of the cycle and typically include depression, pyrexia, inappetance and polydypsia. There may or may not be a continuous discharge of purulent material from the vagina. Where fluid is retained within the uterus varying degrees of abdominal distension may be appre-

ciated. Vomiting may be seen and other signs of toxaemia may develop. Renal damage, both glomerular and tubular, may occur and lead to renal failure in severe cases.

Diagnosis and Treatment

Diagnosis may be made on the basis of the clinical signs, abdominal palpation and where appropriate by radiographic demonstration of an enlarged uterus. Hematological examination invariably reveals a marked neutrophilia with a shift to the left. The use of ultrasound has been reported both in diagnosis and in the monitoring of response to medical treatment.

Treatment of pyometra has traditionally been by ovariohysterectomy. In severely depressed animals this must be combined with, if not preceded by, vigorous supportive treatment including fluid therapy and appropriate antibiotics. Medical treatment of pyometra, using a combination of antibiotics and prostaglandins, has been used more recently and has the advantage of potentially re-establishing fertility. Prostaglandins should be used with care as dose-related side effects such as hypersalivation, vomiting and diarrhoea may occur but success has been achieved using 'low' dose regimes such as $20\ \mu g/kg$ body weight of prostaglandic $F_{2\alpha}$ given intramuscularly three times a day on consecutive days for up to a week. Careful supervision is necessary during treatment.

Complementary References

Andersen, L. J., Jarrett, W. F. H., Jarrett, O. & Laird, H. M. (1971) Feline leukaemia virus infection of kittens: mortality associated with atrophy of the thymus and lymphoid depletion. *J. Nat. Cancer Inst.*, **47**, 807.

Bittle, J. L. & Peckham, J. C. (1971) Genital infection induced by feline rhinotracheitis virus and effects on newborn kittens. *J. Amer. Vet. Med. Assoc.*, **158**, 927–928.

Carmichael, L. E. (1980) Canine herpesvirus infection. Canine brucellosis. In *Current Therapy in Theriogenology*, ed. Morrow, D. A., pp. 631–636. Philadelphia: W. B. Saunders.

Carmichael, L. E. & Kenney, R. M. (1970) Canine brucellosis: the clinical disease, pathogenesis and immune response. *J. Amer. Vet. Med. Assoc.*, **156**, 1726–1734.

Carmichael, L. E., Barnes, F. D. & Percy, D. H. (1969) Temperature as a factor in resistance of young puppies to canine herpesvirus. *J. Infect. Dis.*, **120**, 669–678.

Christianson, I. B. J. (1984) *Reproduction in the Dog and Cat*. London: Baillière Tindall.

Csiza, C. K., de Lahunta, A., Scott, F. W. & Gillespie, J. H. (1972) Spontaneous feline 'ataxia'. *Cornell Vet.* **62**, 300–322.

Darougar, S., Monnickendam, M. A., El-Sheik, H., Treharne, J. D., Woodland, R. M. & Jones, B. R. (1977) Animal models for the study of chlamydial infections of the eye and genital tract. In *Non-gonococcal Urethritis and Related Infections*, eds Hobson, D. and Holmes, K. K., pp. 186–198. Washington, DC: American Society for Microbiology.

Doig, P. A., Ruhnke, H. L. & Bosu, W. T. K. (1981) The genital mycoplasma and ureaplasma flora of healthy and diseased dogs. *Can. J. Comp. Med.*, **45**, 233–238.

Dow, C. (1962) Experimental uterine infection in the domestic cat. *J. Comp. Path.*, **72**, 303–307.

Dubey, J. P. & Johnstone, I. (1982) Fatal neonatal toxoplasmosis in cats. *J. Amer. Anim. Hosp. Assoc.*, **18**, 461–467.

Ellis, T. M. (1981) Jaundice in a cat with *in utero* feline calicivirus infection. *Aust. Vet. J.*, **57**, 383.

Gaskell, R. M. (1984) The natural history of the major feline viral diseases. *J. Small Anim. Pract.*, **25**, 159–172.

Gaskell, R. M. (1985a) Feline panleucopenia. In *Feline Medicine and Therapeutics*, eds Chandler, E. A., Gaskell, C. J. & Hilberry, A. D. R., pp. 251–256. Oxford: Blackwells.

Gaskell, R. M. (1985b) Viral-induced upper respiratory tract disease. In *Feline Medicine and Therapeutics*, eds Chandler, E. A., Gaskell, C. J. & Hilberry, A. D. R., pp. 257–270. Oxford: Blackwells.

Gaskell, R. M. & Povey, R. C. (1982) Transmission of feline viral rhinotracheitis. *Vet. Rec.*, **111**, 359–362.

Gillespie, J. H. & Scott, F. W. (1973). Feline viral infections II. Feline panleucopenia. *Adv. Vet. Sci. Comp. Med.*, **17**, 164–175.

George, L. W., Duncan, J. R. & Carmichael, L. E. (1979) Semen examination in dogs with canine brucellosis. *Amer. J. Vet. Res.*, **40**, 1589–1595.

Hashimoto, A. & Hirai, K. (1986) Canine herpesvirus infection. In *Current Therapy in Theriogenology 2*, ed. Morrow, D. A., pp. 516–520. Philadelphia: W. B. Saunders.

Hashimoto, A., Hirai, K., Okada, K. & Fujimoto, Y. (1979) Pathology of the placenta and newborn pups with suspected intrauterine infection of canine herpesvirus. *Amer. J. Vet. Res.*, **40**, 1236–1240.

Hashimoto, A., Hirai, K., Suzuki, Y. & Fujimoto, Y. (1983) Experimental transplacental transmission of canine herpesvirus in pregnant bitches during the second trimester of gestation. *Amer. J. Vet. Res.*, **44**, 610–614.

Helmsley, L. A. (1956) Abortion in two cats, with the isolation of *Salmonella choleraesius* from one case. *Vet. Rec.*, **68**, 152.

Hill, H. & Mare, C. J. (1974) Genital disease caused by canine herpesvirus. *Amer. J. Vet. Res.* **35**, 669–672.

Hirsh, D. & Wigner, N. (1977) The bacterial flora of the normal canine vagina compared to that of vaginal exudates. *J. Small Anim. Pract.*, **18**, 25–30.

Holzmann, A., Laber, G. & Walzl, H. (1979). Experimentally induced mycoplasma infection in the genital tract of the female dog. *Theriogenology*, **12**, 355–370.

Hoover, E. A. & Griesemer, R. A. (1971) Experimental feline herpesvirus infection in the pregnant cat. *Amer. J. Pathol.*, **65**, 173–184.

Jarrett, J. O. (1985) Feline leukaemia virus. In *Feline Medicine and Therapeutics*, eds Chandler, E. A., Gaskell, C. J. & Hilberry, A. D. R., pp. 271–283. Oxford: Blackwells.

Kane, J. L., Woodland, R. M., Elder, M. G. & Darougar, S. (1985) Chlamydial pelvic infection in cats: a model for the study of human pelvic inflammatory disease. *Genitourinary Med.*, **61**, 311–318.

Kilham, L., Margolis, G. & Colby, E. D. (1971) Cerebellar ataxia and its congenital transmission in cats by feline panleucopenia virus. *J. Amer. Vet. Med. Assoc.*, **158**, 888–901.

Krakowka, S., Hoover, E. A., Koestner, A. & Ketring, K. (1977) Experimental and naturally occurring transplacental transmission of canine distemper virus. *Amer. J. Vet. Res.*, **38**, 919–922.

Laber, G. & Holzmann, A. (1977) Experimentally induced mycoplasmal infection in the genital tract of the male dog. *Theriogenology*, **12**, 177–178.

Lenghaus, C. & Studdert, M. J. (1982) Generalised parvovirus disease in neonatal pups. *J. Amer. Vet. Med. Assoc.*, **181**, 41–45.

Lenghaus, C., Studdert, M. J. & Finnie, J. W. (1980) Acute and chronic canine parvovirus myocarditis following intrauterine inoculation. *Aust. Vet. J.*, **56**, 465–468.

Love, D. (1976) Naturally occurring neonatal canine herpesvirus infection. *Vet. Rec.*, **99**, 501–503.

Norsworthy, G. D. (1974) Neonatal feline infectious peritonitis. *Feline Prac.*, **4(6)**, 34.

Olson, P. N., Jones, R. L. & Mather, E. C. (1986) The use and misuse of vaginal cultures in diagnosing reproductive diseases in the bitch. In *Current Therapy in Theriogenology 2*, ed. Morrow, D. A., pp. 469–475. Philadelphia: W. B. Saunders.

Pacitti, A. M., Jarrett, O. & Hay, D. (1986) Transmission of feline leukaemia virus in the milk of a non-viraemic cat. *Vet. Rec.*, **118**, 381–384.

Pastoret, P.-P. & Henroteaux, M. (1978) Epigenetic transmission of feline infectious peritonitis. *Comp. Immunol. Microbiol. Infect. Dis.*, **1**, 67–70.

Poste, G. & King, N. (1971) Isolation of a herpesvirus from the canine genital tract; association with infertility, abortion and stillbirths. *Vet. Rec.*, **88**, 229–233.

Povey, R. C. (1985) *Escherichia coli* infection. In *Infectious Diseases of Cats. A Clinical Handbook*, pp. FD-1–FD-3. Guelph, Canada: Centaur Press.

Rosendal, S. (1982) Canine mycoplasmas: their ecological niche and role in disease. *J. Amer. Vet. Med. Assoc.*, **180**, 1212–1214.

Sandholm, M., Vasenius, H. & Kivisto, A. K. (1975) Pathogenesis of canine pyometra. *J. Amer. Vet. Med. Assoc.*, **167**, 1006–1010.

Scott, F. W., Geissinger, C. & Peltz, R. (1978) Kitten mortality survey. *Feline Pract.*, **8(6)**, 31–34.

Scott, F. W., Weiss, R. C., Poste, J. E., Gilmartin, J. E. & Hoshino, Y. (1979) Kitten mortality complex (neonatal FIP?) *Feline Pract.*, **9(2)**, 44–56.

Shewen, P. E., Povey, R. C. & Wilson, M. R. (1978) Feline chlamydial infection. *Can. Vet. J.*, **19**, 289–292.

Stewart, S. E., David-Ferreira, J., Lovelace, E., Landon, J. & Stock, N. (1965) Herpes-like virus isolated from neonatal and fetal dogs. *Science*, **148**, 1341–1343.

Tan, R. J. S. & Miles, J. A. R. (1974) Possible role of feline T-strain mycoplasmas in cat abortion. *Aust. Vet. J.*, **50**, 142–145.

Wills, J. M. (1986) Chlamydial infection in the cat. PhD thesis, University of Bristol.

Wills, J. M., Gruffyd-Jones, T. J., Bourne, F. J., Richmond, S. J. & Gaskell, R. M. (1986) Effect of vaccination on conjunctivitis due to feline chlamydia psittaci. In *Chlamydial Infections*, eds Oriel, D., Ridgeway, G., Schacter, J., Taylor-Robinson, D. & Ward, M., pp. 416–419. Cambridge: Cambridge University Press.

Wright, A. I. (1985) Endoparasites. In *Feline Medicine and Therapeutics*, eds Chandler, E. A., Gaskell, C. J. & Hilberry, A. D. R., pp. 352–361. Oxford: Blackwells.

Young, C. (1973) Preweaning mortality in specific pathogen free kittens. *J. Small Anim. Pract.*, **14**, 391–397.

Index